NEONATAL
HEART DISEASE

Progress in
Cardiovascular Diseases

NEONATAL
HEART DISEASE

Edited by

William F. Friedman, M.D.

Chief, Division of Pediatric Cardiology
Associate Professor of Pediatrics and Medicine
University of California, San Diego
School of Medicine
La Jolla, California

Michael Lesch, M.D.

Assistant Professor of Medicine
Harvard Medical School
Boston, Massachusetts

Edmund H. Sonnenblick, M.D.

Director of Cardiovascular Research
Peter Bent Brigham Hospital
Associate Professor of Medicine
Harvard Medical School
Boston, Massachusetts

GRUNE & STRATTON   New York and London

A Subsidiary of Harcourt Brace Jovanovich, Publishers

The chapters of this book originally appeared in the July, September, and November 1972 and January 1973 issues (Vol. XV, Numbers 1, 2, 3, and 4) of *Progress in Cardiovascular Diseases,* a bimonthly journal published by Grune & Stratton, Inc., and edited by Edmund H. Sonnenblick and Michael Lesch.

Library of Congress Cataloging in Publication Data

Friedman, William F   comp.
    Neonatal heart disease.

    Previously published Progress in cardiovascular
diseases, July 1972–Feb., 1973.
    Includes bibliographical references.
    1. Infants (Newborn)—Diseases.   2.   Heart—
Abnormities and deformities.   I.   Lesch, Michael, joint
comp.   II.   Sonnenblick, Edmund H., joint comp.
III.   Progress in cardiovascular diseases.   IV.   Title.
[DNLM: 1.   Heart defects, Congenital.   2.   Heart
diseases—In infancy and childhood.   WS 290 F911n   1973]
RJ421.F75   618.9'21'2   73-4449
ISBN 0-8089-0802-2

Grune & Stratton, Inc.
111 Fifth Avenue
New York, New York 10003

Library of Congress Catalog Card Number 73-4449

International Standard Book Number 0-8089-0802-2

Printed in the United States of America

Contents

Contributors

BRIAN G. BARRATT-BOYES, M.B., Ch.M., F.R.A.C.S., F.A.C.S., F.R.S. (N.Z.): Surgeon-in-Charge, Cardiothoracic Surgical Unit, Green Lane Hospital; and Professor of Surgery, University of Auckland, Auckland, New Zealand

A. G. M. CAMPBELL, M.D., M.R.C.P. (Edin.): Director, Newborn Services, Yale-New Haven Medical Center; and Associate Professor of Pediatrics, Yale University School of Medicine, New Haven, Connecticut

WILLIAM F. FRIEDMAN, M.D.: Chief, Division of Pediatric Cardiology, and Associate Professor of Pediatrics and Medicine, University of California, San Diego, School of Medicine, La Jolla, California

WELTON M. GERSONY, M.D.: Director, Division of Pediatric Cardiology, and Associate Professor of Pediatrics, College of Physicians and Surgeons, Columbia University, New York, New York

IRA H. GESSNER, M.D.: Professor of Pediatrics, J. Hillis Miller Health Center, University of Florida College of Medicine, Gainesville, Florida

THOMAS P. GRAHAM, Jr., M.D.: Associate Professor of Pediatrics, and Director, Division of Pediatric Cardiology, Vanderbilt University Medical Center, Nashville, Tennessee

LEONARD C. HARRIS, M.D.: Professor of Pediatrics, and Director, Division of Pediatric Cardiology, The University of Texas Medical Branch, Galveston, Texas

CONSTANCE J. HAYES, M.D.: Assistant Professor of Clinical Pediatrics, College of Physicians and Surgeons, Columbia University, New York, New York

MICHAEL A. HEYMANN, M.B., B.Ch.: Assistant Professor of Pediatrics in Residence, Cardiovascular Research Institute, University of California, San Francisco, California

JAY M. JARMAKANI, M.D.: Assistant Professor of Pediatrics, Division of Pediatric Cardiology, Duke University Medical Center, Durham, North Carolina

SAMUEL KAPLAN, M.D.: Director, Division of Cardiology, Professor of Pediatrics, and Associate Professor of Medicine, University of Cincinnati, and The Children's Hospital, Cincinnati, Ohio

MAURICE LEV, M.D.: Director, Congenital Heart Disease Research and Training Center, Hektoen Institute for Medical Research; Professor of Pathology, Northwestern University Medical School; Professorial Lecturer, University Of Chicago School of Medicine; Lecturer in Pathology, Abraham Lincoln School of Medicine, University of Illinois; Lecturer in Pathology, The Chicago Medical School, University of Health Sciences; Lecturer, Department of Pathology, Loyola University, Stritch School of Medicine; and Career Investigator and Educator, Chicago Heart Association, Chicago, Illinois

RICHARD A. MEYER, M.D.: Assistant Professor of Pediatrics, University of Cincinnati, and the Children's Hospital, Cincinnati, Ohio

VINCENT N. MILES, M.D.: Fellow in Pediatric Cardiology, University of Colorado Medical Center and affiliated hospitals, Denver, Colorado

ROBERT A. MILLER, M.D.: Chairman, Department of Pediatric Cardiology, Cook County Hospital; and Professor, Department of Pediatrics, Abraham Lincoln School of Medicine, University of Illinois, Chicago, Illinois

WILLIAM W. MILLER, M.D.: Associate Professor of Pediatrics, Department of Pediatrics, The University of Texas Southwestern Medical School, Dallas, Texas

JOHN M. NEUTZE, M.D., F.R.A.C.P.: Cardiologist, Green Lane Hospital, Auckland, New Zealand

QUANG X. NGHIEM, M.D.: Associate Professor of Pediatrics, and Assistant Director, Division of Pediatric Cardiology, The University of Texas Medical Branch, Galveston, Texas

JAMES J. NORA, M.D.: Associate Professor of Pediatrics, and Director of Pediatric Cardiology, University of Colorado Medical Center and affiliated hospitals, Denver, Colorado

ABRAHAM M. RUDOLPH, M.D.: Neider Professor of Pediatrics, and Professor of Physiology, Department of Pediatrics, University of California, San Francisco, California

EVE R. SEELYE, B.A., F.F.A., R.C.S., R.A.C.S.: Anesthetist, Green Lane Hospital, Auckland, New Zealand

MARIE SIMPSON, F.F.A., R.C.S., R.A.C.S.: Anesthetist, Green Lane Hospital, Auckland, New Zealand

NORMAN S. TALNER, M.D.: Director, Pediatric Cardiology, Yale-New Haven Medical Center; and Professor of Pediatrics, Yale University School of Medicine, New Haven, Connecticut

CONSTANTINE J. TATOOLES, M.S., M.D.: Chairman, Department of Cardio-Thoracic Surgery, Cook County Hospital; and Assistant Professor, Department of Surgery and Physiology, Loyola University Medical Center, Chicago, Illinois

L. H. S. VAN MIEROP, M.D.: Professor of Pediatrics and Pathology, J. Hillis Miller Health Center, University of Florida College of Medicine, Gainesville, Florida

ROBERT R. WOLFE, M.D.: Assistant Professor of Pediatrics, and Associate Director of Pediatric Cardiology, University of Colorado Medical Center and affiliated hospitals, Denver, Colorado

Preface

THE RAPID EXPANSION of biomedical investigation in the past 10 yr has contributed significantly to our understanding of the scientific basis of pediatric cardiology and cardiovascular surgery. As a consequence, noticeable improvements have occurred in methods of prevention, detection, and treatment. Moreover, as the discipline of pediatric cardiology continues to evolve, progressively more attention has focused on the challenges presented by the neonate with heart disease. The current emphasis on the newborn period is, in part, a reflection of the excitement felt by cardiologists and their surgical colleagues as they have learned to deal ever more effectively with these fragile patients. Certainly, too, it is in this field where treatment is likely to be most rewarding.

The purpose of this volume is to highlight recent advances in the fields of preventive cardiology, normal and abnormal perinatal physiology, and in the clinical evaluation and management of infants with heart disease.

Thus, Nora and associates summarize current thinking concerning the etiology of congenital heart disease as related to its prevention. A discussion is provided by Van Mierop and Gessner of pathogenetic mechanisms as elucidated by a systematic study of embryologic material, and Maurice Lev has contributed a report of his studies on the pathogenesis of congenital atrioventricular block. A description is supplied by Friedman of the intrinsic physiologic properties of the heart during fetal and postnatal life and the development of myocardial autonomic innervation. Heymann and Rudolph have amplified on their basic studies of the normal fetal circulation and have extended their findings to theorize about the in utero effects of various anomalies and the manner in which subsequent cardiovascular development may be altered. A timely review is given by Miller on the subject of oxygen transport in the normal infant and in infants with cardiovascular disease.

The articles by Talner and Campbell, Graham and Jarmakani, and Meyer and Kaplan are all concerned with the subject of improved detection and diagnosis of congenital heart disease. Thorough descriptions are supplied of the value in patient management of pH and blood gas determinations, newer ultrasound and isotope noninvasive techniques in cardiovascular diagnosis, and current methods for evaluating hemodynamics and cardiac performance in the catheterization laboratory.

In the not too distant past, infants with heart disease were often considered too fragile for diagnostic or surgical intervention, and many potential candidates for palliation or cure were lost. The aggressive approach to these babies by skilled clinicians and surgeons is emphasized in this volume in the reports of Gersony and Hayes, Tatooles and Miller, and Barratt-Boyes and associates. While there is much to be done yet, it would appear that surgical treatment will be undertaken at progressively earlier ages and that the natural history of the operated patient will change accordingly.

Lastly, a comprehensive and scholarly review is provided by Harris and Ng-heim on the important, but often neglected, subject of cardiomyopathies.

It will hopefully be clear to the reader of this volume that fresh insights into neonatal cardiac disease have occurred at a rapid rate and that new ideas are be-

ing tested with appropriate judgment and technical expertise. This is an exciting
and rewarding time for pediatric cardiology and cardiac surgery, and our contributors are, in many ways, responsible for this pleasant state of affairs. Their efforts in supporting the objectives of this book are gratefully acknowledged.

William F. Friedman, M.D.
Associate Professor of Pediatrics and Medicine
Chief of Pediatric Cardiology
University of California, San Diego
School of Medicine
La Jolla, California

Pathogenetic Mechanisms in Congenital Cardiovascular Malformations

L. H. S. Van Mierop and Ira H. Gessner

CONGENITAL ANOMALIES have aroused man's curiosity, superstition, fear, and awe for many centuries. Explanations concerning their etiology and pathogenesis based upon supernatural forces, fatalism, mysticism, philosophy, and scholarly, if not always well founded, scientific reasoning have been offered for almost as long a time. Cardiac anomalies have enjoyed more than their share of interest, either because they are common and usually have profound influence on the life of the individual, or because the heart is an organ which has always had a certain special significance for man, possibly because it seems to have such an obvious, active life of its own within the body and reacts so rapidly and obviously to changes in man's emotional status.

To date, no one has had the opportunity to actually observe the pathogenesis of cardiovascular malformations by systematic study of embryologic material. While it has been possible for many years to induce cardiac (and other) anomalies in experimental animals, the effect of various teratogens appears to be rather nonspecific, and, therefore, the malformations produced by any one agent are not consistently all of the same type. Stockard[1] concluded from his classical work with *Fundulus* that different disturbances applied at the same phase of development would tend to produce the same defects, whereas the same disturbing factor applied at different phases of development produces different defects.

While this may be somewhat of an oversimplification, there seems to be little doubt that in many, if not most cases, the nature of the injurious agent is not as important a determining factor as the precise time in early development at which it is allowed to exert its influence. Such exact timing in administering an experimental insult is virtually impossible, certainly so in mammals.

Thus, it has not been possible as yet to induce transposition complexes, tetralogy of Fallot, or any other specific anomaly reproducibly, and in a high enough percentage of offspring to render embryologic studies practicable and reliable. For this reason, experimental work aimed at producing cardiac anomalies has little or no value for the study of the pathogenesis of such anomalies.

Recently, Gessner[2] has been able to create cardiac anomalies of a fairly uniform type (double outlet right ventricle and double inlet left ventricle) in chick embryos by mechanical means. Undoubtedly, the reason such uniform results

From the Departments of Pediatrics and Pathology, J. Hillis Miller Health Center, University of Florida College of Medicine, Gainesville, Fla.

Supported by USPHS Grant HE 10912.

L. H. S. Van Mierop, M.D.: Professor of Pediatrics (Cardiology) and Pathology, J. Hillis Miller Health Center, University of Florida College of Medicine, Gainesville, Fla.; recipient of NIH Career Development Award 5-KO3-HE 21540. Ira H. Gessner, M.D.: Professor of Pediatrics, J. Hillis Miller Health Center, University of Florida College of Medicine, Gainesville, Fla.; recipient of NIH Career Development Award 1-KO3-HE 35142.

could be obtained is that his method makes possible much more precise timing and duration of the insult. Other methods of producing anomalies involving only a specific region of the heart consist of causing injury to a localized area of the embryonic heart, e.g., by irradiation[3] or application of wire clips on one or more of the aortic arches.[4]

Great promise is also offered by the work of Patterson et al.[5] who, by selective breeding, have been able to acquire colonies of pure-bred dogs, in each of which cardiac anomalies of a certain type occur spontaneously in a very high percentage of offspring.

By correlating observations made on malformed hearts and those made on the cardiovascular system of normal embryos of various ages, it is often possible to arrive at a reasonably plausible explanation as to what might have happened pathogenetically in the case of a particular anomaly. In addition, it is often possible to deduce approximately at which stage of prenatal development, and, therefore, at which gestational age, an anomaly must have made its appearance. It still leaves us in the dark as to exactly when and how the injurious agent, whatever its nature, exerted its influence. In other words, it tells us little or nothing concerning the etiology of the anomaly.

In arriving at any conclusions regarding the possible pathogenesis of congenital cardiac malformations by deductive reasoning, it must be borne in mind that the ability of an embryo to compensate for developmental structural deficiencies is considerable. Valves which, because of such a deficiency, are abnormally formed may have excellent function, e.g., the atrioventricular valve(s) in endocardial cushion defects. Also, structures such as muscle bands in the anomalous heart, which morphologically resemble those present in a normal heart, may not necessarily be identical, and serious errors in interpretation may be made if the spurious nature of the apparent homology is not appreciated. Moreover, abnormal hemodynamic patterns introduced by one or more primary anomalies may have profound influence on the development of other, basically normal structures and may render these secondarily abnormal. For example, the aortic root and ascending aorta in transposition of the great arteries almost never have the same spatial relationships as those of the pulmonary root and trunk of a normal heart but are located slightly further to the right (Fig. 1A). On the other hand, in congenital aortic atresia, the pulmonary trunk arises from a morphologically normal right ventricle, but may, because of altered hemodynamics, resemble in its course the ascending aorta in transposition (Fig. 1B).

For many years congenital anomalies were thought to be due to arrests of development. This idea, first expressed by William Harvey in 1651,[6] but not firmly established until the publication of Meckel's *Handbuch der Pathologischen Anatomie*[7] some 160 yr later, received renewed impetus by the work of Stockard.[1] More recently, it has become recognized that the concept of developmental arrest ("Hemmungsbildungen"), while still constituting an important pathogenetic principle, cannot explain all malformations.

PATHOGENETIC MECHANISMS

One or more of the following developmental errors may play a role in the pathogenesis of cardiovascular anomalies: (1) aplasia or agenesis (complete

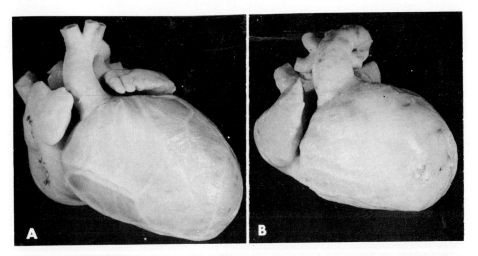

Fig. 1. (A) Transposition of the great arteries. (B) Congenital aortic atresia. Note similarity in origin from right ventricle and course of ascending aorta in (A) and pulmonary trunk and ductus arteriosus in (B).

failure of development); (2) hypoplasia, (incomplete or defective development); (3) dysplasia (intrinsic abnormal development); (4) malposition; (5) dysraphia (failure of fusion of adjoining parts); (6) abnormal fusion; (7) inadequate resorption; (8) excessive resorption; (9) abnormal persistence of patency of vessels; and (10) abnormal (early) obliteration of vessels.

Of these, the first, second, fifth, seventh, and probably in some cases also the third, fourth, and ninth, may be considered instances of developmental arrest in the classical sense.

Let us now consider each of these developmental errors and discuss briefly their role in the pathogenesis of a number of cardiovascular malformations selected here as illustrative examples. A detailed description of normal cardiovascular development and pathogenesis of cardiac malformations falls outside the scope of this paper and will not be given here. Reference is given to previously published accounts concerning these subjects.[8-26]

Aplasia or Agenesis

This term is used to indicate that a particular structure does not develop at all. In the cardiac anomaly known as persistent truncus arteriosus, for example, the truncus septum fails to develop and leaves the embryonic truncus arteriosus undivided. This results in a single arterial trunk, which gives off both the ascending aorta and the short pulmonary trunk, and which arises from the two ventricles over an interventricular communication (Fig. 2B). In many cases of truncus arteriosus, the conus septum is also absent. Associated aplasia of the aortopulmonary septum leads to forms of persistent truncus arteriosus, in which the pulmonary arteries arise independently from the trunk (types 2 and 3 of Collett and Edwards[8]).

Aplasia may also lead to arterial valve anomalies. In the normal heart the posterior (noncoronary) aortic and the anterior pulmonary valve cusps are derived from the intercalated valve swellings. Aplasia of these intercalated

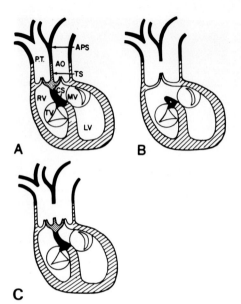

A

B

C

Fig. 2. Diagrammatic representation of atrioventricular valves, ventricles and great arteries. (A) Normal heart. (B) Persistent truncus arteriosus. (C) Aortopulmonary septal defect. AO, aorta; APS, aortopulmonary septum; CS, conus septum, LV, left ventricle; MV, mitral valve; PT, pulmonary trunk; RV, right ventricle; TS, truncus septum; TV, tricuspid valve.

valve swellings results in a type of bicuspid aortic or pulmonary valve in which the coronary cusps are absent (Fig. 3B). Neither of the two remaining cusps, therefore, contains a fibrous ridge or raphe, since such a raphe within a cusp indicates a dual origin from two embryonic anlagen (see below).

Hypoplasia

This term indicates that a particular structure does make its appearance but remains smaller than normal. In cases of anatomical Eisenmenger complex, for example, the conus septum has remained too small, or is even absent in some cases, resulting in a hypoplastic or absent crista supraventricularis. The ventricular septum which normally in part is closed by the conus septum, remains widely patent and the right atrioventricular valve cannot receive its

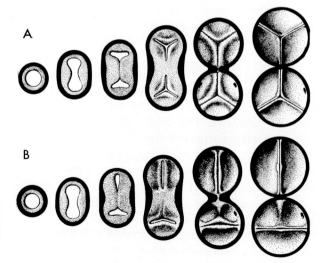

A

B

Fig. 3. (A) Diagram showing septation of truncus arteriosus and formation of arterial valves. (B) Diagram showing formation of a bicuspid valve due to aplasia of intercalated valve swelling (top) or fusion of two valve anlagen (bottom).

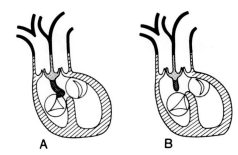

Fig. 4. (A) Infracristal "membranous" ventricular septal defect. (B) Eisenmenger complex.

A   B

contribution from the conus septum. Hence, the medial or conal papillary muscle is absent in Eisenmenger complex, and the anterior cusp of the tricuspid valve is abnormally formed. Furthermore, the aorta overrides the ventricular septal defect (Fig. 4B).

Dysplasia

This term denotes an intrinsic abnormality of development of a particular structure.

A well-known example of dysplasia that occurs in the heart is Ebstein's anomaly of the tricuspid valve. In this condition, the right atrium and right atrioventricular ostium are very large. Of the tricuspid valve cusps, only the anterior cusp originates normally from the annulus. The others appear to take their origin from the right ventricular wall in a more apical position, giving the impression that the right atrioventricular annulus is displaced downward. Thus, a variable part of the right ventricular inflow tract becomes "atrialized." The tricuspid valve cusps are always redundant, often have a crumpled appearance, and the chordae tendinae are usually poorly developed. The tricuspid valve apparatus generally resembles a crumpled sac with an opening generally smaller than the normal tricuspid ostium and is found in a constant position eccentrically near the crista supraventricularis of the right ventricle. Usually multiple smaller openings found elsewhere in the sac represent efforts at formation of chordae tendineae. In milder cases, the wall of the atrialized portion of the right ventricle has retained its musculature; in the severest cases, however, it may be fibrous and extremely thin.

The anomaly appears to be due to an abnormality in the process of undermining the right ventricular wall, which normally leads to the liberation of the inner layer of ventricular muscle. This process should continue until the atrioventricular junction is reached. Much of the apical portion of the valve "skirt" thus formed is normally resorbed until only papillary muscles and narrow muscular strands remain. The latter become fibrous (chordae tendineae) as do the valve cusps themselves. In Ebstein's anomaly, the process of undermining apparently is incomplete and the annulus is not reached (Fig. 5). Resorption takes place very inadequately or not at all, and the result is a valve which is redundant and adherent to the ventricular myocardium to a varying extent, while the chordae tendineae are poorly developed.

In dysplasia of the arterial valves, the cusps are poorly formed, thick and nodular, and look and feel almost cartilaginous. Such valve cusps are nearly

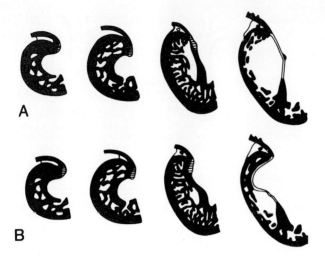

A

B

Fig. 5. (A) Diagram show-
ing formation of a normal atrioventricular valve cusp. (B) Ebstein's anomaly.

immobile and functionally result in stenosis, even though the commissures between the dysplastic cusps are not necessarily fused.

Another type of dysplasia involves the ventricular myocardium. In early embryos, the free lumen of the ventricle is comparatively small, while the trabeculated portion of the myocardium is very thick and has a sponge-like appearance. While such a thick spongy myocardium is normal in lower vertebrates, in mammals most of the trabeculae disappear, thus greatly enlarging the free lumen of the ventricles, particularly that of the left ventricle. Occasionally, however, the embryonic trabecular pattern persists and is commonly associated with an element of endocardial fibroelastosis. The result is a very poorly functioning ventricle.

Malposition

Malposition may involve the whole heart, or it may involve segments of the embryonic bulboventricular loop or the cardiac septa.

In ectopia cordis, the heart may lie outside the thoracic cavity, or it may occupy an abnormal position in the upper abdomen or in the neck. None of these represent primary anomalies of the cardiovascular system, although such anomalies may be, and usually are, associated. The cardiac malposition is due to a deficiency of the ventral body wall, or diaphragm, or both.

Malposition of one or more segments of the bulboventricular loop leads to two of the more interesting and commonly seen severe cardiac anomalies: double inlet left ventricle (both atrioventricular valves enter into what appears to be a morphologic left ventricle [Fig. 6A]), and double outlet right ventricle (both great arteries arise from the right ventricle [Fig. 6B]). In order to be able to understand the nature of these two malformations, it is necessary to discuss briefly some pertinent aspects of normal cardiac development.[18]

In the 20-somite embryo, after formation of the cardiac loop, the heart is still little more than a simple, albeit convoluted, tube. Local expansions of this convoluted tube give rise to the formation of the common atrium, the primitive left ventricle (earlier the embryonic ventricle) and the primitive right ven-

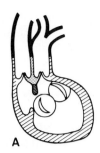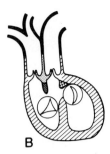

Fig. 6. (A) Double inlet left ventricle. (B) Double outlet right ventricle.

A   B

tricle (the expanding proximal one-third of the bulbis cordis; the remaining two-thirds constitute the truncoconal portion of the bulboventricular loop). The atrioventricular canal, the narrow segment which connects the common atrium with the primitive left ventricle, is located far to the left. On the other hand, the truncoconal portion of the bulboventricular loop, which, after partitioning, will form the outflow portions of both definitive ventricles and the pulmonary and aortic roots, arises from the primitive right ventricle and is located far to the right. The two primitive ventricles communicate with each other by way of the primary interventricular foramen.

In normal development, there is a medial shift of both the atrioventricular canal (to the right) and the truncoconal portion (to the left) of the developing heart. This makes it possible for the still undivided atrium to discharge its blood directly into both primitive ventricles, while at the same time it becomes possible for both ventricles to eject their blood directly into the truncoconal portion of the heart. After partitioning of the atrioventricular canal by the superior and inferior atrioventricular endocardial cushions, the left atrioventricular ostium empties into the left ventricle, while the right atrioventricular ostium and its surrounding area become incorporated into the primitive right ventricle to form its atrioventricular valve and inflow portion. After partitioning of the truncus and conus, the posteromedial portion of the conus cordis becomes the left ventricular outflow tract, while the anterolateral portion is incorporated into the right ventricle to become its outflow portion, commonly referred to as the right ventricular infundibulum.

Normally, therefore, the definitive right ventricle is derived from the primitive right ventricle, the right side of the primitive left ventricle, and the anterolateral part of the conus cordis. The definitive left ventricle is derived from the left and major portion of the primitive left ventricle and the posteromedial part of the conus cordis.

Failure of the medial rightward shift of the atrioventricular canal will result, after its partitioning, in both atrioventricular ostia communicating with the primitive left ventricle only. The end product is a heart that has one large ventricle, which generally has the characteristics of a morphologic left ventricle, and into which both atrioventricular valves enter; hence, the aptly descriptive, if somewhat inaccurate, term double inlet left ventricle. In the complete form of this anomaly, both atrioventricular valves structurally resemble a mitral valve, one the mirror image of the other. Commonly, the right atrioventricular valve overrides the small muscular ventricular septum, i.e., the anomaly is "incomplete" or "partial." The right ventricle remains small since it does not receive the right atrioventricular ostium and surrounding area which normally form its inflow portion. Usually the aorta arises from this small "outflow chamber" while the pulmonary trunk originates from the left ventricle, i.e., transposition of the great arteries is associated. Double inlet left ventricle with normally interrelated great arteries is known by the eponym "Holmes heart." It is not understood why transposition of the great arteries is such a commonly associated anomaly in double inlet left ventricle. The reason, in the complete form of the anomaly, that both atrioventricular valves structurally resemble a mitral valve, one the mirror image of the other, is that the right atrioventricular valve fails to gain relationships with either the muscular ventricular septum or the conus septum, and therefore does not receive its normal contribution from the latter to form the medial-most part of the anterior cusp and the medial or conal papillary muscle. Consequently, both valves develop in a fashion similar to the normal mitral valve.

If the medial shift of the truncoconal part of the heart does not occur, this part of the heart retains its original connection with the primitive right ventricle only, and the sole outlet for the left ventricle is formed by the primary interventricular foramen. The result is that the embryonic conoventricular fold is retained, and that both portions of the conus cordis, after formation of the conus septum, become part of the right ventricle. Both great arteries, therefore, continue to arise from that ventricle, a condition aptly, but again somewhat inaccurately, called double outlet right ventricle, and both atrial valves remain separated from the atrioventricular valves by a band of muscle. Transposition of the great arteries may or may not be associated; usually it is not.[19]

A special type of malposition involving the bulboventricular loop results in the interesting anomaly known as ventricular inversion with transposition of the great arteries, or "corrected" transposition of the great arteries. In this condition, the atria are normal, but the atrioventricular valves and ventricles are inverted, the morphologic tricuspid valve and right ventricle being on the left, and the morphologic mitral valve and left ventricle being on the right. The aorta almost always arises anteriorly from the morphologic right ventricle, while the pulmonary trunk springs from the morphologic left ventricle posteriorly. It is generally agreed at present that the anomaly is due to inverted development of the bulboventricular loop, i.e., to the left instead of to the right. The associated transposition is not the result of an additional developmental error but is a necessary sequel, since the aortopulmonary septum develops normally, while the truncus septum is formed in the mirror image of normal.[20]

Probably the best known example of an anomaly caused by malposition of one of the embryonic cardiac septa is tetralogy of Fallot. In this condition there is a large interventricular communication, a right ventricular outflow obstruction of varying degree from mild stenosis to atresia at the infundibular level, and the aorta arises from both ventricles (dextroposed or overriding aorta [Fig. 7D]). The pulmonary valve may or may not be bicuspid and/or stenotic, but is almost always more or less hypoplastic because of reduced blood flow. The commonly associated right aortic arch is probably also a secondary anomaly induced by the altered hemodynamics.

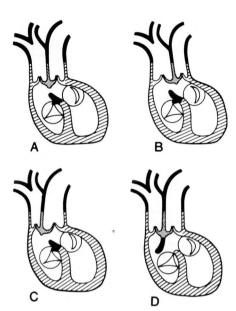

Fig. 7. (A) Supracristal ventricular septal defect without displacement of truncus septum. (B) Supracristal ventricular septal defect with posterior displacement of truncus septum. (C) Supracristal ventricular septal defect with anterior displacement of truncus septum. (D) Tetralogy of Fallot.

In normal development the truncus and conus septum divide the respective portions of the heart into two equal parts. The normal conus septum helps to close the primary interventricular foramen and also contributes to the formation of the tricuspid valve, specifically the medial-most portion of the anterior cusp and the medial or conal papillary muscle. In tetralogy of Fallot, the anteriorly displaced conus septum divides the conus cordis into two unequal portions at the expense of the anterolateral part, normally destined to become the right ventricular outflow tract. If the anterior displacement only involves the proximal portion of the conus septum, the result will be stenosis of the infundibular ostium. In such cases there is a distinct infundibular chamber, and the pulmonary root and pulmonary trunk may be well developed and of nearly normal size. If all of the conus septum is displaced anteriorly, the result is a long, narrow infundibulum. In such cases, the truncus septum is probably always displaced anteriorly also, and the pulmonary root and trunk are severely hypoplastic. Anterior displacement of the conus septum makes it impossible for this septum to contribute to the closure of the interventricular foramen, and this results in a large ventricular septal defect. Since the displaced conus septum is far removed from the right atrioventricular ostium, it also cannot contribute to the formation of this valve. This valve is, therefore, structurally abnormal, while the medial or conal papillary muscle characteristically is absent. Even though the tricuspid valve in tetralogy of Fallot is anatomically abnormally formed, it is almost never incompetent, another illustration of the ability of the embryo to make do with whatever material is available to it from a well-functioning structure.

Malposition of one of two adjoining embryonic cardiac septa makes it difficult or impossible for such septa to fuse with each other. For example, if the conus septum develops normally, but the truncus septum is displaced posteriorly, the result is a type of supracristal ventricular defect in which the large pulmonary trunk and valve override the defect (Fig. 7B). This type of ventricular septal defect is extremely uncommon as an isolated malformation, but, in our experience, is seen in most, if not all, cases of true interruption of the aortic arch. This, incidentally, might suggest the interesting possibility that true aortic arch interruption is a secondary rather than a primary abnormality.

If the truncus septum is displaced anteriorly, then the result again is a supracristal ventricular septal defect but with the aorta overriding the defect (Fig. 7C). The pulmonary trunk is quite narrow and the valve may be bicuspid, but the crista supraventricularis, the tricuspid valve, and the medial papillary muscle are normal. Physiologically, this uncommon cardiac malformation mimics tetralogy of Fallot and is usually misdiagnosed as such.

Failure of Fusion

It is unlikely that very many cardiac anomalies are simply due to failure of fusion of opposing or adjoining structures; an element of hypoplasia is probably almost always present. One of the best-known examples of this type of defect is persistent atrioventricular canal in its various forms, also known by the term endocardial cushion defect. The heart in the complete form of the anomaly so obviously resembles that of a young (6–9 mm C-R [crown-rump] length) embryo that the pathogenesis of the condition has been recognized for many years. In fact, it is the only cardiac anomaly of which the name (endocardial cushion defect) indicates its pathogenesis, and it is one of the few cardiac defects named with an embryologic term (others: persistent truncus arteriosus, patent ductus arteriosus, aortopulmonary septal defect). This curious circumstance is undoubtedly due to lack of communication between embryologists and clinicians. The former have had little opportunity to study anomalous hearts, and the latter generally have only a rudimentary grasp of cardiac embryology.

In endocardial cushion defects, partial or complete failure of fusion of the superior and inferior endocardial cushions is the principal pathogenetic feature. Normally, the superior and inferior atrioventricular endocardial cushions fuse in embryos of about 10 mm C-R length. At the same time, the fusing cushions bend to form an arch or bay, which is convex towards the atrial side and concave towards the ventricular side. Subsequently, the atrial septum primum fuses with the dorsal or convex aspect of the fused endocardial cushions midway between their right and left extremities. The ventricular septum in turn blends with the right extremity of the fused cushions over a rather broad area. The left half of the fused endocardial cushions develops into the central portion of the anterior cusp of the mitral valve. The part between the areas of fusion of septum primum and the ventricular septum becomes the atrioventricular part of the cardiac septum. The extreme right side, by a process of undermining which takes place in the ventricles, and which normally leads to the formation of the atrioventricular valve cusps, chordae tendineae, papillary muscles, and trabeculae carneae, develops into the anterior half of the septal cusp of the tricuspid valve and the adjacent part of the ventricular septum, the anterior-most portion of which eventually becomes thin and fibrous to form the interventricular part of the membranous septum.

In endocardial cushion defects, in addition to the partial or complete failure of fusion of the two major endocardial cushions, the arch or bay is usually not formed. This results in an apparent downward or apical displacement of the atrioventricular valve cusps medially. Furthermore, the free border of the atrial septum primum cannot fuse with the endocardial cushions, so that an inter-atrial communication remains, and the atrioventricular part of the cardiac septum is not formed. In addition, the upper portion of the ventricular septum remains deficient to a greater or lesser degree, resulting in either an inter-ventricular communication or a large area of fibrous tissue. The cleft in the anterior mitral valve cusp seen in nearly all forms of endocardial cushion defects is a result of failure of fusion of the left halves of the endocardial cushions.

Even though the anomaly is a severe one, the function of the abnormal atrio-ventricular valve may be quite good, even in the complete form of the defect, and particularly in infants and young children. This is again an example of the rather amazing ability of the embryo to compensate for deficiencies. Incompetence does tend to develop sooner or later, however, and, once initiated, may rapidly increase in severity.

Undoubtedly, many basilar, "membranous," ventricular septal defects (Fig. 4A) are due to failure of fusion of those portions of the embryonic heart which normally execute the closure of the interventricular foramen, i.e., the atrio-ventricular endocardial cushions, the fused atrioventricular endocardial cushions, and the conus septum, although a certain amount of hypoplasia of one or more of these contributors probably plays an important role in many cases. The exact size and location of the defect depends upon which of the contributors is mainly at fault.

Other cardiac anomalies which are probably mainly due to failure of fusion are the type of supracristal ventricular septal defect in which neither the aorta nor the pulmonary trunk overrides the defect (there is no associated displacement of the truncus septum [Fig. 7A]) and the anomaly known as aortopulmonary septal defect or aortopulmonary window, in which the aortopulmonary septum has failed to fuse with the distal face of the truncus septum (Fig. 2C). One might ask why defects of this sort are more or less circular rather than slit-shaped, as one might expect when nonfusion of adjoining structures is the underlying pathogenetic mechanism. Two reasons may be postulated: it is likely, as we already mentioned above, that some degree of hypoplasia plays a role, and, in addition, it might be expected that continued flow of blood through an originally slit-shaped orifice will eventually change its shape to a more circular one.

Abnormal Fusion

The best known and most common anomalies, which are due to abnormal fusion, are stenoses or atresias of the atrioventricular and arterial valves. Commissures between adjoining valve cusps may become partially or completely fused. When such fusion involves one of the commissures of an arterial valve, the result commonly is a "bicuspid valve," actually an incompletely tricuspid valve, in which one of the cusps is somewhat larger than the other and contains a raphe indicating the position where the commissure separating the two embryonic valve anlages should have been. Such a valve initially is not hemodynamically stenotic, i.e., there is no demonstrable pressure gradient. It does, however, interfere with the smooth flow of blood and causes turbulence. This, in turn, damages the cusps, which later in life often become calcified and secondarily stenotic. Fusion of two commissures always causes significant stenosis; if all three are fused completely the valve obviously is atretic.

Fusion of the left extremity of one of the atrioventricular endocardial cushions (usually the inferior one) with the left lateral cushion results in the anomaly known as "double mitral valve," an unfortunate misnomer. The papillary muscles and chordae tendineae of such a mitral valve with two orifices are normal, and, as Whimsatt[25] has pointed out, the ostium is simply divided by a bridge of valve tissue.

Inadequate Resorption

One of the most common examples of inadequate resorption is seen in cases of partial or total retention of the right sinus valve. This valve is very large in young embryos and aids in diverting part of the systemic venous blood to the left atrium across the foramen ovale. Only a relatively narrow opening allows blood to enter the right atrium. Normally the right sinus valve, by a process of resorption (due to necrobiosis), is greatly reduced in size, leaving a vestigial, sickle-shaped fold, the Eustachian valve, flanking the ostium of the inferior vena cava. Occasionally, all or nearly all of the valve persists and may cause more or less significant obstruction to blood flow. This condition has been referred to as right-sided tri-atrial heart. Occasionally, multiple resorption sites convert the valve into a delicate lace or netlike structure known as Chiari's network.

The left sinus valve is normally also reduced in size, and what is left fuses with the atrial septum. In rare cases, it may persist as a thin fold of variable width just to the right of the atrial septum, giving the impression that there is a double septum primum, one in either atrium.

Other examples of inadequate resorption have been referred to above in connection with Ebstein's anomaly of the tricuspid valve (inadequate resorption of valve tissue), and dysplasia of the ventricles (inadequate resorption of embryonic ventricular trabeculae).

Excessive Resorption

This process is responsible for one of the commonest forms of congenital cardiac disease: the atrial septal defect at the fossa ovalis, or so-called "secundum" type atrial septal defect. Normally, in embryos of about 7–8 mm C-R length, local resorption of septum primum prior to closure of ostium primum leads to the formation of ostium secundum. If this process is carried to excess, or if there are multiple, ectopic resorption sites, an extremely large ostium secundum is produced which cannot be guarded by septum secundum, resulting in an interatrial communication.

Defects in the muscular portion of the ventricular septum may also be thought of as due to excessive resorption. Such resorption takes place normally in the ventricular portion of the heart and leads to the formation of trabeculae carneae. Excessive resorption of the ventricular septum could lead to communication between the two ventricles and could also explain why muscular ventricular septal defects are so often multiple.

Abnormal Persistence of Patency

Abnormal persistence of patency of arterial and venous channels, or segments thereof, is extremely common. One of the best known and most common anomalies of this sort is continued patency of the ductus arteriosus after birth. The ductus arteriosus, derived from the distal portion of the left sixth brachial arterial (aortic) arch of the embryo, is the only portion of the aortic arch system which is a muscular rather than an elastic type artery. It is, therefore, able to contract to occlusion, and normally does so within hours or days after birth, thus physiologically interrupting blood flow between the pulmonary trunk and aorta. Anatomical closure follows and eventually the ductus arteriosus is reduced to a fibrous strand. It is not well understood at present as to why, in some cases, the ductus arteriosus remains patent. On the other hand, the tendency for the ductus arteriosus to close is so strong that it almost always does so even in cases where continued patency would be of great benefit to the individual, e.g., in cases of severe reduction of pulmonary blood flow due to pulmonary valvar stenosis or atresia.

An equally well-known but rare anomaly, in which there is pathologic patency of an arterial channel, is bilateral persistence of the dorsal aorta beyond the subclavian artery, resulting in a double aortic arch. Normally, this segment of the dorsal aorta involutes on the right side so that the right subclavian artery comes to arise from the brachiocephalic trunk, its first portion being formed by the right fourth aortic arch and the proximal segment of the right dorsal aorta.

A common systemic venous anomaly resulting from abnormal persistence of an embryonic venous channel is the persistent left superior vena cava. This condition, normally present in many lower mammals but not seen in man, is the result of continued patency of the left common cardinal vein–left sinus horn complex. It causes no hemodynamic embarrassment, and it is almost always found as an incidental finding, either isolated or associated with other cardiovascular anomalies.

Abnormal Obliteration

Abnormal total regression of the left embryonic fourth arch, in addition to the normal obliteration of the right dorsal aorta, leads to the anomaly known as interruption of the aortic arch. There is no trace of any connection between the aortic arch beyond the left common carotid artery and the descending aorta, which receives its blood from the pulmonary trunk by way of the ductus arteriosus. An associated anomalous right subclavian artery arising from the descending aorta, indicating disappearance of the right fourth arch as well, is very common. The possibility that the anomaly secondarily is the result of abnormal hemodynamics associated with the type of supracristal ventricular septal defect with overriding pulmonary trunk has been alluded to above.

Very often abnormal persistence of an arterial channel, or segment thereof, is associated with abnormal involution of another. For example, in cases of

Table 1

Streeter's Horizon	Crown-Rump (C-R) Length	Ovulation Age (Days)	Normal Developmental Events	Anomalies Becoming Manifest	Developmental Error
IX-X	1.5–1.8mm late presomite to two somite embryo	20–21	Development of bilaterally symmetrical vascular system	None known in man	—
X	2.0–2.2 mm 4–7 somite embryo	22–23	Fusion of segments of left and right vascular system ventral to foregut to form single heart tube which comes to lie intrapericardially First pair of aortic arches Vitelline (omphalomesenteric) veins	None known in man	—
XI–XII	2.4–3.3 mm 8–22 somite embryo	23–26	Formation of bulboventricular loop with convexity to the right Early ventricular trabeculation Breakdown of mesocardium Second pair of aortic arches Umbilical veins Cardinal venous system	Ventricular inversion with transposition of the great arteries ("corrected" transposition of the great arteries)	Inverted development of the bulbo-ventricular loop with normal development of atrium and truncoaortic sac
XII–XIV	3.5–6 mm	26–29	Medial shift of atrioventricular canal (to the right) and of the trunco conal portion of the bulboventricular loop (to the left) Development of extensive sponge-like ventricular trabeculae Appearance of atrioventricular endocardial cushions	Double inlet left ventricle Double outlet right ventricle Muscular ventricular septal defect	Failure of medial shift of atrioventricular canal Failure of medial shift of truncoconal portion of the heart Excessive resorption of ventricular septum resulting in perforation

Stage	Size	Normal development	Malformation	Abnormal development
		Appearance of truncus swellings	Persistent truncus arteriosus	Aplasia (hypoplasia) of truncus swellings
		Appearance of conus swellings		
		Appearance of septum primum	Common atrium	Aplasia (hypoplasia) of septum I
		Appearance of common pulmonary vein	Total anomalous pulmonary venous connection	Aplasia (early obliteration?) of common pulmonary vein
		Third, fourth (fifth) and sixth pair of aortic arches		
		Appearance of subcardinal veins		
		Involution of first and second pair of aortic arches		
		Involution of left proximal vitelline vein	Left common hepatic vein	Persistence of left proximal vitelline vein
XVI–XV	7–8 mm	Fusion of truncus swellings to form truncus septum	Transposition of the great arteries	Early appearance and dominance of intercalated valve swellings which execute division of truncus arteriosus instead of truncus swellings. These in turn remain small and form a valve cusp each
		Formation of aortopulmonary septum by invagination of trunco aortic sac	Persistent truncus arteriosus types 2 and 3	Aplasia of truncus swellings and of aortopulmonary septum
XVI–XVII	9–13 mm	Fusion of atrioventricular endocardial cushions	Endocardial cushion defect (persistent atrioventricular canal)	Failure of fusion (total or in part) of atrioventricular endocardial cushions
		Fusion of aortopulmonary septum with truncus septum, establishing arterial roots, ascending aorta and pulmonary trunk	Aortopulmonary septal defect (aortopulmonary window)	Failure of fusion of aortopulmonary septum with truncus septum
		Appearance of intercalated valve swellings and early development of arterial valves	True bicuspid aortic or pulmonary valve	Aplasia of intercalated valve swellings

(Continued)

Table 1 (Cont'd)

Streeter's Horizon	Crown-Rump (C-R) Length	Ovulation Age (Days)	Normal Developmental Events	Anomalies Becoming Manifest	Developmental Error
			Fusion of conus swellings towards end of period to form conus septum	Tetralogy of Fallot	Unequal partitioning of conus at the expense of the right ventricular outflow tract
			Fusion of conus septum with truncus septum	Eisenmenger complex	Hypoplasia of conus septum
				Supracristal ventricular septal defect, 3 types	Failure of fusion (with or without displacement of truncus septum) of conus and truncus septa
			Establishment of ostium secundum	Atrial septal defect at fossa cvalis	Excessive resorption of septum primum, too large ostium secundum
			Closure of ostium primum		
			Involution of right and proximal left umbilical veins		
			Establishment of intersubcardinal anastomosis and subcardinohepatic anastomosis		
			Early involution of left proximal common cardinal vein		
			Appearance of the spleen on left side of dorsal mesogastrium	Asplenia syndrome*	Aplasia of the spleen
				Polysplenia syndrome*	Appearance of a spleen on both sides of dorsal mesogastrium
XVIII–XX	14–23 mm	37–42	Closure of interventricular foramen by endocardial cushions, conus septum and ventricular septum	Infracristal ("membranous") ventricular septal defects	Failure of fusion between (and hypoplasia of) endocardial cushions, conus septum and ventricular septum

Early elaboration of posterior mitral and posterior tricuspid valve cusps	Atrioventricular valve stenosis or atresia	Abnormal partial or complete fusion between two or more cusp anlagen
Involution of right distal sixth aortic arch, right and left ductus caroticus (segment of dorsal aorta between third and fourth aortic arches) and right dorsal aorta distal to right seventh intersegmental artery, establishing normal adult aortic arch pattern	Aortic arch anomalies (double aortic arch, right aortic arch with ipsi—or contralateral ductus arteriosus, anomalous subclavian artery arising from descending aorta, double ductus, absent proximal pulmonary artery, etc.)	Abnormal persistence with or without abnormal involution of various components of the embryonic aortic arch system
Incorporation of common pulmonary vein and its primary branches into the embryonic left atrium	Cor triatriatum	Failure of expansion of junction of common pulmonary vein with embryonic left atrium (failure of incorporation of common pulmonary vein and its primary branches into the embryonic left atrium
Development of supracardinal (azygos) venous system		
Involution of posterior cardinal veins (except proximal segment)		
Establishment of definitive inferior vena cava		
Formation of left renal, adrenal and gonadal veins from subcardinal venous system		

*None of the cardiovascular anomalies occurring in asplenia and polysplenia syndrome, which become manifest in this period of development, is unique for either syndrome. Total absence of a splenic anlage, or appearance of two such anlagen, one on either side of the dorsal mesogastrium in embryos larger than 10 mm C-R length, should be diagnostic.

right-sided aortic arch, the entire right-sided dorsal aorta persists to form part of the thoracic aorta, whereas most of the left-sided dorsal aorta disappears. It is, of course, difficult to say in a situation of this sort whether the abnormal persistence of patency is the primary anomaly, or whether patency is retained as a compensatory mechanism necessitated by abnormal involution of the normal channel.

Total anomalous pulmonary venous connection may be thought of as being due to aplasia or abnormal early obliteration of the common pulmonary vein. One or more embryonic venous connections between the pulmonary venous plexus and the systemic veins are retained as alternate drainage routes for the pulmonary venous return.

At this point we would like to make some comments concerning a cardiovascular anomaly which appears to be somewhat of an enigma, namely, transposition of the great arteries. No cardiovascular anomaly has received more attention and generated more discussion and controversy for as long a time. In fact, even the validity of its name has recently been questioned,[27] and no one as yet has been able to define it to everyone's satisfaction. To this date, there continues to be a singular lack of agreement among experts in the field concerning its pathogenesis. Certainly there is no stage of development in which the embryonic heart resembles the great vessel–ventricular relationships seen in transposition, and it cannot, therefore, be considered due to a simple arrest of development. The fact that the anomaly is common, and, in more than half the cases, not associated with other defects, while its great vessel interrelationship is almost always present in ventricular inversion, strongly suggests that it is due to a single, fundamental aberration in development, which deserves to occupy its very own niche within the framework of congenital malformations of the heart.

Finally, it might be of interest to give a chronological overview of the periods of development at which times various forms of cardiovascular anomalies might be expected to become manifest (not induced). This we have attempted to do in Table 1.

REFERENCES

1. Stockard, C. R.: Developmental rate and structural expression: An experimental study of twins, "double monsters" and single deformities, and the interaction among embryonic organs during their origin and development. Amer. J. Anat. 28:115, 1921.

2. Gessner, I. H., and Van Mierop, L. H. S.: Experimental production of cardiac defects: The spectrum of dextroposition of the aorta. Amer. J. Cardiol. 25:272, 1970.

3. Le Douarin, G.: Malformations résultant d'irradiations localisées de différentes parties de l'ébauche cardiaque chez l'embryon de poulet. J. Embryol. Exp. Morph. 9:556, 1961.

4. Rychter, Z.: Experimental morphology of the aortic arches and the heart loop in chick embryos. Advances Morph. 2:333, 1962.

5. Patterson, D. F.: Epidemiologic and genetic studies of congenital heart disease in the dog. Circ. Res. 23:171, 1968.

6. Harvey, W.: De Generatione Animalium. Translation by R. Willis In The works of William Harvey. London, 1847.

7. Meckel, J. F.: Handbuch der Pathologischen Anatomie. Leipzig, Reclam, 1812.

8. Collett, R. W., and Edwards, J. E.: Persistent truncus arteriosus: Classification according to anatomic types. Surg. Clin. N. Amer. 29:1245, 1949.

9. De la Cruz, M. V., Espino-Vela, J., Attie, F., and Munoz, L. C.: An embryologic theory for ventricular inversions and their classification. Amer. Heart J. 73:777, 1967.

10. — , and DaRocha, J. P.: An ontogenetic

theory for the explanation of congenital malformations involving the truncus and conus. Amer. Heart J. 51:782, 1956.

11. —, and Miller, B. L.: Double inlet left ventricle: Two pathological specimens with comment on the embryology and on its relation to single ventricle. Circulation 37:249, 1968.

12. Grant, R. P.: The morphogenesis of transposition of the great vessels. Circulation 26:819, 1962.

13. Kramer, T. C.: The partitioning of the truncus and conus and the formation of the membranous portion of the interventricular septum in the human heart. Amer. J. Anat. 71:343, 1942.

14. Patten, B. M.: Human Embryology. New York, Blakiston, 1953.

15. Stewart, J. R., Kincaid, O. W., and Edwards, J. E.: An Atlas of Vascular Rings and Related Malformations of the Aortic Arch System, Springfield, Ill., Charles C Thomas, 1964.

16. Tandler, J.: Anatomie des Herzens. In Bardeleben's Handbuch der Anatomie des Menschen. Jena, Gustav Fischer, 1913.

17. Van Mierop, L. H. S., Alley, R. D., Kausel, H. W., and Stranahan, A.: The anatomy and embryology of endocardial cushion defects. J. Thorac. Cardiovasc. Surg. 43:71, 1962.

18. —, Alley, R. D., Kausel, H. W., and Stranahan, A.: Pathogenesis of transposition complexes. I. Embryology of the ventricles and great arteries. Amer. J. Cardiol. 12:216, 1963.

19. —, and Wiglesworth, F. W.: Pathogenesis of transposition complexes. II. Anomalies due to faulty transfer of the posterior great arteries. III. True transposition of the great vessels. Amer. J. Cardiol. 12:226, 1963.

20. — : Section III: Embryology, and Section IV: Diseases-congenital anomalies. In Netter, F. H. (Ed.): The Ciba Collection of Medical Illustrations, Volume V. The Heart. New York, Ciba Foundation, 1969.

21. — : Pathology and pathogenesis of the common cardiac malformations. Cardiovasc. Clinics 2:27, 1970.

22. Van Praagh, R., Van Praagh, S., Vlad, P., and Keith, J. D.: Anatomic types of congenital dextrocardia. Diagnostic and embryologic implications. Amer. J. Cardiol. 13:510, 1964.
Van Praagh, S., Vlad, P., and Keith, J. D.: Anatomic types of congenital dextrocardia. Diagnostic and embryologic implications. Amer. J. Cardiol. 13:510, 1964.

23. —, and Van Praagh, S.: Isolated ventricular inversion. A consideration of the morphogenesis, definition and diagnosis of nontransposed and transposed great arteries. Amer. J. Cardiol. 17:395, 1966.

24. Wakai, C. S., and Edwards, J. E.: Developmental and pathologic considerations in persistent common atrioventricular canal. Proc. Staff Meet. Mayo Clinic 31:487, 1956.

25. Whimsatt, W. A., and Lewis, F. T.: Duplication of the mitral valve and a rare apical interventricular foramen in the heart of a yak calf. Amer. J. Anat. 83:67, 1948.

26. Witham, A. C.: Double outlet right ventricle. Amer. Heart J. 53:928, 1957.

27. Van Praagh, R., et al.: Transposition of the great arteries with posterior aorta, anterior pulmonary artery, subpulmonary conus and fibrous continuity between aortic and atrioventricular valves. Amer. J. Cardiol. 28:621, 1971.

The Intrinsic Physiologic Properties
of the Developing Heart

William F. Friedman

I T HAS BECOME INCREASINGLY CLEAR that an understanding of the changes in cardiovascular structure and function that accompany growth is a prerequisite to a proper comprehension of the clinical consequences of congenital heart lesions throughout life. Although certain intrinsic structural, chemical, mechanical, and pharmacologic properties of heart muscle may be age dependent, many difficulties have surrounded previous efforts to analyze these properties in the fetal or neonatal heart in situ. Accordingly, the objective of the studies described in the present report was to define more clearly the mechanics of myocardial contraction as a function of age; the passive pressure-volume or compliance characteristics of each ventricle of the developing heart; some of the relations between age and myocardial energy metabolism; and the development of sympathetic and parasympathetic innervation of the mammalian heart.

INTRINSIC MECHANICAL PROPERTIES

In order to assess the mechanics of myocardial contraction as a function of age, while obviating the technical difficulties that complicate efforts to study the fetal or neonatal heart in situ, an isolated heart muscle preparation was em-employed in most of our studies to provide quantitative comparisons of the hearts of fetal and newborn lambs and adult sheep. After hysterotomy under local anesthesia, right ventricular moderator bands were removed rapidly from the hearts of fetal lambs in the last 15 days of gestation, and from newborn and adult animals after pentathol anesthesia. Muscles were placed in a myograph and studied under identical conditions of temperature (30°C), pH (7.4), and frequency of stimulation (12/min). The mechanical arrangement of the muscle in the myograph permitted the study of either isometric, or isotonic afterloaded contractions, so that one could define length-tension and force-velocity relations.

One of the advantages of studying isolated heart muscle in the perinatal period, rather than the heart in situ, is illustrated in Fig. 1. This is an isometric tension tracing showing the effects of paired electrical stimulation on fetal ventricular myocardium. During the course of cardiac catheterization studies in infants under 2 wk of age, several investigators[1] were unable to identify any rise in ventricular pressure in the beat following a premature ventricular contraction. This finding suggested that some intrinsic difference might exist in the

From the Division of Pediatric Cardiology, and the Department of Pediatrics, University of California, San Diego, School of Medicine, La Jolla, Calif.

Supported by USPHS Grant HE 12373.

William F. Friedman, M.D.: Chief, Division of Pediatric Cardiology, and Associate Professor of Pediatrics and Medicine, University of California, San Diego, School of Medicine, La Jolla, Calif.; recipient of National Heart and Lung Institute Research Career Development Award 5 KO4 HE41737.

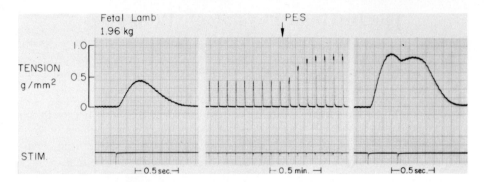

Fig. 1. Isometric tension tracing of a right ventricular moderator band isolated from the heart of a fetal lamb. Note the marked augmentation In cardiac contractility associated with onset of paired electrical stimulation (PES). STIM, stimulus artifact.

newborn heart in contractility, or in the excitation-contraction process. Our studies do not support this view because we were always able to demonstrate poststimulation potentiation or augmented myocardial contractility after paired electrical stimulation in the fetus or newborn of many mammalian species.

The dependence of developed myocardial force on initial muscle length is the basis of the well-known Frank-Starling principle. In our studies, isometric, passive, and active length-tension curves of cardiac muscle from fetal lambs were compared to those obtained from adult sheep (Fig. 2). At all muscle lengths along the length-tension curve, there is a significant reduction in the active tension generated by fetal muscles when compared to the adult. Figure 2 also demonstrates that resting, or passive tension, is higher in the fetus than the adult at any muscle length along the length-tension curve. The steeper slope of

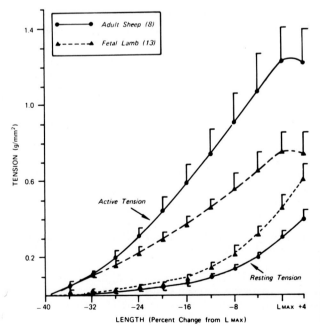

Fig. 2. Isometric passive and active length-tension curves from the fetus and adult. Numbers in brackets refer to numbers of animals studied. Each point and the vertical bars represent the mean ± SEM.

the fetal resting tension curve suggests a reduced compliance of these muscles when compared to the adult, and this difference is most pronounced as L_{max} is approached. In these isolated muscle experiments, it is important to recognize that developed tension is normalized for the cross-sectional area of the isolated muscles.

In order to evaluate more thoroughly these age-dependent differences, a number of muscles were fixed with glutaraldehyde at the apex of their length-tension curves, and then prepared for electron microscopic examination. It was of considerable interest that the length of sarcomeres at L_{max} for both fetal and adult cardiac muscle was similar, and averaged 2.18 μ. It has been shown previously that it is at this length that the two sets of myofilaments of the sarcomere are most ideally situated to provide the greatest area for their interaction.[2] The electron micrographs did, however, reveal a major difference between the fetus and adult. First, it was evident that the diameter of the fetal cell was smaller than that of the adult. Further, in fetal ventricular myocardium, the proportion of noncontractile mass (primarily nuclei, mitochondria, and surface membranes) to the number of myofibrils is significantly higher than in the adult. Approximately 60% of the adult muscle consists of contractile mass, in contrast to a value of about 30% of the fetus. Therefore, in our length-tension studies, if the tension data is normalized, not only for the cross-sectional area, but also for the higher fetal ratio of noncontractile/contractile mass, the results suggest that individual myofilaments in both the fetal and adult hearts are capable of similar force generation. In other words, a gram of fetal ventricle contains significantly fewer sarcomeres than a gram of adult ventricle. While the intrinsic strength of the sarcomeres appears to be similar at both ages, the adult ventricular muscle generates significantly more force per unit area.

By studying the relation between load and velocity of shortening, Hill[3] described what has been termed the most fundamental property of a muscle's contractile elements, the force-velocity relation. Thus, in order to characterize developing muscle more completely, isotonic afterloaded contractions were studied at a similar length relative to L_{max}. Figure 3 illustrates the relations between both extent and velocity of shortening and tension. As would be expected from the age-related differences observed in the isometric length-tension curves, the extent of shortening was less in the fetus at any level of tension when compared to the adult (Fig. 3A). This finding supports and provides an explanation for Downing's past observation that a depression in stroke volume occurs in intact newborn lambs at levels of afterload that would be considered quite low for an adult animal.[4] Of special interest was the observation that the force-velocity curve of fetal muscle was also shifted to the left of the adult curve (Fig. 3B). The intercept on the horizontal axis, which is isometric tension, is reduced in the fetus. Moreover, at any given tension the velocity of shortening is diminished in the fetus when compared to the adult. The force-velocity relation is of special interest because the velocity of the unloaded muscle (V_{max} or intrinsic velocity) is a reflection of the cyclic force-generating processes within the sarcomere, and alterations in contractile state may be detected by observing changes in V_{max}.[5] In our experiments, when maximum velocity at zero load is estimated by extrapolating the curves to the velocity intercept, it can been seen that the fetal and

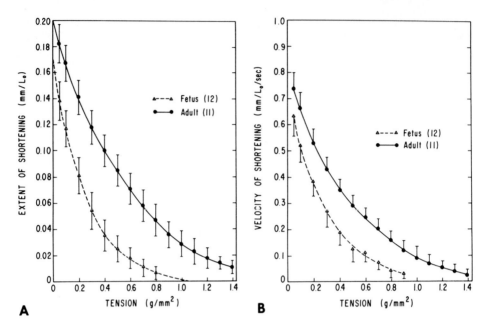

Fig. 3. Relationships between the extent (A) and velocity (B) of shortening and developed tension. Numbers in brackets reflect numbers of lambs and sheep from which heart muscle was isolated. Each point and the vertical bars represent the mean ± SEM.

adult curves tend to converge, and that no significant differences exist in V_{max} between fetus and adult (Fig. 3B). In this analysis, both the velocity and extent of shortening have been corrected for muscle length, while tension has been normalized for cross-sectional area. Once again, it must be recognized that additional normalization of the tension data for the noncontractile/contractile mass differences, which are greater in the fetus, would shift both fetal curves to the right (Fig. 4). Thus, one can interpret this data as also being consistent with a decrease in the young hearts in the number of contractile units or sarcomeres, in keeping with the electron microscopic findings. It would appear, therefore, that the intrinsic velocity of contraction of each fetal sarcomere is not significantly different from the adult.

Support for the above interpretation may be found biochemically. Hill has described the theoretical relationship that exists between the rate of turnover of energy-yielding processes and the velocity of contraction.[3] Since the ATPase activity of the contractile proteins may be an index of energy release, this activity should be related to contractile velocity. An excellent correlation has been shown between the ATPase activity of myosin and the maximum speed of shortening of a host of different muscle types.[6] As shown in Fig. 5, when ATPase activity was assessed in myofibrils obtained from fetal and adult hearts, no age-related differences were observed, and the pattern of magnesium activation was similar in the fetus and adult. In these experiments, ATPase activity was assessed in myofibrils, rather than in a more pure preparation, such as myosin or actomyosin, in order to take advantage of the higher level of structural organization.[7] The myofibrils were inspected periodically during preparation by phase

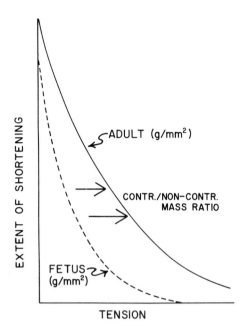

Fig. 4. A diagrammatic representation of the relations between the extent of shortening and tension showing the shift of the fetal curve if normalization of the tension data takes into account the higher fetal ratio of noncontractile to contractile mass. Similar shifts would occur in the length-active tension or force-velocity curves.

contrast microscopy to insure morphologic consistency in the final preparation, and mitochondrial ATPase activity was inhibited by the addition of sodium azide.

Despite the fact that the ultrastructural differences were the most likely explanation for the age-dependent, mechanical findings, we felt it was necessary to explore other possible explanations. Therefore, a glycerinated cardiac muscle fiber preparation was developed for the study of both the fetal and adult heart.[39] A myograph was constructed and was linked to a Zeiss microscope and a polaroid camera such that sarcomere lengths of the glycerinated fibers could be controlled by altering preload. The bath fluid could be recovered quantitatively. Figure 6 shows the reproducibility of sequential contractions of a glycerinated fiber at a controlled sarcomere length. When cardiac muscle fibers are glycerinated, the contributions to contraction of mitochondria, sarcolemma, and sar-

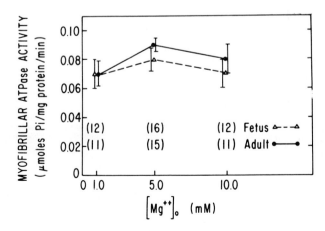

Fig. 5. Myofibrial ATPase activity of ventricular myocardium at different levels of magnesium activation. Numbers in brackets refer to numbers of lamb and sheep hearts studied. Each point and the vertical bars represent the mean ± SEM.

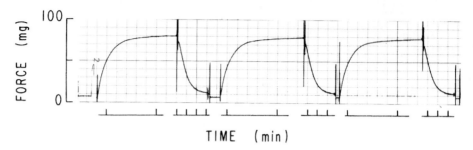

Fig. 6. Sequential contractions of a glycerinated cardiac muscle fiber. Contractions were obtained by alternating contraction solution (pCa^{++} = 5.4) with relaxation solution (pCa^{++} = 9). The initial sarcomere length was 2.2 μ.

coplasmic reticulum are lost. When the fiber is made to contract by adding calcium and isotopically labeled ATP, the tension-generating capabilities of the contractile apparatus are observed in a system lacking the normal mechanism for excitation–contraction coupling. It was of great interest in these glycerinated fiber studies that at identical sarcomere lengths, identical tensions were generated by both fetal and adult glycerinated fibers at different levels of calcium concentration (Table 1). At first glance, these findings appear to be in sharp contrast to the differences in force generation that were seen in the corresponding, intact, nonglycerinated ventricular muscles. However, these results are not necessarily inconsistent. If the contractile apparatus of the fetus is capable of generating normal tension, then the source of decreased active tension in the intact muscle preparations may either be the ultrastructural differences, or may involve a preceding mechanism, perhaps excitation–contraction coupling. It remains to be determined if excitation–contraction coupling differences exist between the fetus and adult heart, and this should be a challenging, but worthwhile, area for investigation.

Since labeled ATP was used in these experiments to elicit fiber contraction, and the bath fluid could be recovered quantitatively, one may calculate the ATP hydrolized by the fiber during contraction. It was of great interest to find that the fetus and adult showed identical ATPase activities (Table 1). Thus, it would appear that the utilization of energy by the contractile apparatus was also virtually identical in the fetus and adult.

On the basis of the experiments cited above, we can state that isometric force development, and both the extent and velocity of shortening at any load are reduced in the fetus when compared to the adult. These differences may be ex-

Table 1. Glycerinated Fiber Studies of Tension at Varying Levels of Calcium Concentration

Glycerinated Fiber	Fetus	Adult
Tension (mg/mm^2)		
pCa 9.0	383 + 14	390 + 42
PCa 5.4	2369 + 34	2383 + 74
ATP Hydrolysis (nmole/mg/min)	123 + 5	126 + 6

plained, at least in part, by age-related changes in the proportion of myo-cardial tissue consisting of myofilaments. The results suggest that the intrinsic speed and strength of contraction of individual sarcomeres are similar in the fetus close to term and the adult.

The isolated muscle studies suggested also that age-dependent differences exist in the force required to distend the ventricular chambers. If such differences exist, they must be considered in assessing and comparing the responses of the premature, newborn, and adult hearts to normal or disease-induced alterations in ventricular volume. Of course, changes in ventricular volume are associated with many cardiovascular malformations and invariably accompany corrective or palliative cardiac operations. Thus, the purpose of the investigations to be described was to analyze and compare the distensibility or compliance of the right and left ventricles in hearts obtained from fetal and newborn lambs and adult sheep.[8] Pressure-volume characteristics of each ventricle were analyzed (Fig. 7). Moreover, in order to assess the influence of filling of the controlateral chamber on compliance, the distensibility of each ventricle was determined with the opposite ventricle empty and at several fixed pressures. Using various models of left and right ventricular geometry, the pressure-volume data was converted to units of wall tension and percentage change in internal radius, allowing a direct comparison of all of the age groups studied. In addition, the concentrations of ventricular hydroxyproline were determined to evaluate the contribution of connective tissue to compliance at each age level.

The results of these studies indicate that the pressure-volume and wall tension —radius relations of both the left and right ventricles are comparable in the fetal lamb close to term. In the early newborn period (1–18 days), the right ventricle has compliance characteristics similar to the right ventricle of the fetus, and

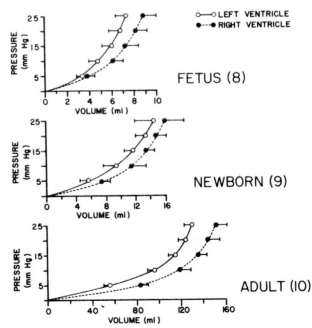

Fig. 7. Average left and right ventricular pressure-volume curves for each age group. Numbers in brackets are numbers of animals studied. Each point and the horizontal bars are mean values ± SEM. Note differences in horizontal volume scale. No significant differences were observed between the two ventricles in fetus. In newborn, left ventricular pressure-volume curve was significantly shifted to left of right ventricular curve at 15 and 20 mm Hg ($p < 0.05$). In adult, significantly greater left ventricular pressures existed at every level of volume when compared to right ventricle ($p < 0.001$).

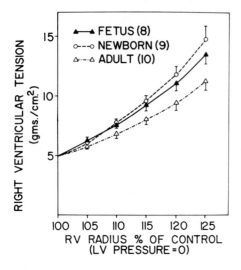

Fig. 8. Right ventricular wall tension–radius relations with left ventricle empty. Control right ventricular radius (100%) was defined as radius corresponding to 5g/cm² right ventricular wall tension. At any radius, right ventricular wall tension was significantly higher in both fetus and newborn than in adult ($p < 0.05$). No significant differences existed between fetus and newborn. Numbers in brackets are number of hearts studied.

the adult right ventricle is significantly more compliant than either the fetal or newborn right ventricle (Fig. 8). In the early postnatal period, the left ventricle alters its pressure-volume and stress-strain characteristics and assumes an intermediate position between fetus and adult (Fig. 9). At all ages, the right ventricle is more compliant than the left ventricle. When one evaluates the influence of filling one ventricle on reducing the distensibility of the opposite ventricle, the most profound effect is observed in the fetus, followed by the newborn and then the adult (Fig. 10). This increased sensitivity of the fetal ventricle to filling of the contralateral chamber may explain the ease with which the premature and newborn human infant exhibits sytemic venous congestion in the presence of lesions primarily deranging left ventricular volume or pressure.

A number of factors may be responsible for the distensibility differences ob-

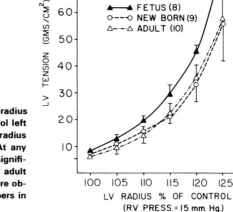

Fig. 9. Left ventricular wall tension—radius relations with right ventricle empty. Control left ventricular radius (100%) corresponds to radius at a calculated wall tension of 5g/cm². At any radius, left ventricular wall tension was significantly greater in fetus than in newborn or adult ($p < 0.025$). No significant differences were observed between newborn and adult. Numbers in brackets are number of hearts studied.

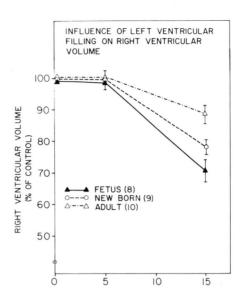

Fig. 10. Influence of filling left ventricle on right ventricular volume. Change in right ventricular volume is expressed as % of control volume. Control volume (100%) is defined as that volume that produces 5 mm Hg intracavitary pressure with an empty contralateral chamber. Similar values existed at 5 mm Hg left ventricular pressure. However, at 15 mm Hg left ventricular pressure, reduction in fetal right ventricular volume is significantly greater than in newborn ($p < 0.01$), and reduction in newborn is greater than in adult ($p < 0.01$). Numbers in brackets are number of hearts studied.

served between the young and old hearts. Well-known differences exist in various mammalian species in the mass relationships between the two ventricles in the perinatal period when compared to the adult.[9] The perinatal changes in right and left ventricular mass undoubtedly reflect the cardiocirculatory transition associated with the transfer from placental to pulmonary gas exchange, and the accompanying changes in systemic and pulmonary venous return and vascular resistance.[10] The cardiac chamber weights and dimensions that were obtained in our studies reveal a disproportionate rate of change of chamber size and wall thickness between the two ventricles after birth (Fig. 11).[8] Thus, in the newborn, the left ventricle gets larger and thicker-walled faster than the right ventricle gets larger and thinner-walled. Since the calculation of wall tension is inversely proportional to wall thickness,[11,12] the rapidly thickening newborn left ventricle begins to approximate the adult in its stress-strain relations, while the right ventricular wall thickness and stress-strain relations are still similar to the fetus.

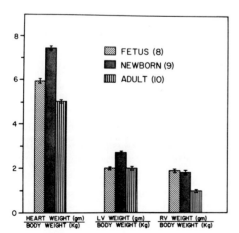

Fig. 11. Relations between heart weight, chamber weight, and body weight in fetal and newborn lamb and adult sheep. Columns represent average values ($\pm$ SEM). The significantly higher newborn heart weight/body weight ratio ($p < 0.001$) results from a higher LV weight/body weight ratio ($p < 0.001$) than either the fetus or adult. For both fetus and newborn, the RV weight/body weight ratio was higher than the adult ($p < 0.001$). Thus, the fetus has a greater heart weight/body weight ratio than the adult ($p < 0.001$) because of a greater RV mass.

Since we have also found reduced compliance in cardiac muscle that is *isolated* from the fetal heart when compared to the adult (Fig. 2), it must be pointed out that the isolated muscle differences cannot be accounted for by the alterations in the mass relationships between the ventricles, since the curves relating resting tension to muscle length are significantly steeper in the fetus and newborn, even when the tensions generated by the isolated muscles are corrected for cross-sectional area. The ultrastructural differences that exist between fetal and adult myocardium may also help explain the reduced compliance in the young hearts since relatively increased amounts in the fetus and newborn of noncontractile cellular elements, including surface membranes, may contribute to the decrease in ventricular distensibility.

There are several factors that may be excluded as accounting for the apparent stiffness of the fetal and newborn hearts. Experiments demonstrating changes in pressure-volume relations following coronary perfusion with collagenase indicate that passive ventricular distensibility may be influenced by interstitial connective tissue.[13] In our studies there were no significant differences in cardiac hydroxyproline concentration when the data were corrected for dry weight.[8] However, when corrected for wet weight, there was significantly more hydroxyproline found in the adult because the young heart has a higher water content. Since our compliance and connective tissue findings are directionally opposite, the age-related changes in collagen concentration cannot offer an explanation for the reduced compliance found in the youngest hearts. Moreover, no apparent geometrical differences in left ventricular shape existed between the three age groups to account for the results obtained.

IN SITU PHYSIOLOGIC STUDIES

Most recently, we have devoted our efforts to developing methods appropriate to assess left ventricular function in situ in the chronically instrumented fetal and neonatal lamb.[40] These studies were prompted by the fact that indirect measurements of fetal myocardial performance estimated from acute, exteriorized fetal lamb experiments are associated with multiple problems and may be decidedly unphysiologic. The important studies of Drs. Abraham Rudolph and Michael Heymann and their associates[41,42] employing chronic techniques of fetal cardiovascular study have pioneered in pointing out the advantages of studying the intact, undisturbed fetal lamb. Borrowing many of Rudolph's surgical techniques, we have adapted sonocardiometry methods recently utilized in the study of the intact adult heart.[43] Figure 12 diagrammatically illustrates the general experimental situation. Time-dated, pregnant ewes were operated upon at known fetal-gestational ages of 110–124 days. Under spinal anesthesia, hysterotomy is performed and the instrumentation accomplished. Systemic arterial pressure is recorded with a catheter inserted in the fetal carotid artery. A balloon catheter with lumen is placed in the superior vena cava for measurement of central venous pressure and also for producing acute alterations in loading conditions by inflation of the balloon. In addition, after left thoracotomy, bipolar pacing wires are sutured to the left atrial appendage for cardiac pacing or for recording the electrocardiogram. A left atrial catheter is inserted both for recording pressure and for volume infusion to allow the study of pressure–volume

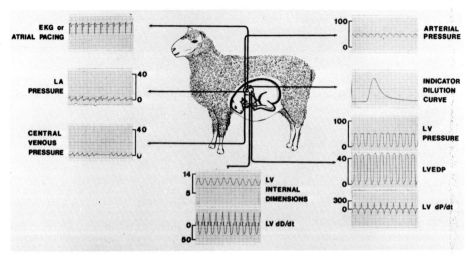

Fig. 12.   The instrumentation for the chronic study of the fetal lamb heart is illustrated. See text for details.

relations. A solid-state micromanometer pressure transducer is inserted into the cavity of the left ventricle. This transducer is calibrated using the systemic arterial and left atrial pressures. A zero pressure reference is provided by a catheter sutured to the fetal precordium. This same zero reference catheter also allows the measurement of intrauterine pressure, which is subtracted from all fetal pressure data. Lastly, two $3\frac{1}{2}$-mm piezoelectric crystals are placed opposite one another on the endocardial surface of the left ventricle. These crystals are placed perpendicular to the longitudinal axis of the left ventricle and across its greatest internal diameter. The sonomicrometer used to measure left ventricular internal diameter is a modification of the one described previously by Stegall et al.[44] In order to measure distance linearly to 3 mm with a 1% error, one endocardial piezoelectric transducer is shock excited at a high repetition rate (5000/sec), and the time required for each ultrasonic burst to pass from one transducer to the other is converted into a voltage suitable for recording. Since sound velocity in blood is known to be 1.5×10^3 m/sec, the readings may be converted into distance. Differentiating circuits are employed to derive the first derivatives of both left ventricular pressure and left ventricular internal dimensions. In order to determine left ventricular cardiac output, indicator-dilution curves were obtained with injection of dye into the left atrium and sampling from the carotid artery.

One of the exciting advantages of the above technique is that physiologic observations could be made throughout labor and delivery, since the instrumentation does not prevent the normal vaginal delivery of the animal. Thus, data could be recorded during passage through the birth canal, concurrent with the first breath of life, and then postnatally.

Figure 13 shows recordings obtained from a fetal lamb at 131 days gestation. The figure demonstrates the fidelity of the diameter tracing. Vertical lines are drawn at the onset of isovolumetric contraction. The velocity trace (dD/dt) shows that peak velocity is reached shortly after the onset of ejection. The small-

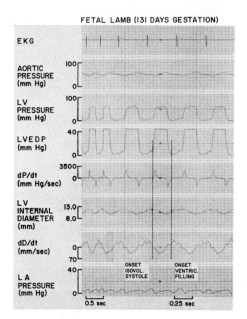

FETAL LAMB (131 DAYS GESTATION)

EKG

AORTIC PRESSURE (mm Hg)

LV PRESSURE (mm Hg)

LVEDP (mm Hg)

dP/dt (mm Hg/sec)

LV INTERNAL DIAMETER (mm)

dD/dt (mm/sec)

LA PRESSURE (mm Hg)

ONSET ISOVOL. SYSTOLE   ONSET VENTRIC. FILLING

0.5 sec   0.25 sec

Fig. 13. The fidelity of the sonomicrometer tracings is demonstrated in a fetal lamb at 131 days gestation. The vertical dotted lines are drawn through the onset of isovolumetric contraction and through the onset of ventricular filling. See text for further details.

est internal diameter is reached at end systole. With the onset of isovolumetric relaxation, there is an increase in internal diameter. Passive ventricular filling and active atrial contraction are detected clearly in the velocity tracing. There is a slight diminution in internal diameter during isovolumetric contraction, which most likely reflects ballooning of the mitral valve superiorly while left ventricular wall thickness increases.

One of the more striking findings observed in these studies was a doubling of left ventricular output in the immediate postnatal period. As seen in Fig. 14, this is associated with a remarkable increase in cardiac dimensions. Figure 14 shows the changes in ventricular dimensions in a representative animal that was studied from 124 days of gestation to 41 days of postnatal life. At the moment of birth, there is a sharp increase in both end-diastolic and end-systolic dimensions. An initial increase in dimensions was observed when the thorax was delivered, and a further increase was noted with the onset of pulmonary ventilation. In the en-

Fig. 14. Internal left ventricular transverse dimensions in a fetal lamb studied from 124 days gestational age through delivery, and up to 41 days of postnatal life. The instrumentation was placed operatively at 114 days gestation.

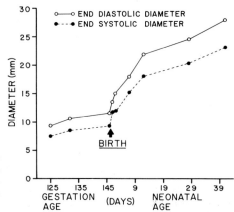

suing 10 days of life, internal left ventricular dimensions increased at a greater rate than that observed prior to birth, or in the period beyond 10 days of life.

Data utilizing the above methods is currently being accumulated. The sono-cardiometry techniques permit calculations of left ventricular volume, ejection fraction, velocity of circumferential fiber shortening, myocardial pressure–volume and force–velocity relations, and peripheral resistance. New information may be anticipated concerning the manner in which the developing myocardium reacts to altered physiologic conditions, specific cardiovascular deformities created by in utero surgery, prolonged and complicated labor and delivery, a variety of other neonatal abnormalities, and the administration of pharmacologic agents to the mother, fetus, and neonate.

CARDIAC ENERGY METABOLISM

The influence of growth on myocardial energy metabolism has not yet been thoroughly elucidated, although age-related variations in aerobic and anaerobic metabolism of many organs and of the entire organism have been observed in several mammalian species.[14–17] Mitochondria are the main source of production of myocardial ATP, and the heart is dependent primarily upon aerobic

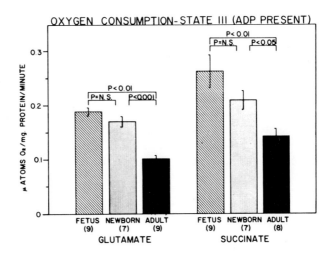

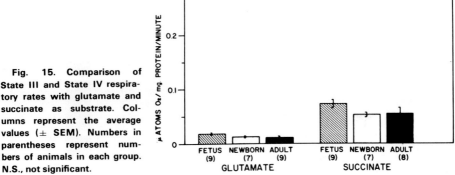

Fig. 15. Comparison of State III and State IV respiratory rates with glutamate and succinate as substrate. Columns represent the average values (± SEM). Numbers in parentheses represent numbers of animals in each group. N.S., not significant.

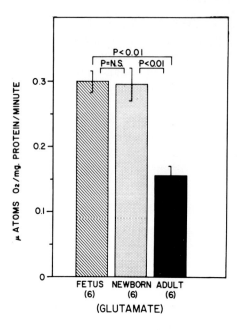

Fig. 16. Comparison of mitochondrial oxygen consumption with glutamate as substrate after uncoupling by dinitrophenol (DNP). The numbers in parentheses represent the numbers of animals in each group. N.S., not significant.

metabolism. Because little is known about the relationship between oxidative metabolism in heart muscle and age, studies were designed to characterize and compare oxidative phosphorylation in mitochondria from the hearts of fetal and newborn lambs and sheep.[18] No age-related differences were found in P/O ratios, a measure of efficiency of ATP production with either succinate or glutamate as substrate, or in ATPase activity, another index of mitochondrial functional integrity, in the presence or absence of dinitrophenol (DNP). However, mitochondria from fetal and newborn animals had significantly increased oxygen consumption/mg protein in the presence of ADP (state III respiration) com-

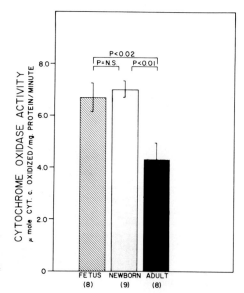

Fig. 17. Comparison of cytochrome c oxidase activity. The columns represent average values (± SEM). N.S., not significant. The numbers in parentheses represent the numbers of animals in each group.

pared to the adult (Fig. 15). As a result, respiratory control ratios, a measure of the dependence of respiratory rate on ADP, were increased significantly in the fetus and newborn compared to the adult. In addition, oxygen consumption in mitochondria uncoupled by DNP was higher in the fetus and newborn compared to the adult (Fig. 16), suggesting that the augmented respiratory rates in mitochondria from the hearts of the youngest animals are a reflection of increased electron transport. This view was consistent with the finding of significantly greater cytochrome c oxidase activities in fetal and newborn mitochondria, respectively, when compared to the adult (Fig. 17). It is possible that the increase in the aerobic capacity of mitochondria from the hearts of both the fetus and newborn may provide an important margin of tolerance to hypoxia for the developing organism, especially when coupled with the known increased anaerobic capacity of hearts from young animals.[17] Moreover, the age-related differences in mitochondrial oxidative phosphorylation may contribute to meeting the additional energy requirements related to rapid growth of the heart in early life.

DEVELOPMENT OF SYMPATHETIC AND PARASYMPATHETIC INNERVATION

Thus far, physiologic and pharmacologic studies undertaken to assess the maturation of the autonomic control of the circulation have been largely concerned with the ability of young animals to respond to various physiologic stimuli, such as hypoxemia, acidosis, and carotid sinus hypotension, or to the injection of catecholamines.[19,23] Although the autonomic nervous system plays an important role in cardiocirculatory control in the mature mammal, the precise mechanisms and degree of neural control of the circulation of the fetus and newborn are not clear. There remains a lack of quantification of the development of the separate factors constituting an integrated circulatory response: the afferent, central, and efferent components of a vascular reflex, the responsiveness of the peripheral vasculature, and the direct inotropic and chronotropic effects on the myocardium of the sympathetic and parasympathetic neurotransmitters. Accordingly, the objective of the following studies was to define more clearly the development of sympathetic and parasympathetic innervation of the mammalian heart.

Pharmacologic Studies

As already mentioned, a variety of technical difficulties have surrounded previous efforts to analyze myocardial contractility in the fetal or neonatal heart in situ. Thus, there is an absence of meaningful comparisons of fetal, neonatal, and adult cardiac tissue response to the sympathetic neurotransmitter, norepinephrine, and to the parasympathetic neurotransmitter, aceytlcholine. We believe we have obviated many of these technical difficulties in our laboratory by isolating myocardium from fetal and newborn lambs and adult sheep, and studying its pharmacologic responsiveness to the adrenergic and cholinergic neurotransmitters in a myograph under identical conditions. Other pharmacologic stimuli have also been employed to further understand age-related differences in responsiveness. As in the studies on muscle mechanics, a single right ventricular papillary muscle or moderator band was removed rapidly from the heart of either a fetal lamb in the last 15 days of gestation by hysterotomy under local anesthesia, or from a newborn lamb or an adult sheep, and suspended in a myograph in oxygenated Ringer's solution at 30°C and pH 7.4, and stimulated at 12 contractions/min. The muscle was stretched to the apex of its length-active tension curve, and the changes in isometric tension were recorded after addition to the bathing medium of the appropriate pharmacologic stimulus. In certain experiments, atrial tissue rather than ventricular myocardium was studied in a similar manner.

Figure 18A shows the average dose response curves of fetal and adult ventricular myocardium to norepinephrine. It is quite clear that fetal cardiac tissue has a much lower threshold to the inotropic effects of norepinephrine, the sympathetic neurotransmitter, and is also about threefold more sensitive to norepinephrine throughout the dose response curve when compared to the adult. Figure 18B shows a similar but less marked contrast in sensitivity to norepinephrine when ventricular myocardium from newborn lambs younger than 3 days of age was compared to that obtained from lambs ranging in age from 4 days to 3 wk.

Supersensitivity to norepinephrine would be expected if the fetal and early newborn myocardium lacked a complete development of sympathetic innervation, or if sympathetic nerves within these young hearts had a reduced capacity to take up and bind catecholamines. Uptake and binding represent an important mechanism for the inactivation of norepinephrine, and it would be anticipated that reduction in the heart's ability to utilize this mechanism of inactivation would permit a higher concentration of the neurotransmitter to reach and activate the heart's beta receptors, and thereby render the heart supersensitive. In order to evaluate more completely this hypothesis, the pharmacologic responsiveness of fetal and adult ventricular muscle to isoproterenol was determined. Isoproterenol is a direct acting beta-adrenergic agonist that is not taken up and stored in sympathetic nerves. In contrast to the findings with norepinephrine, equal responsiveness of fetal and adult myocardium was observed (Fig. 19). This finding indicates that beta-receptor sensitivity to catecholamines is similar in adult and fetal myocardium, and supports the notion that sympathetic innervation is incomplete or functionally immature in the heart of the fetus or early newborn.

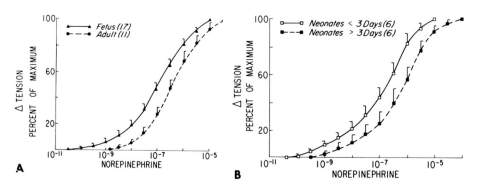

Fig. 18. (A) Average norepinephrine dose response curves of isolated right ventricular myocardium obtained from 17 fetal lambs and 11 adult sheep. Vertical bars, SEM. (B) Average norepinephrine dose response curves of isolated right ventricular myocardium obtained from six newborn lambs less than 3 days of age and six newborns ranging in age from 3 days to 3 wk. Vertical bars, SEM.

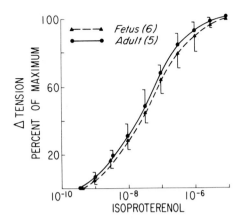

Fig. 19. Average isoproterenol dose response curves showing equal responses for fetal and adult ventricular tissue. Numbers in brackets are numbers of animals from which cardiac tissue was obtained. Vertical bars, SEM.

Vagal stimulation or administration of the parasympathetic neurotransmitter, acetylcholine, depresses atrial contractions. Figure 20A illustrates our data concerning the effects of acetylcholine on myocardial contractility. These dose response curves demonstrate that the negative inotropic effects of acetylcholine on isolated atrial myocardium is similar in the fetal lamb when compared to the adult sheep. Furthermore, when the atria are pretreated with atropine (Fig. 20B), the responsiveness to acetylcholine is different at the two different ages. In this circumstance, we are looking at the composite result of a number of acetyl-

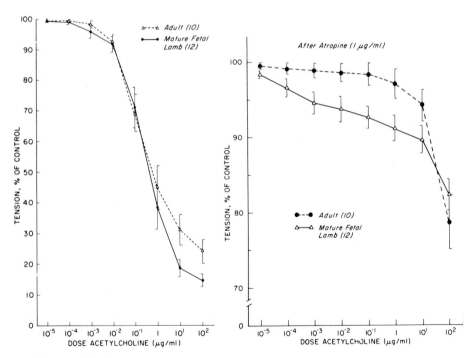

Fig. 20. (A) Average acetylcholine dose response curves of isolated right atrial myocardium stimulated at 30 contractions/min (B) Average acetylcholine dose response curves of isolated right atrial myocardium after pretreatment with atropine. Numbers in parentheses are numbers of animals from cardiac tissue was obtained. Vertical bars, SEM.

choline effects. First, the muscarinic depression of contractility, which is inhibited competitively by atropine. Second, in high concentrations, acetylcholine may produce a positive inotropic effect by releasing catecholamines from sympathetic nerve endings in the heart. The separation after atropine of the fetal acetylcholine dose-response curve from the adult curve may be another reflection of reduced or functionally immature sympathetic innervation in the fetus, and reduced norepinephrine release by acetylcholine.

It has been suggested that acidosis does not depress cardiac function in the newborn animal in the presence of an intact sympathetic nervous system unless hypoxemia supervenes.[24] Figure 21 is representative of a number of experiments in which force-velocity curves were constructed from isotonic, afterloaded contractions at a high pO_2 before the addition of norepinephrine at a normal pH, and at a reduced pH of 7.1. Acidosis was produced by either increasing the pCO_2 in the muscle bath or by adding lactic or hydrocholoric acid. Raising the pCO_2, analogous to respiratory acidosis, always depressed contractility more than by simulating metabolic acidosis. As Fig. 21 illustrates, when the pH is lowered, the force-velocity curve is depressed and shifted downward and to the left. At all ages studied, for both normal and acidotic muscles, norepinephrine produced a marked increase in tension and in the velocity of shortening at any tension, and the absolute increase in both was similar. However, despite this marked augmentation in contractility, when the pH was reduced there was substantially less force generation and velocity of shortening than heart muscle at a normal pH. These findings indicate clearly that acidosis produces a shift in norepinephrine dose responsivess, even in the absence of hypoxia.

Since age-related differences in myocardial responsiveness to norepinephrine were observed, it was considered important to examine the age dependency of the effects of a beta-adrenergic antagonist, propranolol. Propranolol possesses

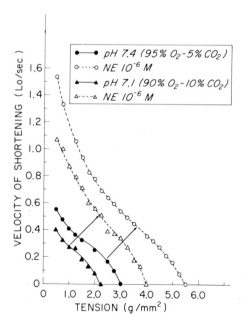

Fig. 21. A typical experiment in which force velocity curves were constructed from isotonic, afterloaded contractions of right ventricular myocardium isolated from a fetal lamb in the last week of gestation. The pH was reduced from 7.4 to 7.1 by increasing the CO_2 tension of bathing medium. Acidosis depressed both velocity of shortening and tension development, and although norepinephrine augmented both velocity and force, levels achieved were not comparable to those when muscle was bathed at a normal pH.

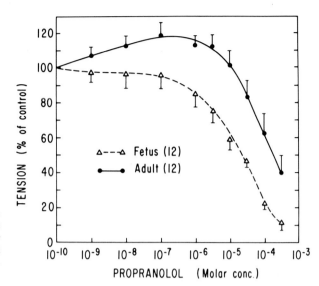

Fig. 22. Average propranolol dose response curves of isolated right ventricular myocardium obtained from 12 fetal lambs and 12 adult sheep. Vertical bars, SEM.

other actions besides producing blockade of beta receptors.[25] Examination of the fetal curve in Fig. 22 reveals especially the direct depressant effects of propranolol on the myocardium. This negative inotropic action is also seen in the adult curve, but, in the adult, propranolol exerts a small, direct, positive inotropic action before its depresses contractility. Thus, at any concentration of the beta blocker, the fetal heart is significantly more depressed than the adult. Despite this age-related difference in sensitivity to the inotropic effects of propranolol, we observed that the beta blocking action of the drug is the same for fetus and adult. Figure 23 shows dose-response curves of fetal and adult heart muscles to isoproterenol, constructed in the absence of beta blocker (the curves labeled Control), and in the presence of two different molar concentrations of propranolol (3×10^{-8} and 3×10^{-6}). As would be expected, propranolol reduced the response to isoproterenol in a dose-related manner and displaced the curves to the right. Thus, in the presence of beta blocker, a higher concentration of iso-

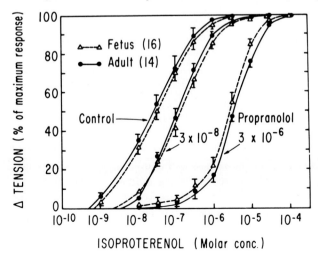

Fig. 23. Average dose response curves of ventricular myocardium to isoproterenol in absence of propranolol (control) and in presence of two different molar concentrations of beta blocker. Numbers in parentheses refer to numbers of animals studied. Vertical bars, SEM.

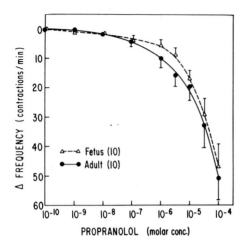

Fig. 24. Dose response curves of spontaneously beating SA node–right atrial myocardium obtained from ten fetal lambs and ten adult sheep. Vertical bars, SEM.

proterenol was required to achieve a given increase in tension. Note, however, that the degree of blockade was the same for the fetus and the adult.

Interestingly, in contrast to the age-dependent differences that existed in the inotropic actions of propranolol, we did not uncover a difference in the chronotropic actions of the beta blocker. A spontaneously beating SA node—right atrial preparation was employed to study the effect on intrinsic heart rate. In Fig. 24 the absolute change in the frequency of contraction is plotted against the concentration of propranolol. Both the fetus and adult were slowed to the same extent.

Biochemical Studies

In order to describe the development of the heart's ability to synthesize, store, and metabolize catecholamines, we have measured the myocardial norepinephrine stores and the critical enzymes in norepinephrine biosynthesis and degradation. These studies were also undertaken to understand more completely the mechanism of the age-dependent differential sensitivity to norepinephrine described above.

The cardiac concentration of norepinephrine in fetal, neonatal, and adult animals may be employed as an index of the magnitude of sympathetic innervation because the heart's stores of norepinephrine are localized almost exclusively in intracellular storage sites within the terminations of the sympathetic nerves.[26] Norepinephrine was determined spectrophotofluorometrically by the trihydroxyindole method after alumina absorption.[27] Figure 25 compares the cardiac norepinephrine stores in lambs and sheep at different stages of development. Myocardial concentrations of norepinephrine in the fetus within several wks of term was significantly lower than in the newborn lamb less than 3 days old, and there was no difference between older newborns and adult sheep. Similar results were observed when other mammalian species were studied. Thus, a gradual increase with advancing age was observed in the myocardial norepinephrine stores of the rabbit (Fig. 26) and substantial age-related differences were also observed in swine (Fig. 27).

The rate of formation of norepinephrine is determined by tyrosine hydroxy-

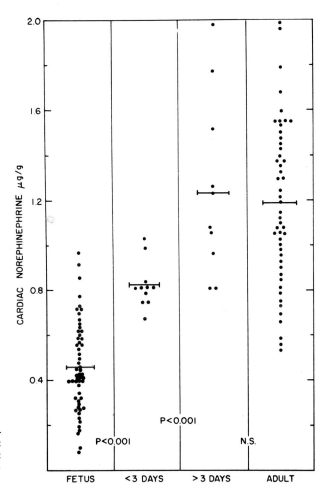

Fig. 25. Myocardial nor-
epinephrine concentrations at
different stages of development
in the lamb and sheep. Horizontal bars, mean values.

lase. This intraneuronal enzyme catalyzes the first transformation in catecholamine biosynthesis.[28] Its activity was determined by measuring the formation of
tritiated water from 3,5-ditritiotyrosine.[29] In the fetal lamb, as compared to the
adult sheep, tyrosine hydroxylase activity and the cardiac stores of norepinephrine were reduced (Fig. 28). It was of particular interest that the adrenal glands

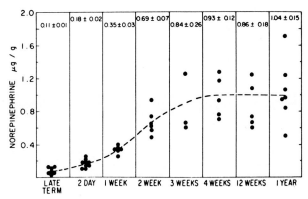

Fig. 26. Gradual increase
with advancing age in myocardial norepinephrine stores
in rabbit. Mean values are
joined by dash line. (By permission.[32]

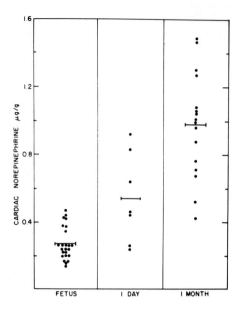

Fig. 27. Myocardial norepinephrine concentrations at different stages of development of swine. Fetal values were obtained within 2 wk of term. Horizontal bars, mean values.

of these same fetal lambs showed equal activities of tyrosine hydroxylase and abundant catecholamine stores when compared to adult sheep (Fig. 29). These findings suggest that the low myocardial activity of the enzyme is related to delayed development of sympathetic innervation, rather than to a generalized immaturity of enzyme synthesis.

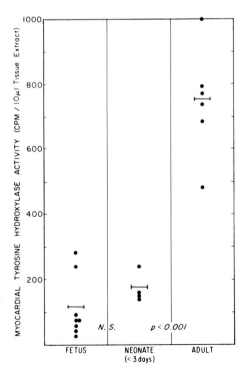

Fig. 28. Myocardial tyrosine hydroxylase activities at different ages in the lamb and sheep. Horizontal bars, mean values.

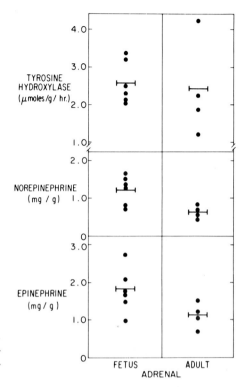

Fig. 29. Adrenal tyrosine hydroxylase activities and norepinephrine and epinephrine concentrations in the fetal lamb and adult sheep. Horizontal bars, mean values.

Monoamine oxidase is a catabolic enzyme that catalyzes the oxidative deamination of norepinephrine, and the enzyme is located in part within sympathetic nerves. When this enzyme's activity was determined by measuring the deaminated ^{14}C metabolites of ^{14}C-tryptamine,[30] we observed a reduced activity in the fetal heart when compared to the adult (Fig. 30).

In contrast to norepinephrine and the intraneuronal enzymes, tyrosine hydroxylase and monoamine oxidase, catechol-o-methyl transferase metabolizes norepinephrine outside the nerve only. The activity of catechol-o-methyl transferase was determined by measuring the ^{14}C normetanephrine formed from norepinephrine and ^{14}C-S-adenosylmethionine in the presence of divalent cations.[30] The activity of this enzyme was significantly higher in fetal than in adult myocardium (Fig. 31), and significant inverse relationships were evident when the catechol-o-methyl transferase activity was correlated with cardiac norepinephrine concentration, tyrosine hydroxylase activity, and monoamine oxidase activity. All of the above biochemical observations are compatible with the concept that a significant increase in the magnitude of sympathetic innervation occurs postnatally.

Histochemical Observations

The monoamine fluorescence technique of Falck and Owman[31] was employed to evaluate histochemically the distribution of sympathetic nerves within the hearts of the differently aged animals. These studies provided final confirmation that sympathetic innervation is incomplete in the fetal and early newborn

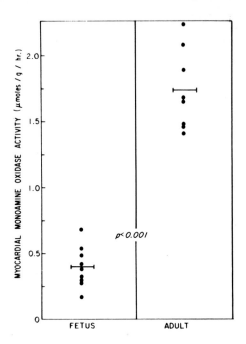

Fig. 30. Myocardial monoamine oxidase activities in the fetal lamb and adult sheep. Horizontal bars, mean values.

heart, or that uptake and binding are immature. In these studies, the myocardium is treated in such a way that the norepinephrine within the adrenergic nerves fluoresce, and the fluorescence is visualized microscopically. As Fig. 32 shows, in the adult the heart is innervated by a dense network of intensely flourescent, varicose nerve fibers. At all ages, there appear to be more adrener-

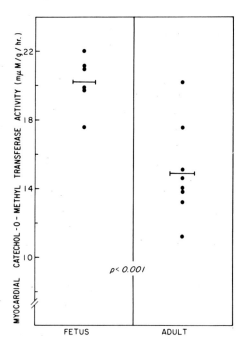

Fig. 31. Myocardial catechol-o-methyl transferase activities in the fetal lamb and adult sheep. Horizontal bars, mean values.

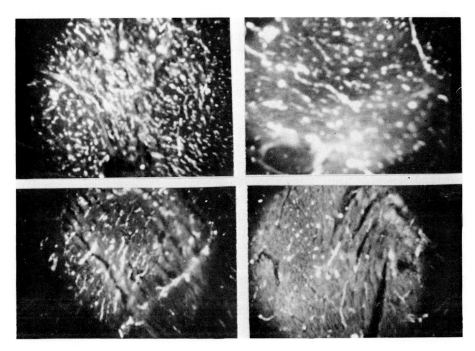

Fig. 32. Histochemical appearance (at same magnification) of atrial (left) and ventricular (right) myocardium obtained from a 2-yr-old sheep (top) and a term fetal lamb (bottom). The Falck technique was employed.

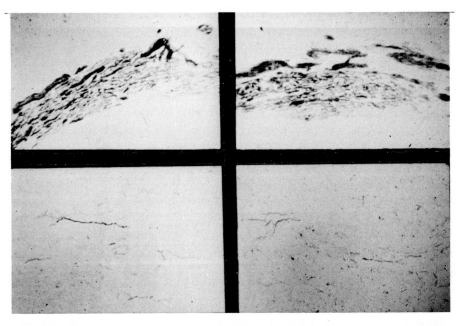

Fig. 33. Cholinergic fibers at same magnification in AV mode (top) and interventricular septum (bottom) of the fetal lambs close to term (left) and adult sheep (right). No apparent age-related differences were observed.

gic fibers in the atria than in the ventricles, but, more importantly, there is a reduced density of neurons in both fetal chambers when compared to the adult.
Similar findings were observed in the rabbit heart.[32] In both the lamb and the
rabbit, the fetal myocardium contained large, intensely fluorescent, preterminal
nerve trunks in the epicardium and the tunica adventia surrounding coronary
arteries, and coursing in the connective tissue between cardiac muscle bundles.
In these younger animals, intense fluorescence resided only in terminal varicosities within the large nerve trunks. In contrast, the nerve trunks in the older
sheep or rabbits did not contain terminal varicosities and fluoresced only weakly.
The appearance of large preterminal nerve trunks enclosing intensely fluorescent, catecholamine-containing terminal varicosities suggests that the latter
move into the heart during early development, perhaps in response to an increase in sensory input, and branch out and arborize to form the autonomic
ground plexus. Since norepinephrine storage granules flow down cardiac adrenergic nerves from neuronal cell bodies in the cervical and thoracic sympathetic ganglia, the intense preterminal fluorescence suggests that these ganglia
are quite prepared to respond appropriately to central efferent impulse traffic.
Moreover, it appears that a significant proportion of the norepinephrine
measured in the fetal and newborn heart resides in the preterminal nerve trunks,
and therefore may not be in close anatomic proximity to the adrenergic receptors
of the myocardial cell.

While one cannot stain specifically for acetylcholine in tissues, it is possible
to localize acetylocholinesterase histochemically, and it has been shown that
reasonably good correlations exist between the concentrations of acetylcholine,
acetylcholinesterase, and choline acetylase in various regions of the peripheral
and central nervous systems. The photomicrograph shown in Fig. 33 has been
stained for acetylocholinesterase by the thiocholine technique after selective inhibition of pseudocholinesterase.[33] It would appear that the density of stained
cholinergic fibers present in atrial, SA and AV nodal, and ventricular tissue is
comparable in the fetus and the adult.

The findings of these latter investigations illustrate that dynamic changes in
the anatomic, biochemical, and physiologic disposition of cardiac catecholamines occur in the perinatal period and allow an explanation for age-dependent differences in the pharmacologic responsiveness of ventricular myocardium
to norepinephrine, the sympathetic neurotransmitter. The hearts of the fetuses
close to term and youngest neonates were found to be supersensitive to norepinephrine. The histochemical findings supported the view that these hearts were
partially innervated with a good deal of the visualized norepinephrine residing
in preterminal nerve trunks, rather than in terminal nerve endings. Beta-receptor sensitivity was similar in fetal and adult myocardium, indicating that catecholamine receptor sites are fully functional before the complete development of
an extrinsic nerve supply. At a comparable stage of development, the adrenal
glands, unlike the heart, were found to contain abundant catecholamine stores.
Moreover, at a stage in development when a reduction exists in sympathetic
nerves and in cardiac norepinephrine stores and the intraneuronal enzymes concerned with norepinephrine biosynthesis and degradation, there appear to be
no age-related differences in parasympathetic innervation.

The heart of the adult mammal is richly supplied with sympathetic nerves, and the release of norepinephrine from the endings of these nerves provides one of the fundamental mechanisms for the modulation of cardiac contractility.[34] Although there is evidence to suggest that regulation of the heart rate and arterial blood pressure in the newborn is under some autonomic control,[19-22] the extent to which sympathetic nerves contribute to the contractile state of the heart at this stage of development has not been previously defined. It has been shown that the ordinary activity of the adrenergic nervous system may have minimal effects on the normal heart, and that the intrinsic contractile state of the myocardium may not be influenced by alterations in endogenous catecholamine stores.[35] The force of contraction of the heart may be stimulated profoundly by an increase in the number of impulses traversing the sympathetic nerves whenever an imbalance exists between the cardiac output and the perfusion requirements of the peripheral tissues. When the latter occurs in the perinatal period, the interaction between a supersensitive myocardium and the adrenal release of catecholamines may play a more critical, compensatory role in maintaining ventricular contractility than in the adult. In adult animals, it is evident that only a small fraction of the normal cardiac stores of norepinephrine is necessary to elicit a functional response to adrenergic nerve stimulation[36] or tyramine,[37] although the magnitude and perhaps the duration of the response may be reduced.[38]

It is clear that a more complete understanding of the normal development of the heart and autonomic influences is necessary to provide a framework within which the effects of a variety of disease states can be elucidated. In this regard, a host of interesting questions remain unsolved, most especially concerning the influence on subsequent autonomic development of such factors as premature delivery, nutrition, and cardiac decompensation. Of interest also will be the study of the influence on the fetal heart of drugs including reserpine and ganglionic-blocking agents, commonly administered to hypertensive or toxemic mothers. These and other questions are currently under investigation.

ACKNOWLEDGMENT

A number of individuals have participated in a major way in various aspects of these studies, including Drs. Charles Cooper, Stanley Kirkpatrick, Tomas Romero, Burton Sobel, Robert Wells, James Covell, Philip Henry, Edmund Sonnenblick, Judith Su, David Jacobowitz, and Peter Pool. I am especially grateful to Dr. Eugene Braunwald for creating an environment in which the highest priorities exist for the advancement of the cardiovascular sciences.

REFERENCES

1. Arcilla, R. A., Lind, J., Zetterquist, P., and Oh, W.: Hemodynamic features of extrasystoles in newborn and older infants. Amer. J. Cardiol. 18:191, 1966.

2. Sonnenblick, E. H., Spiro, D., and Spotnitz, H.: Ultrastructural basis of Starling's law of the heart. Amer. Heart J. 68:336, 1964.

3. Hill, A. V.: Heat of shortening and dynamic constants of muscle. Proc. Roy. Soc. London (Biol.) 126:136, 1938.

4. Downing, S. E., Talner, N. S., and Gardner, T. H.: Ventricular function in the newborn lamb. Amer. J. Physiol. 208:931, 1965.

5. Brutsaert, D. L., Claes, V. A., and Sonnenblick, E. H.: Velocity of shortening of unloaded heart muscle and the length-tension relation. Circ. Res. 29:63, 1971.

6. Barany, M.: ATPase activity of myosin correlated with speed of muscle shortening. J. Gen. Physiol. 50:197, 1967.

7. Seagren, S. C., Skelton, L. C., and Pool, P. E.: Relation of cardiac myofibrillar ATPase activity to increased contractile state. Amer. J. Physiol. 220:847, 1971.

8. Romero, T., Covell, J., and Friedman, W. F.: A comparison of the pressure-volume relations of the fetal, newborn and adult heart. Amer. J. Physiol. In press.

9. Hort, W.: The normal heart of the fetus and its metamorphosis in the transition period. *In* Cassels, D. E. (Ed.): The Heart and Circulation in the Newborn and Infant. New York, Grune & Stratton, 1966, p. 210.

10. Rudolph, A.: The changes in the circulation after birth. Circulation 41:343, 1940.

11. Gault, J. H., Ross, J., Jr., and Braunwald, E.: Instantaneous tension-velocity-length relations in patients with and without disease of the left ventricular myocardium. Circ. Res. 22:451, 1968.

12. Sandler, H., and Dodge, H. T.: Left ventricular tension and stress in man. Circ. Res. 23:91, 1963.

13. O'Brien, L. J., and Moore, C. M.: Connective tissue degradation and distensibility characteristics in the non-living heart. Experientia 22:845, 1966.

14. Beatty, C. H., Besinger, G. M. and Bocek, R. M.: Oxygen consumption and glycolysis in fetal, neonatal, and infant muscle of the rhesus monkey. Pediatrics 42:5, 1968.

15. Shelley, H. J.: Blood sugars and tissue carbohydrates in foetal and infant lambs and rhesus monkeys. J. Physiol. 153:527, 1960.

16. Gregson, N. P., and Williams, P. L.: A comparative study of brain and liver mitochondria from newborn and adult rats. J. Neurochem. 16:617, 1969.

17. Jolley, R. L., Cheddely, V. H., and Newburgh, R. W.: Glucose catabolism in fetal and adult heart. J. Biol. Chem. 233:1289, 1958.

18. Wells, R. J., Friedman, W. F., and Sobel, B. E.: Increased oxidative metabolism in the fetal and newborn lamb heart. Amer. J. Physiol. In press.

19. Downing, S. E., Milgram, E. A., and Halloran, K. H.: Cardiac responses to autonomic nerve stimulation during acidosis and hypoxia in the lamb. Amer. J. Physiol. 220: 1956, 1971.

20. —, Gardner, T. H., and Solis, R. T.: Autonomic influences on cardiac function in the newborn lamb. Circ. Res. 19:947, 1966.

21. Dawes, G. S., Handler, J. J., and Mott, J. C.: Some cardiovascular responses in fetal, newborn and adult rabbits. J. Physiol. 139:123, 1957.

22. Born, G. V. R., Dawes, G. S., and Mott, J. C.: Oxygen lack in autonomic nervous control of the fetal circulation in the lamb. J. Physiol. 134:149, 1956.

23. Talner, N. S., Gardner, T. H., and Downing S. E.: Influence of acidemia on left ventricular function in the newborn lamb. Pediatrics 38:457, 1966.

24. Downing, S. E., Talner, N. S., and Gardner, T. H.: Influences of arterial oxygen tension and pH on cardiac function in the newborn lamb. Amer. J. Physiol. 211:1203, 1966.

25. Parmley, W. W., and Braunwald, E.: Comparative myocardial depressant and antiarrythmic properties of d-propranolol, dl-propranolol and quinidine. J. Pharmacol. Exp. Ther. 158:11, 1967.

26. Dahlstrom, A., Fuxe, K., Mya-tu, M., and Zetterstrom, B. E. M.: Observations on adrenergic innervation of dog heart. Amer. J. Physiol. 209:689, 1965.

27. Crout, J. R., Creveling, C. R., and Udenfriend, S.: Norepinephrine metabolism in rat brain, heart. J. Pharmacol. Exp. Ther. 132: 269, 1961.

28. Levitt, M., Spector, S., Sjoerdsma, A., and Udenfriend, S.: Elucidation of the rate-limiting step in norepinephrine biosynthesis in the perfused guinea pig heart. J. Pharmacol. Exp. Ther. 148:1, 1965.

29. —, Gibb, J. W., Daly, J. W., Lipton, M., and Udenfriend, S.: A new class of tyrosine hydroxylase inhibitors and a simple assya of inhibition in vivo. Biochem. Pharmacol. 16:1, 1967.

30. Krakoff, L. R., Buccino, R. A., Spann, J. F., Jr., and DeChamplain, J.: Cardiac catechol-o-methyl transferase and monoamine oxidase activity in congestive heart failure. Amer. J. Physiol. 215:549, 1968.

31. Falck, B., and Owman, C.: A detailed methodological description of the flourescence method for the cellular demonstration of biogenic monoamines. Acta Univ. Lund. II:7, 1965.

32. Friedman, W. F., Pool, P. E., Jacobowitz, D., Seagran, S. C., and Braunwald, E.: Sympathetic innervation of the developing rabbit heart: biochemical and histochemical comparisons of fetal, neonatal, and adult myocardium. Circ. Res. 23:25, 1968.

33. Jacobowitz, D., and Koelle, G. B.: Histochemical correlations of acetylocholine-esterase and catecholamines in post ganglionic autonomic nerves of the cat, rabbit and guinea pig. J. Pharmacol. Exp. Ther. 148:225, 1965.

34. Braunwald, E., Chidsey, C. A., Harrison, D. C., Gaffney, T. E., and Kahler, R. L.:

Studies on the function of the adrenergic nerve endings in the heart. Circulation 28:958, 1963.

35. Spann, J. F., Jr., Sonnenblick, E. H., Cooper, T., Chidsey, C. A., Willman, V. L., and Braunwald, E.: Cardiac norepinephrine stores and the contractile state of heart muscle. Circ. Res. 19:317, 1966.

36. Anden, N. E., Magneusen, T., and Waldeck, B.: Correlation between noradrenaline uptake and adrenergic nerve function after reserpine treatment. Life Sci. 3:19, 1964.

37. Crout, J. R., Muskus, A. J., and Trendelenburg, U.: Effect of tyramine on isolated guinea pig atria in relation to their noradrenaline stores. Brit. J. Pharmacol. 18:600, 1962.

38. Covell, J. W., Chidsey, C. A., and Braunwald, E.: Reduction of the cardiac response to post-ganglionic sympathetic nerve stimulation in experimental heart failure. Cir. Res. 19:51, 1966.

39. Henry, P. B., Ahumada, G. G., Friedman, W. F., and Sobel, B. E.: Simultaneous isometric tension and ATP hydrolysis in glycerinated fibers from normal and hypertrophied rabbit heart. Circ. Res. 31:740, 1972.

40. Kirkpatrick, S. E., Covell, J. W., and Friedman, W. F.: The continuous assessment of left ventricular performance in the fetal and neonatal lamb. Amer. J. Obstet. Gynec. In press.

41. Barrett, C. T., Heymann, M. A., and Rudolph, A. M.: Alpha and beta adrenergic receptor activity in fetal sheep. Amer. J. Obstet. Gynec. 112:1114, 1972.

42. Creasy, R. K., Barrett, C. T., DeSuiet, M., Kahanga, K. V., and Rudolph, A. M.: Experimental intrauterine growth retardation in the sheep. Amer. J. Obstet. Gynec. 112:567, 1972.

43. Horowitz, L. D., and Bishop, V. S.: Left ventricular pressure dimension relationships in the conscious dog. Cardiovasc. Res. 6:163, 1972.

44. Stegall, H. F., Kardon, M. B., Stone, H. L., and Bishop, V. S.: A portable, simple sonomicrometer. J. Appl. Physiol. 23:289, 1967.

Effects of Congenital Heart Disease on Fetal and Neonatal Circulations

Michael A. Heymann and Abraham M. Rudolph

P REVIOUSLY, THE HEMODYNAMIC EFFECTS of congenital heart malformations generally have been considered only after birth. Little attention has been given to the possibility that these malformations may considerably alter the development of the circulation in the fetus, despite the fact that many congenital heart malformations are compatible with apparently normal fetal somatic development. Although minimal documentation is available regarding these effects in the fetus, it is possible, on the basis of studies of the development of the normal fetal circulation, to hypothesize how different congenital heart malformations might influence the fetal circulation. We have reviewed the normal fetal circulation and the mechanisms by which congenital heart malformation may influence the normal physiology and structure of the fetal circulation. We have also reviewed the circulatory changes after birth and the possible means by which abnormal development of the circulation in utero may effect circulatory adjustments after birth.

THE FETAL CIRCULATION

General Circulation

The general course of the flow of blood in the fetus and many aspects of fetal cardiovascular function have been extensively studied by several groups of investigators.[1-3] Barclay et al.[2] first defined clearly the direction of flow in fetal lambs with angiographic techniques, but they, like most of the earlier investigators, made anatomical descriptions and demonstrated only the general properties of flow within the fetal circulation.

The general arrangement of the fetal circulation is shown in Fig. 1. Umbilical venous blood returns from the placenta and, after joining with portal venous return from the gastrointestinal tract, passes into the inferior vena cava either directly through the ductus venosus, thereby bypassing the liver, or through the hepatic circulation. The inferior vena caval return from the lower body and the placenta then enters the right atrium, and because of the position of the foramen ovale a large proportion of this inferior vena caval stream is directed preferentially into the left atrium (Fig. 2). The foramen ovale is situated very low in the interatrial septum close to the inferior vena cava. The superior margin of the foramen ovale lies on the right side of the atrial septum and is formed by the

From the Cardiovascular Research Institute and Department of Pediatrics, University of California, San Francisco, Calif.

Supported by Program Project Grant HL 06285 from the National Heart and Lung Institute.

Michael A. Heymann, M.B., B.Ch.: *Assistant Professor of Pediatrics in Residence, Cardiovascular Research Institute, University of California, San Francisco, Calif; recipient of Research Career Development Award HD 35398 from the National Institute of Child Health and Human Development.* Abraham M. Rudolph, M.D.: *Neider Professor of Pediatrics, and Professor of Physiology, Department of Pediatrics, University of California, San Francisco, Calif.*

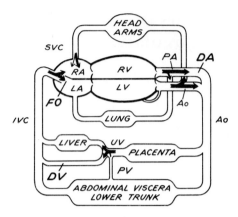

Fig. 1. Diagrammatic representation of the fetal circulation. UV, umbilical vein; PV, portal vein; DV, ductus venosus; IVC, inferior vena cava; SVC, superior vena cava; FO, foramen ovale; RA, right atrium; LA, left atrium; RV, right ventricle; LV, left ventricle; PA, pulmonary artery; DA, ductus arteriosus; and Ao, aorta.

lower, free edge of the septum secundum. This free margin is called the crista dividens, and it lies in such a manner that it overrides the opening of the inferior vena cava into the right atrium. The valve of the foramen ovale, which forms the inferior margin of the foramen, is derived from the septum primum, and lies with its free edge on the left side of the atrial septum. The crista dividens, therefore, effectively splits the inferior vena caval stream into an anterior and rightward stream that enters the right atrium, and a posterior and leftward stream that passes through the foramen ovale into the left atrium. The more posterior stream does not enter the right atrial chamber but flows directly from the inferior vena cava into the left atrium across the valve of the foramen ovale. This blood, after entering the left atrium, mixes with pulmonary venous return, enters the left ventricle, and is ejected by the left ventricle into the ascending aorta.

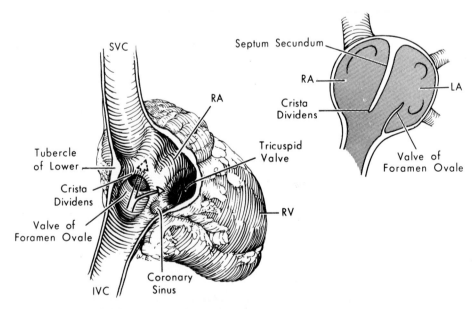

Fig. 2. Anatomical arrangement of foramen ovale, right atrium, and vena cavae, which allows for preferential flow within the fetal heart (see text for details). SVC, superior vena cava; IVC, inferior vena cava; RA, right atrium; LA, left atrium; and RV, right ventricle.

From the ascending aorta, blood is distributed to the heart and upper body, and a portion traverses the aortic isthmus to the descending aorta.

Superior vena caval return also streams preferentially as shown in Fig. 2. The tubercle of Lower (crista interveniens) is situated in the posterolateral aspect of the right atrial wall and effectively directs superior vena caval return towards the tricuspid valve. The tubercle of Lower becomes confluent with the crista dividens, and, therefore, to enter the left atrium superior vena caval blood would have to cross this ridge into the inferior vena cava and then pass through the foramen ovale. The coronary sinus drains into the right atrium between the crista dividens and the tricuspid valve, and consequently coronary venous return is also preferentially directed towards the tricuspid valve. Blood enters the right ventricle and is then ejected into the main pulmonary trunk. From there, blood flows either to the lungs through the main left and right pulmonary arteries or through the ductus arteriosus into the descending aorta.

The earliest quantitative measurements of flow in various parts of the fetal circulation were those made in exteriorized fetal lambs by Dawes et al.[4] They obtained blood samples for O_2 saturation determinations from numerous cardiac chambers and vessels and estimated the cardiac output and the respective volumes ejected by the left and right ventricles. Assali et al.[5] subsequently placed electromagnetic flow transducers on the ductus arteriosus, main pulmonary artery and aorta and, like Dawes et al.[4], calculated that the ventricles ejected similar volumes. It has been customary to express the cardiac output in the fetus as the combined output of both ventricles, since the pulmonary and systemic circulations are in parallel. This differs from the usual manner in which cardiac output is expressed postnatally when the pulmonary and systemic circulations are in series and the cardiac output indicates the volume ejected by each ventricle. Recently, we have measured organ blood flows, cardiac output, and the distribution of blood ejected by the left and right ventricles in fetal lambs using the injection of radionuclide-labeled microspheres.[6-8] Although the proportions of combined ventricular output ejected by the left and right ventricles in our studies were similar to those of Dawes et al.[4] and Assali et al.,[5] the actual levels of output from each ventricle that we measured were somewhat higher, probably since our studies were on unanesthetized fetal lambs in utero. On the basis of these and previous observations, the proportions of flow through the heart and major arteries have been delineated, as shown diagrammatically in Fig. 3.

The main pulmonary trunk receives from the right ventricle about 50% of the combined ventricular output. Forty-two per cent of the combined ventricular output passes across the ductus arteriosus to the descending aorta; the lungs, therefore, receive only about 8% of the combined ventricular output. The ascending aorta receives from the left ventricle about 50% of the combined ventricular output. About 21% of the combined ventricular output is distributed through the brachiocephalic vessels to the brain, head, neck, and upper extremities, and about 4% of combined ventricular output, is distributed to the left and right coronary arteries. Therefore, only about 25% of combined ventricular output traverses the aortic isthmus to the descending aorta. Descending aortic flow, which comprises both ductus arteriosus and aortic isthmus flow, therefore accounts for about 67% of combined ventricular output. Of this amount, the ma-

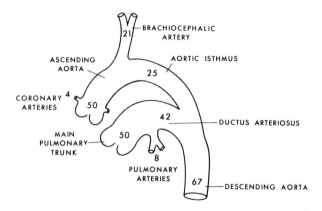

Fig. 3. Diagram showing the percentages of combined ventricular output traversing the major vessels in a normal fetal lamb.

jority, about 40%–45% of combined ventricular output is distributed to the umbilical placental circulation. The average percentages of the combined ventricular output distributed to the major organs in term fetal lambs are shown in Fig. 4.[8] From these values, it can be seen that the total inferior vena caval return accounts for about 70% of the total venous return to the heart, whereas superior vena caval return accounts for only about 20%. Although these figures are based on studies on fetal lambs, recent studies on fetal monkeys[9] as well as pre-viable human fetuses[10] have shown similar patterns of distribution.

The proportions of combined ventricular output carried by the various major fetal arteries are reflected in their relative size. The importance of the magnitude of flow through these arteries in determining the diameter of each vessel will be discussed in detail later in relationship to specific congenital heart malformations. In normal fetal lambs, the diameter of the ductus arteriosus, ascending aorta, and descending aorta are similar. The aortic isthmus is about 20% less in diameter than the descending aorta (Fig. 5). McNamara[11] has made similar observations in postmortem specimens obtained from human fetuses and neonates without cardiovascular malformations. We have confirmed these observations cineangiographically in 16 premature or full-term infants, in whom

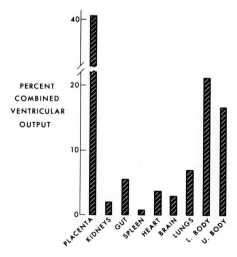

Fig. 4. Percentages of combined ventricular output distributed to various organs in normal full-term fetal lambs. L Body, lower body; and U Body, upper body.

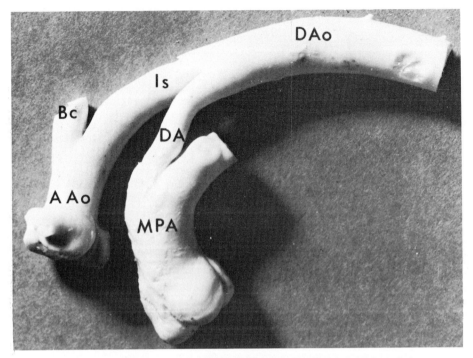

Fig. 5.   Silicone rubber cast demonstrating the relative diameter of the major vessels in a normal-term fetal lamb. AAo, ascending aorta; Bc, brachiocephalic artery; MPA, main pulmonary trunk; DA, ductus arteriosus; Is, aortic isthmus; and DAo, descending aorta.

cardiac catheterization was performed to exclude congenital heart disease because of the presence of severe cardiorespiratory distress. An example of an aortogram from one of these infants is shown in Fig. 6.

The design of the fetal circulation provides the most advantageous distribution of oxygenated and deoxygenated blood to the various fetal organs (Fig. 7). Umbilical venous blood has a P_{O_2} of about 28–30 mm Hg, a P_{CO_2} of 37–38 mm Hg, a pH of 7.36–7.38, and an oxygen saturation of 75%–80%. This highly saturated blood mixes with desaturated blood returning from the lower body to give a saturation of about 70% in the inferior vena cava. This well-saturated blood is largely diverted across the foramen ovale into the left atrium. Here it mixes with pulmonary venous return that is relatively small and then passes into the left ventricle and out the ascending aorta. This then provides the coronary and cerebral circulations with blood of the highest possible P_{O_2}. Carotid arterial P_{O_2} is generally 23–26 mm Hg, P_{CO_2}, 39–42 mm Hg, pH, 7.34–7.36, and oxygen saturation about 65%.

Superior vena caval blood, which is relatively desaturated with an oxygen saturation of about 40%, and coronary sinus blood are directed into the right ventricle, main pulmonary trunk, and across the ductus arteriosus to the descending aorta and towards the placenta for gas exchange. The P_{O_2} of blood in the main pulmonary trunk is usually about 17–20 mm Hg and the oxygen saturation about 55%, and, as this stream mixes with that traversing the aortic isthmus from the ascending aorta, the resultant descending aortic blood P_{O_2} is slightly

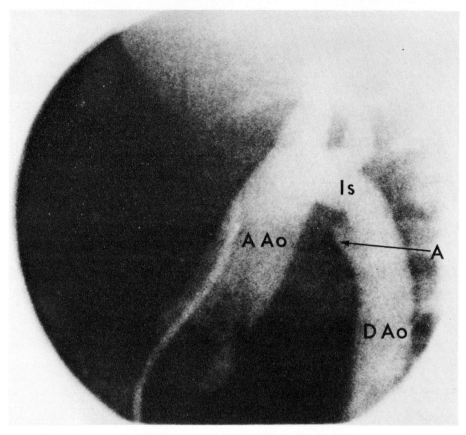

Fig. 6. Aortogram from a 2-day-old full-term infant without heart disease. The relatively narrow aortic isthmus is well shown. AAo, ascending aorta; Is, aortic isthmus; DAo, descending aorta; and A, ductal ampulla.

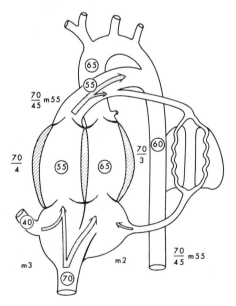

Fig. 7. Diagrammatic representation of patterns of blood flow within the normal fetal heart and great vessels. Numbers in circles are per cent oxygen saturations; other numbers are pressures in mm Hg; m, means pressure.

higher, usually 19–23 mm Hg. The P_{CO_2} in descending aortic blood is usually 42–45 mm Hg, the pH, 7.32–7.34, and the oxygen saturation, 60%.

The ductus arteriosus diameter is as large as that of the descending aorta, and this allows for equalization of pressures in the aorta and pulmonary artery and the left and right ventricles (Fig. 7). In these circumstances, the distribution of blood flow to all fetal organs and the lungs will depend on the local vascular resistance within each organ. Placental vascular resistance is very low; hence the distribution of 40%–45% of combined ventricular output to the placenta for gas and nutrient exchange. The lungs, however, receive only about 8% of combined ventricular output, reflecting a fairly high pulmonary vascular resistance.

Fetal Pulmonary Circulation

Diversion of the right ventricular output away from the lungs through the ductus arteriosus is due to the high fetal pulmonary vascular resistance and low placental vascular resistance. Reynolds[12] suggested that this high pulmonary vascular resistance is due to tortuosity and kinking of the small pulmonary vessels, but this theory has been largely discounted as the major responsible mechanism. More recent evidence suggests that the resistance in the small pulmonary arterioles is largely regulated by the P_{O_2} to which they are subjected. However, other mechanisms such as pH and P_{CO_2} levels, nervous influences, and the presence of circulating vasoactive substances such as catecholamines and bradykinin also play a role in the regulation of pulmonary vascular resistance in the fetus.

Several authors[13–17] have shown that, in fetal lambs, pulmonary vasodilatation is produced by increasing P_{O_2} or by decreasing P_{CO_2} or pH. These changes were effected either by altering the pH, P_{O_2} or P_{CO_2} in the gas or fluid mixture expanding the lungs or in the blood perfusing the lungs. However, the exact patterns of response to changes in blood gases perfusing the fetal lungs are, as yet, not fully established. In some recent preliminary studies in fetal lambs, we have found a curvilinear relationship between P_{O_2} and pulmonary vascular resistance similar to that seen in newborn calves.[18] A fall of 2–3 mm Hg in the P_{O_2} of blood perfusing the pulmonary arteries markedly increased pulmonary vascular resistance. The P_{O_2} of blood normally perfusing the lungs is about 17–20 mm Hg. This low P_{O_2}, to which the pulmonary arterioles are exposed, is probably primarily responsible for maintaining a constant degree of pulmonary vasoconstriction with a consequent high pulmonary vascular resistance.

Colebatch et al.[19] and Campbell et al.[20] have shown, particularly in term fetal lambs, that the pulmonary arterioles are also partly under direct control of the sympathetic nervous system. Sectioning the sympathetic nerve supply to the lung produced mild vasodilatation. Production of systemic hypoxemia in the fetus, while maintaining the P_{O_2} of blood perfusing the lungs at a normal level by cross circulation from another fetus, produced an increase in pulmonary vascular resistance, and this was thought to represent a direct sympathetic nervous effect on the lungs.

Injection of epinephrine[14] or methoxamine[21] directly into the pulmonary artery produces a fall in pulmonary blood flow indicating an increase in pulmonary vascular resistance. Conversely, the injection of bradykinin,[22] acetylcholine or isoproterenol directly into the pulmonary artery produced a fall in pulmonary vascular resistance.

Fig. 8 is a schematic representation of some of the changes in the pulmonary circulation that take place during gestational development. Based on our studies in fetal lambs[8] before 120 days of gestation, pulmonary blood flow accounts for only 3%–4% of combined ventricular output. At term (150 days), 8% of combined ventricular output is distributed to the lungs. Actual calculated pulmonary vascular resistance falls markedly during advancing gestation. However, when related to fetal body weight the pulmonary vascular resistance is fairly constant with only a minimal decrease near term. During the same period of gestation there is an increase in the amount of smooth muscle in the medial layer of the walls of the small pulmonary vessels.[23] The fall in pulmonary vascular resistance in the face of this increase in the amount of muscle indicates that there is an overall increase in the total cross-sectional area of the pulmonary vascular bed, due either to an increase in the number of vessels or to an enlargement of the lumen of existing vessels.

POSTNATAL CIRCULATORY CHANGES

General

Although individual organ resistances may change considerably following birth, the most dramatic alterations in vascular resistances are the elimination of the very low resistance placental vascular bed and the marked pulmonary vasodilatation produced by concurrent initiation of ventilation. As a result

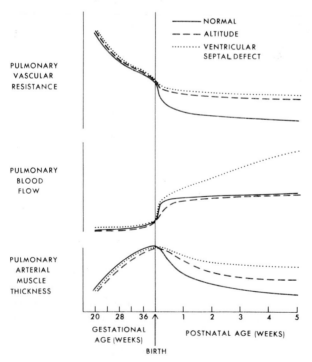

Fig. 8. Schematic representation of fetal and postnatal developmental changes in pulmonary vascular resistance, pulmonary blood flow, and thickness of medial muscle in the pulmonary arterioles. These changes are shown for a normal fetus and infant at sea level, a normal fetus and infant at altitude, and a fetus and infant with a ventricular septal defect at sea level.

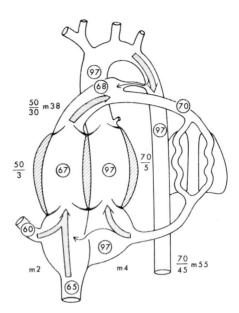

Fig. 9. Diagrammatic representation of the patterns of blood flow within the heart and great vessels of a normal newborn infant. Numbers in circles are per cent oxygen saturations; other numbers are pressures in mm Hg; m, mean pressure.

of these changes, systemic vascular resistance increases markedly whereas pulmonary vascular resistance falls. This produces a reorientation of flow patterns within the heart and circulation (Fig. 9). While the ductus arteriosus remains widely patent, pressures in the pulmonary and systemic circulations will remain similar, and distribution of flow will still be related to local organ resistances. As pulmonary vascular resistance falls, there will be preferential flow through the lungs with the direction of flow from the descending aorta into the main pulmonary artery. This is in the reverse direction of flow in the fetus, which is from the main pulmonary trunk through the ductus arteriosus into the descending aorta. However, the ductus arteriosus generally is functionally closed within 10–15 hs after birth, and left-to-right shunting is minimal in the period before that.

Whereas in the fetus right atrial exceeds left atrial pressure, with the elimination of the placental circulation and the subsequent decrease in inferior vena caval return, right atrial pressure falls; with the almost simultaneous establishment of pulmonary circulation, pulmonary venous return increases, and this, in turn, results in an increase in left atrial pressure, which now exceeds right atrial pressure. As a result, there is functional closure of the foramen ovale as the valve of the foramen ovale is forced closed against the septum secundum. Closure of both the ductus arteriosus and foramen ovale within the first day after birth effectively separates the pulmonary and systemic circulations, which are now in series and not in parallel as in the fetus. Cardiac output now reflects the volume ejected by each ventricle separately, and these are equal.

Pulmonary Circulation

Expansion and ventilation of the lungs is associated with a dramatic fall in pulmonary vascular resistance and increase in pulmonary blood flow (Fig. 8). Physical expansion of the lungs by introduction of air alone into the alveoli is responsible for some of this change;[16,17,19] however, the major factor in re-ducing pulmonary vascular resistance is an increase in the P_{O_2}, to which the pulmonary vessels are exposed.[13,17] The relationships between the level of ar-terial P_{O_2} and pulmonary vascular resistance in newborn calves is shown in Fig. 10.[18] As the P_{O_2} rises to a level of about 30 mm Hg, there is a marked decrease in pulmonary vascular resistance. The effect of acidemia is also shown. A fall in pH alone produces some increase in resistance, and in the presence of acidemia a fall of P_{O_2} produces an even greater increase in pulmonary vascular resistance than at a normal pH.

The exact mechanisms by which alteration in the oxygen environment, to which pulmonary vessels are exposed, produces changes in pulmonary vascu-lar resistance are not yet clearly defined. Lloyd[24] has suggested the possibil-ity that some mediator may be released from lung parenchyma, which acts on the walls of the small pulmonary vessels. He showed that isolated strips of pulmonary arteries, when suspended in a tissue bath, failed to constrict when P_{O_2} was decreased. However, when surrounded by a cuff of lung paren-chymal tissue, they demonstrated the expected constriction.

Since bradykinin is a potent pulmonary vasodilator in the fetus, we have en-tertained the possibility that the effect of O_2 could be due to the release of bradykinin. We demonstrated in term fetal lambs that on expansion of the lungs with oxygen, but not N_2, bradykinin becomes detectable in left atrial blood, suggesting that it is produced in the lungs. In addition, on exposing pregnant ewes to hyperbaric oxygenation without ventilation of the fetal lungs, the fetal P_{O_2} increased and there was an associated significant produc-tion of bradykinin.[25]

Following the initial dramatic fall in pulmonary vascular resistance, there is a more gradual decrease related to the regression of the medial smooth muscle in the pulmonary arterioles (Fig. 8[23,26]). Since the ductus arteriosus is by now normally closed, the systemic and pulmonary circulation are sep-arated, and associated with this decrease in medial muscle mass and pul-monary vascular resistance is a fall in pulmonary arterial and right ventricu-

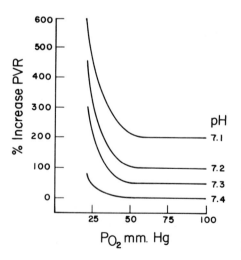

Fig. 10. Patterns of responses of pulmon-ary vasculature of newborn calves to changes in levels of P_{O_2} and pH. The average increase of pulmonary vascular resistance associated with a decrease in pH or P_{O_2} are expressed as percentage increases from the resistance at pH 7.4, and P_{O_2} 100 mm Hg.

lar pressure[27] (Fig. 8). The rate of decrease in muscle mass is fairly rapid within the first 5 days after birth and is more gradual thereafter. In normal infants living at sea level the histologic appearance of the vessels is similar to that in the adult within 3–5 wk after birth.

A decrease in oxygen environment such as occurs at altitude may be expected to interfere with the normal maturation of the pulmonary arterioles with persistence of the medial muscle component. This would lead to a delayed fall in pulmonary vascular resistance and pulmonary arterial pressures (Fig. 8). Evidence to indicate that this occurs has been provided by Arias-Stella and Saldana,[28] who have shown increased amounts of smooth muscle in the pulmonary vessels of individuals native to high altitudes. Also Sime et al.[29] showed that children born and living at altitudes have higher pulmonary vascular resistances and pulmonary arterial pressures than those at sea level. A decrease in P_{O_2} resulting from disease states that cause alveolar hypoxia in infants may also interfere with normal pulmonary vascular maturation as has been shown by Naeye and Letts.[30]

Infants born prematurely follow a pattern of postnatal maturation of the pulmonary arterioles somewhat different from those born at full term. Related to body weight, pulmonary vascular resistance would be about the same as that in a full-term infant. However, if the development of medial muscle in the pulmonary arterioles in the fetus follows the normal pattern, at the time of premature birth the actual amount of muscle present would not be as great as that in a full-term infant (Fig. 11). The 26–28-wk-gestation premature infant may, therefore, have relatively little medial muscle. Postnatal regression of the muscle would be expected to occur at the same rate regardless of the gestational age of the infant, and, since there may be considerably less muscle present in premature infants (the amount depending on gestation), the adult vascular pattern would be developed much more rapidly. It is, therefore, likely that pulmonary vascular resistance might fall much more rapidly

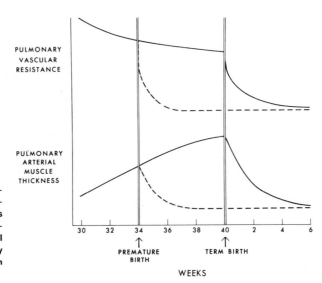

Fig. 11. Schematic representation of fetal and postnatal developmental changes in pulmonary vascular resistance and thickness of medial muscle in the pulmonary arterioles in prematurely born and full-term infants.

after birth than in the mature infant. The importance of this relationship to left-to-right shunts and particularly to the ductus arteriosus will be discussed later.

Branch Pulmonary Arteries

In addition to maturational changes in the small pulmonary arterioles, there are also alterations in the configuration of the main pulmonary trunk and the main left and right pulmonary arteries after birth.[31] As shown in Fig. 12A, in the fetus the ductus arteriosus is a direct continuation of the main pulmonary trunk, with the main left and right pulmonary arteries arising as considerably smaller branches from the trunk. Following birth and closure of the ductus arteriosus, the discrepancy between the sizes of the main pulmonary arterial trunk and the main left and right branches persists. The main branches arise from the postero-inferior aspect of the main pulmonary trunk, and there is an area of doming in the antero-superior portion of the

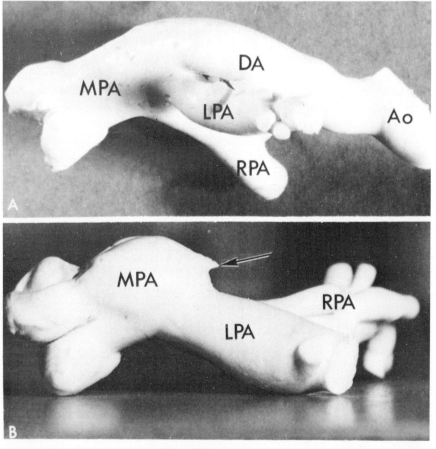

Fig. 12. Silicone rubber casts of the main (MPA) and left (LPA) and right (RPA) branch pulmonary arteries, ductus arteriosus (DA) and descending aorta (Ao) in a stillborn term human fetus (A), and 3-mo-old infant (B), both without congenital cardiac malformations. Arrow indicates area of doming of the main pulmonary artery in the region of the closed ductus arteriosus.

main pulmonary trunk in the region of the ductus arterosus (Fig. 12B). In many instances, a pressure difference may exist between the main and branch pulmonary arteries during the first several months after birth.[31] With growth, the acute angulation of the origin of the main branch pulmonary arteries disappears, and they enlarge to produce the adult contour by about 3–4 mo of age; associated with these normal maturational changes, the pressure difference also disappears.

THE DUCTUS ARTERIOSUS

The ductus arteriosus generally is functionally closed within 10–15 hr after birth in normal full-term infants. Previous studies have demonstrated that an increase in P_{O_2}, to which it is exposed, produced constriction of the ductus arteriosus.[32–35] The actual level of P_{O_2}, to which the muscle layer of the ductus arteriosus is exposed in the fetus in vivo, is still unclear. The ductus receives a direct arterial blood supply from the ascending aorta via branches from the left coronary and first intercostal arteries; this blood would have a P_{O_2} of 23–26 mm Hg. However, it is not known whether the ductus muscle is subjected to this level of P_{O_2}, or rather to the P_{O_2} of the blood flowing within its lumen, which would have a P_{O_2} the same as that in the main pulmonary trunk (17–20 mm Hg). After birth, the P_{O_2} of blood in both the pulmonary artery and aorta is usually increased to levels over 40 mm Hg.

The actual level of P_{O_2} required to produce initial constriction of the ductus arteriosus and the relationship between increasing the level of P_{O_2} and further constriction were not previously known. We have recently studied these relationships in fetal lambs in an vitro preparation by perfusing the isolated ductus arteriosus with Tyrode solution at constant pH and P_{CO_2} and by varying the P_{O_2}.[36] The degree of ductus constriction was assessed by calculating ductal resistance from the pressure difference across it and the flow. The responses of the ductus arteriosus to O_2 were dependent on the gestational age of the fetuses. The less mature the fetus the greater was the level of P_{O_2} re-

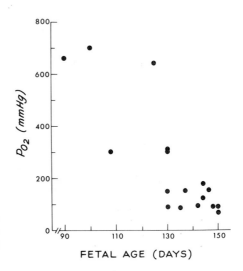

Fig. 13. Initial level of P_{O_2} at which constriction first occurred in the perfused ductus arteriosus from fetal lambs of increasing gestational age.

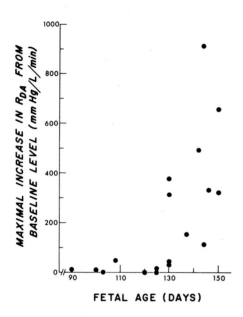

Fig. 14. Maximal constriction developed expressed as increase in resistance (RDA) of isolated perfused ductus arteriosus from fetal lambs of advancing gestational age following exposure to P_{O_2} levels of over 600 mm Hg. Zero resistance is that at P_{O_2} levels of 25–35 mm Hg.

quired to produce constriction, and in lamb fetuses under 90 days gestation no response to P_{O_2} levels of even 600 mm Hg could be elicited (Fig. 13). In addition, the maximal amount of constriction that occurred on exposure to high P_{O_2} was much greater in the mature fetuses than in the immature (Fig. 14). The responses of the ductus arteriosus to O_2 at different gestational ages are summarized in Fig. 15.

Although little or no response to O_2 occurred in the immature fetal lamb, ductus arteriosus constriction did occur in response to the addition of acetylcholine. Similar observations have been made in the ductus arteriosus obtained from midterm, previable human fetuses (10–20 wk).[37]

The mechanisms responsible for the O_2 constrictor response have not been previously delineated. In recent studies on the isolated ductus arteriosus from

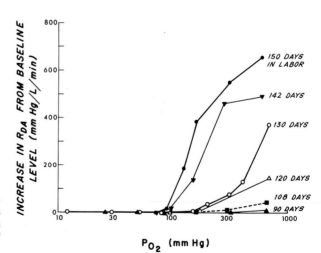

Fig. 15. Patterns of response to increasing P_{O_2} levels of isolated perfused ductus arteriosus from fetal lambs of advancing gestational ages.

fetal lambs, we have confirmed that alpha and beta sympathetic blockade did not interfere with the constrictor response to O_2, but that atropine consistently prevented constriction with O_2 or relaxed the ductus arteriosus constricted by exposure to high P_{O_2}. Acetylcholinesterase also relaxed the ductus arteriosus constricted by O_2. When the ductus arteriosus was relaxed at a P_{O_2} level of about 35 mm Hg, addition of an anticholinesterase, edrophonium (Tensilon), produced constriction of the ductus arteriosus. These studies suggested that the response of the ductus arteriosus to changes in O_2 environment is mediated through the local release of acetylcholine[38] and showed that the response could be prevented by atropine.

EFFECTS OF CONGENITAL HEART MALFORMATIONS ON THE FETAL CIRCULATION

Abnormalities of Development of the Great Arteries

In many congenital malformations associated with anomalies of the aorta and pulmonary artery, somatic fetal growth is apparently unaltered and it is probable that blood flows to the placenta and the various fetal organs are similar to those in normal fetuses. It is, therefore, possible to speculate what the hemodynamic effects of various congenital malformations might be on the development of the pulmonary artery and the aorta in the fetus.[39]

Increased Aortic Isthmus Flow: This would be present in lesions in which blood flow from the right ventricle to the main pulmonary trunk is compromised; this would occur in lesions such as tetralogy of Fallot, tricuspid atresia, and pulmonary atresia. In order to maintain descending aortic and thereby placental flow, blood flow normally carried by the main pulmonary trunk (50% of combined ventricular output) and the ductus arteriosus (about 42% of combined ventricular output) would now be handled by the left ventricle, ascending aorta, and aortic isthmus, in addition to the flow usually carried by them. The aortic arch, therefore, would be expected to have a wider diameter than in the normal fetal circulation; this is illustrated diagrammatically in Fig. 16. Pulmonary blood flow would be expected to be approximately the same as normal (8% of combined ventricular output), but the ductus arteriosus would now carry only this small volume of flow from the aorta

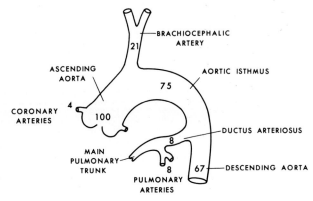

Fig. 16. Diagram showing percentages of combined ventricular output traversing the major vessels in pulmonary atresia.

to the pulmonary arteries, that is, in the reverse direction from normal. Due to this reorientation of flow patterns, the angle of connection of the ductus arteriosus with the aorta is also abnormal.

This is well shown in Fig. 17, which shows an aortogram from a 1-day old infant with pulmonary atresia. The acute inferior angle between the ductus arteriosus and the descending aorta can be contrasted with the obtuse angle found in normal infants (Fig. 6). This realignment of the ductus arteriosus is not well recognized, and it is often referred to as an abnormally high bronchial vessel arising from the aortic arch.

Normal Aortic Isthmus Flow: In lesions such as hypoplastic left ventricle or aortic atresia, little or no blood is ejected by the left ventricle into the ascending aorta. In aortic atresia, therefore, coronary, cerebral, and upper body flow must be provided in a retrograde manner from the main pulmonary trunk through the ductus arteriosus (Fig. 18). Since it appears that flow to these organs is normal in the fetus (20%–25% of combined ventricular output) the volume of flow through the aortic isthmus will be similar to that in the normal fetus but in the reverse direction. The ascending aorta now carries only the coronary blood supply and is markedly underdeveloped.

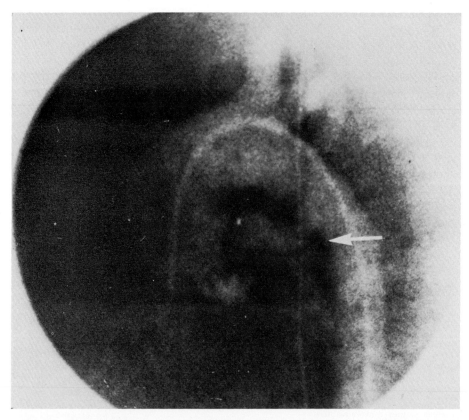

Fig. 17.   Aortogram from a 1-day-old infant with pulmonary atresia. Arrow indicates the acute inferior angle between ductus arteriosus and descending aorta.

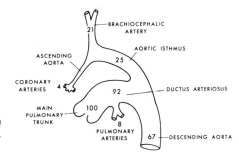

Fig. 18. Diagram showing percentages of combined ventricular output traversing the major vessels in aortic atresia.

Decreased Aortic Isthmus Flow: This flow may occur in lesions in which a moderate proportion of left ventricular output is diverted away from the ascending aorta and is carried by the pulmonary artery. If left ventricular output is sufficient to supply flow to the coronary arteries, brain, and upper body, aortic isthmus flow may be extremely low and lead to underdevelopment of that portion of the aorta. This might occur in lesions such as endocardial cushion defect with left-ventricular-to-right-atrial shunting (Fig. 19), large ventricular septal defects, double-outlet right ventricle, and tricuspid atresia with aortopulmonary transposition.

Development of the Pulmonary Circulation

As discussed previously, the pulmonary circulation in the fetus is normally perfused by blood with a P_{O_2} of 17–20 mm Hg. This low level of P_{O_2} is largely responsible for the fetal pulmonary arteriolar constriction and the development of the thick medial muscle layer in the fetal pulmonary vessels. If these vessels are subjected to a higher than normal P_{O_2} during fetal life, it is possible that the degree of pulmonary vasoconstriction would be decreased, and that the stimulus for the development of the medial muscle thereby would be reduced (Fig. 20). Many congenital cardiac malformations alter the patterns of blood flow within the fetal heart and may produce an increase in the P_{O_2} of blood perfusing the lungs. This would occur when complete admixture

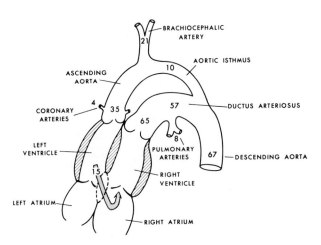

Fig. 19. Diagram showing percentages of combined ventricular output traversing the heart and major vessels in endocardial cushion defect.

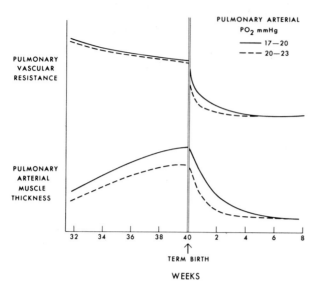

PULMONARY VASCULAR RESISTANCE

PULMONARY ARTERIAL MUSCLE THICKNESS

PULMONARY ARTERIAL PO$_2$ mmHg
—— 17—20
- - - 20—23

32   34   36   38   40   2   4   6   8
↑
TERM BIRTH
WEEKS

Fig. 20. Schematic representation of fetal and postnatal developmental changes in pulmonary vascular resistance and thickness of medial muscle in the pulmonary arterioles in normal fetus and infant at sea level (P$_{O_2}$ of blood perfusing fetal lungs 17–20 mm Hg) and in a fetus and infant with a congenital heart malformation that produced an increase in P$_{O_2}$ of blood perfusing the fetal lungs (P$_{O_2}$ 20–23 mm Hg).

of inferior and superior vena caval streams is produced in lesions such as hypoplastic left ventricle and mitral, tricuspid, pulmonary or aortic atresia. Other lesions in which complete admixture may not necessarily occur but in which the preferential streaming of the normal fetal circulation could be disturbed are double outlet right ventricle or complete aortopulmonary transposition. In complete aortopulmonary transposition, the arrangement of preferential shunting of oxygenated blood into the left atrium and left ventricle is retained. However, with the pulmonary artery arising directly from the left ventricle, the P$_{O_2}$ of blood perfusing the lungs might be expected to be higher than normal (Fig. 21). In certain other lesions without aortopulmonary transposition, either partial or complete, there may also be an increase in the P$_{O_2}$ of blood perfusing the lungs. In the presence of an endocardial cushion defect with predominant direct left-ventricular-to-right-atrial shunting (Fig. 22), blood with a higher P$_{O_2}$ would be shunted to the right side and the P$_{O_2}$ of blood perfusing the lungs may also be expected to be somewhat higher than normal. Roberts[40] has reported a group of patients with ventricular septal defects in whom the defects were situated more anteriorly than usual. In the presence of this type of ventricular septal defect, there may be interference with the normal flow pattern from the left ventricle into the aorta. A fetus with this type of lesion could possibly have predominant left-to-right shunting, and the pulmonary artery may be expected to be perfused with blood having a P$_{O_2}$ higher than normal. Flow into the ascending aorta could also be reduced with consequent changes in the development of the aortic arch as described earlier.[39]

General Organ Development

Redistribution of blood flow in the fetus in the presence of a congenital cardiac malformation, in addition to changing the levels of P$_{O_2}$ in blood perfusing the lungs, may also change the level of P$_{O_2}$ in blood perfusing the rest of the fetal body.

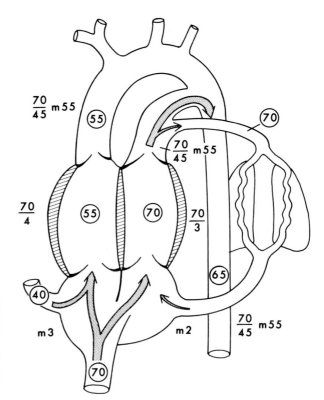

Fig. 21. Diagrammatic representation of the patterns of blood flow within the heart and great vessels in a fetus with aortopulmonary transposition. Numbers in circles are percent oxygen saturations; other numbers are pressures in mm Hg; m, mean pressure.

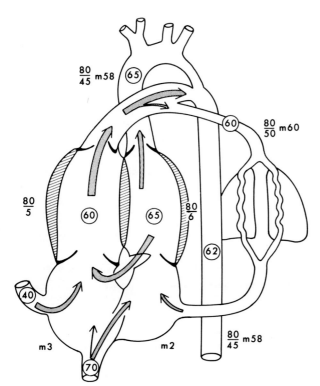

Fig. 22. Diagrammatic representation of the patterns of blood flow within the heart and great vessels in a fetus with endocardial cushion defect. Numbers in circles are per cent oxygen saturations; other numbers are pressures in mm Hg; m, mean pressure.

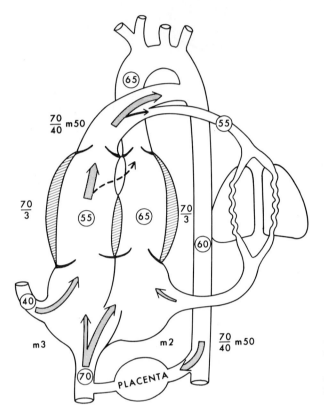

Fig. 23. Diagrammatic representation of the patterns of blood flow within the heart and great vessels in a fetus with ventricular septal defect. Numbers in circles are per cent oxygen saturations; other numbers are pressures in mm Hg. m, mean pressure.

In aortopulmonary transposition (Fig. 21) the P_{O_2} of blood perfusing the heart, brain, and upper body would be lower than normal. In a fetus with a large ventricular septal defect in the usual position, shunting in either direction is potentially possible. With the high pulmonary vascular resistance normally present in the fetus, right-to-left shunting would possibly be expected (Fig. 23). This too could produce a small decrease in the P_{O_2} of blood leaving the left ventricle and perfusing the coronary arteries and brain from the ascending aorta.

Fetal development does not seem to be impaired in these situations although the effects of a persistently lowered arterial P_{O_2} on myocardial function in the fetus are not yet known. There is a suggestion that alterations in the P_{O_2} of blood perfusing various endocrine organs may alter their function, as Naeye reported [41] the presence of both pancreatic islet cell and adrenal cortical hyperplasia in infants with aortopulmonary transposition.

The effects on the functional development of other organs such as aortic or carotid chemoreceptors and systemic arterioles is quite unknown.

Ductus Arteriosus

Congenital heart lesions producing reorientation of the distribution of left and right ventricular outputs may alter the normal development of the ductus arteriosus. The extreme situations would be aortic and pulmonary atresia.

In aortic atresia, the ductus arteriosus carries flow to the whole fetus and placenta with the exception of pulmonary blood flow (Fig. 18). This would be considerably greater than the normal volume handled by the ductus arteriosus. In pulmonary atresia, the ducuts arteriosus carries only pulmonary blood flow, and this in a retrograde manner for the fetus (Fig. 16). Alterations in the flows carried by the ductus arteriosus as well as in the P_{O_2} of the blood supplying the ductus arteriosus, either from within its lumen or by branches from the aorta, may well change the structural development of the ductus. At present, there are no studies to substantiate this theory.

CONGENITAL HEART MALFORMATIONS AND POSTNATAL CIRCULATORY CHANGES

After birth, the major circulatory changes are removal of the placenta, development of the pulmonary circulation, and closure of the ductus arteriosus and foramen ovale, thereby effectively separating the pulmonary and systemic circulations into circulations in series. Removal of the placenta markedly increases systemic vascular resistance and decreases inferior vena caval return. Onset of ventilation produces a marked fall in pulmonary vascular resistance.

Changes in Pulmonary Circulation

In the presence of a patent ductus arteriosus, ventricular septal defect, truncus arteriosus communis, double outlet right ventricle, and several other lesions that allow for free communication between the systemic and pulmonary arterial circuits, equalization of pulmonary and systemic arterial pressures persists following birth. The hemodynamic changes will be determined largely by the relationship between the pulmonary and systemic vascular resistances. The fall in pulmonary vascular resistance following expansion of the lungs will favor flow into the pulmonary circulation and away from the systemic circulation. The resultant increase in pulmonary venous return to the left atrium and left ventricle will produce an elevation in diastolic volume of the left ventricle. This, in turn, based on the Frank-Starling mechanism, produces an increase in left ventricular stroke volume. The importance of the pulmonary vascular resistance in regulating the amount of systemic-to-pulmonary or left-to-right shunting that occurs has been well documented in experimental animals.[27,42] When an artificial aortopulmonary shunt was produced in adult dogs, opening the shunt produced a large left-to-right shunt with the development of acute left ventricular failure. However, in newborn calves that had not yet undergone the normal maturation of the pulmonary arterioles, and in which pulmonary vascular resistance was still elevated, opening the artificial shunt produced little left-to-right shunting and no cardiac failure.

Based on this relationship between the pulmonary and systemic vascular resistances in full-term infants with large systemic to pulmonary communications, it might be expected that significant left-to-right shunting with cardiac failure would develop within the first and second wks after birth, if the pulmonary vascular resistance follows the normal postnatal pattern of maturation. However, it is unusual to find evidence of a large left-to-right shunt with left ventricular failure before the ages of 4–12 wk.[43] This apparent delay in the

onset of cardiac failure in the nature infant may be explained by alterations
in the postnatal development of the pulmonary vasculature in the presence of
a large systemic to pulmonary communication (Fig. 8). Although the small
pulmonary vessels appear normal in fetuses with ventricular septal defects,
following birth there is an abnormal persistence of the medial smooth
muscle.[44] This increased amount of muscle is probably responsible for the delay in the normal fall in pulmonary vascular resistance. The possible mechanisms responsible for the retention of the muscle have been presented previously, but no precise cause has yet been determined.[27]

Another mechanism responsible for a delayed fall in pulmonary vascular
resistance after birth is hypoxia (Fig. 8), which, in turn, will also effect the
postnatal development of left-to-right shunting. The causes of hypoxia are
varied and include pulmonary disease, cerebral disease producing alveolar
hypoventilation, or chronic upper airway obstruction. Infants with large left-
to-right shunts and who develop intercurrent pulmonary disease frequently
show clinical improvement with regard to the amount of shunting and cardiac
failure, and then become progressively worse as the lung disease improves.
The effects of moderate hypoxia due to altitude have also been well documented.[45] Infants with large ventricular septal defects in Denver tend to have
smaller left-to-right shunts and a more benign clinical course than those at sea
level.[46]

In premature infants in whom there is a lesion such as a patent ductus arteriosus or ventricular septal defect that will allow left-to-right shunting, cardiac
failure tends to occur sooner after birth than in mature infants. Although not
clearly documented, there is considerable evidence to suggest that the variations in onset of symptoms are related to differences in the development and
postnatal changes in the pulmonary vessels. Since the amount of pulmonary
vascular smooth muscle increases during the last trimester, an infant born
prematurely will have less muscle than a full-term infant at the time of birth
(Fig. 11). If the rate of decrease in muscle mass after birth is the same as that
in a full-term infant, then low levels of pulmonary vascular resistance would be
reached far more rapidly (Fig. 11). However, many premature infants have
associated idiopathic respiratory distress syndrome and consequently, due to
the effects on the pulmonary vessels of hypoxia and frequently acidosis, do not
show evidence of significant left-to-right shunting until they are recovering
from the lung disease.[47] A more detailed discussion of these findings will be
presented later in relationship to persistent patency of the ductus arteriosus
in premature infants.

A similar pattern might be observed in infants with lesions that could have
been associated with an increased level of P_{O_2} in blood perfusing the lungs
during fetal life. As shown in Fig. 20, if the development of medial smooth
muscle were less than normal, then after birth full-term infants with lesions
such as aortopulmonary transposition and the others mentioned above would
tend to behave like premature infants in regard to pulmonary vascular
changes, left-to-right shunting and clinical symptomatology. However, no
data are currently available to substantiate this hypothesis.

Left-to-right shunting in atrial septal defects is also probably directly related to the decrease in pulmonary vascular resistance, and not only to the relative compliances of the ventricles as previously held. A fall in impedance against which the ventricle ejects produces an increase in stroke volume of that ventricle.[48] Therefore, as pulmonary vascular resistance falls, the right ventricle will increase its stroke volume, and systolic emptying will be greater. In the presence of a large interatrial communication with equal atrial pressures, the right ventricle would therefore tend to fill preferentially. The lower the pulmonary vascular resistance, the greater will be the stroke volume of the right ventricle and the greater ventricular emptying. As a result, the progressive fall in pulmonary vascular resistance will result in an increasing left-to-right atrial shunt. The importance of the relationship between pulmonary and systemic vascular resistances in shunting in atrial septal defects has recently been shown experimentally.[49] It is apparent that the pulmonary vascular resistance plays a critical role in determining the hemodynamic and subsequently the clinical course of infants with various lesions that allow left-to-right shunting. It is appropriate to term this group of lesions *dependent* shunts.[27]

As opposed to this group, there are certain left-to-right shunt lesions in which decreasing pulmonary vascular resistance is not crucial in determining the magnitude of shunting or the onset of cardiac failure. These are lesions in which there is a left-to-right shunt directly from the left ventricle or systemic artery into a systemic vein or the right atrium. This group of lesions has been termed *obligatory* (independent) shunts.[27] and includes systemic arteriovenous communications, sinus of Valsalva communications with the right atrium, and left ventricular to right atrial communications.

These concepts of dependent and obligatory shunting are of great importance in the management of patients, particularly when banding of the pulmonary artery is being considered. They are particularly well demonstrated in patients with endocardial cushion defects. In some of these, the shunting is either predominantly from the left to the right atrium or from the left to the right ventricle. In these patients, the shunting would be of the dependent type. If pulmonary arterial banding is indicated when there is a large ventricular shunt, pulmonary blood flow would be decreased by increasing the right ventricular outflow resistance with a good clinical result. However, if, as frequently occurs, there is predominant shunting from the left ventricle directly into the right atrium or through a cleft mitral valve into the right atrium (Figs. 19 and 22), this would behave as an obligatory shunt. In these circumstances, banding the pulmonary artery would not be expected to alter the amount of left-to-right shunting. Since an additional impedance would be placed on the right ventricle without reducing the volume ejected by that ventricle, right ventricular work would be markedly increased and failure aggravated.

Another lesion in which postnatal development is dependent on changes of pulmonary vascular resistance is anomalous origin of the left coronary artery from the pulmonary artery. In fetal life, pulmonary arterial and aortic pressures are equal, so that left coronary artery perfusion would be adequate albeit with blood of a slightly lower P_{O_2} than normal. After birth, as pulmonary vascular resistance and pulmonary arterial pressure fall normally, perfusion pressure will fall and coronary blood flow to the left ventricular myocardium may be decreased resulting in myocardial ischemia. If adequate collateral anatomoses develop between the left and right coronary arteries, blood would flow from the aorta to the right coronary artery, into the left coronary artery, and then into the pulmonary artery, effectively producing a left-to-right shunt.

The Ductus Arteriosus

Importance in the Premature Infant: In full-term infants, the ductus arteriosus is generally functionally closed within 10–15 hs after birth. However, in premature infants, delayed closure of the ductus arteriosus may occur.[50] A recent survey of deliveries in our institution shows an incidence of 15.3% in infants under 1750g.[47] This is possibly due to the recent advent of methods for more readily overcoming ventilatory problems in premature infants.[51] With the resultant increased survival of small premature infants, the number of infants with patent ductus arteriosus has therefore increased.

Since the incidence of patent ductus arteriosus in infants born at altitude is much greater than in those born at sea level,[52] it was previously thought that one of the major reasons for delayed closure of the ductus arteriosus in premature infants was a low arterial P_{O_2}. However, since many of the premature infants with persistent patency of the ductus arteriosus we have followed were well oxygenated, the experimental studies discussed above suggest the high incidence of patent ductus arteriosus in premature infants is related to the inadequate development of the constrictor response to oxygen of the ductus in these infants.

In fetal lambs as well as in midterm human fetuses, the ductus arteriosus, which does not constrict in response to oxygen, does constrict when exposed to acetylcholine[36,37] indicating that the ductus arteriosus muscle is capable of contracting. We are, therefore, currently investigating the possibility of utilizing acetylcholine as a therapeutic pharmacologic agent at the time of cardiac catheterization. We have demonstrated that infusion of acetylcholine into the aorta at the site of ductal attachment produces definite constriction of the ductus, and in several infants permanent closure has ensued. Unfortunately, in many instances the effect on the ductus was only transient. This is not a recommended form of therapy at present since there are potentially harmful side effects that have not yet been fully evaluated.

Clinical evidence of ductal shunting and symptomatology in any individual premature infant may be quite variable. Although it is possible that these variations could be due to changes in the degree of constriction of the ductus arteriosus, it is probable that alterations in the pulmonary vascular resistance are largely responsible for the changes in the amount of left-to-right shunting. Major changes in pulmonary vascular resistance are likely to occur in infants with respiratory distress syndrome.

Importance in Congenital Cardiac Malformations; Postnatal pulmonary blood flow: As mentioned previously, flow through the ductus arteriosus in fetal life may be considerably less than normal in those lesions such as pulmonary atresia (Fig. 16), which produce either complete or partial obstruction to right ventricular outflow. It is probable, therefore, that the ductus arteriosus is not normally developed in infants with these lesions. Since survival following birth may be dependent on adequate patency of the ductus arteriosus, it may not be large enough to carry sufficient flow to the lungs, and the establishment of pulmonary blood flow would be inadequate.

A delicate balance exists between the increased pulmonary blood flow while the ductus remains open and the increased arterial P_{O_2} resulting from the increased pulmonary flow. As P_{O_2} increases, the ductus may constrict, thereby decreasing pulmonary flow with a resultant fall in P_{O_2}. The ductus will then dilate, and pulmonary flow will increase once again. Although infants with lesions, such as pulmonary atresia, have significantly decreased pulmonary blood flow and are, therefore, severely hypoxic, the ductus arteriosus usually tends to close, although closure may be somewhat delayed. The reason for this is not yet understood. The initial smaller diameter may allow for slight constriction to occur in response to O_2 or other agents such as circulating catecholamines that are elevated in hypoxia. This, coupled with thrombosis within the vessel and within the vessel wall, may then produce eventual complete closure. Since closure of the ductus arteriosus is not predictable, infants with these lesions are, therefore, at extreme risk and should be diagnosed by catheterization and treated promptly.

Since we have shown that in fetal lambs atropine completely relaxes the constriction of the ductus arteriosus in response to oxygen, it is possible that atropine may be a useful therapeutic agent in the temporary management of the infants who may be dependent on patency of the ductus for survival.

Postnatal systemic blood flow: In infants with hypoplastic left ventricle, aortic atresia, or mitral atresia with intact ventricular septum, the ductus arteriosus is responsible in the postnatal period for supplying the complete systemic output (Fig. 24). In infants with interrupted aortic arch, it is responsible for supplying the lower body. After birth, the increase in P_{O_2} associated with ventilation will tend to produce ductal constriction thereby interfering with the systemic blood flow, which is derived from the pulmonary artery. Furthermore, the postnatal fall in pulmonary vascular resistance will allow blood to flow preferentially through the pulmonary circulation, particularly if ductal and systemic vascular resistances are increased. The combined effect of low pulmonary vascular resistance and ductal constriction will result in a severe reduction in systemic blood flow with low blood pressure, poor tissue perfusion, and severe acidemia. The use of oxygen therapy in these infants may be questioned, since it might accelerate both the fall in pulmonary vascular resistance and ductal constriction. As in the previous group of infants, atropine may be useful as a temporary therapeutic agent to prevent ductal closure.

Postnatal development of coarctation of the aorta: Several theories have previously been proposed invoking the role of the ductus arteriosus in the clinical presentation of localized coarctation of the aorta.[39] It had been suggested that there was abnormal extension of ductus muscle into the aortic wall that, when constricted, produced coarctation. We have recently described a new concept relating normal closure of the ductus arteriosus and the development of symptoms in infants with aortic coarctation.[39]

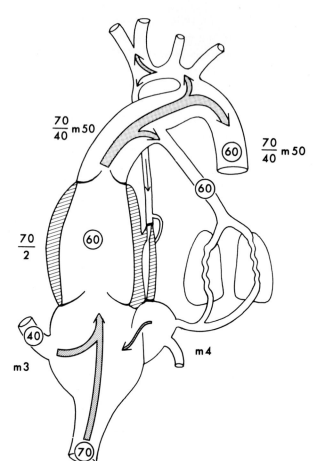

$\frac{70}{40}$ m 50

$\frac{70}{40}$ m 50

60

60

$\frac{70}{2}$

60

40

m 3

m 4

70

Fig. 24. Diagrammatic representation of the patterns of
blood flow within the heart and
great vessels in a neonate with
aortic atresia. Numbers in circles are per cent oxygen saturations; other numbers are
pressures in mm Hg; m, mean
pressure.

Localized coarctation morphologically presents as a well-circumscribed
posterior shelf that protrudes into the aortic wall directly opposite the ductus
arteriosus.[53] During fetal life, while the ductus arteriosus is widely patent,
this shelflike juxtaductal protrusion will not offer any obstruction. Due to the
arrangement of the junction of the ductus arteriosus with the descending
aorta, the direction of flow from the main pulmonary trunk through the
ductus arteriosus into the descending aorta is such that the coarctation does
not interfere with the usual pattern of this flow (Fig. 25). It is probable too that
there is little or no interference with flow from the aortic isthmus into the
descending aorta, since this flow can readily bypass the coarctation by flowing
through the aortic end of the ductus arteriosus. Following birth and constriction
of the ductus arteriosus, the aortic end of the ductus often remains dilated for a
variable period forming a ductal dimple or ampulla. It is, therefore, possible
that in the presence of this ampulla no obstruction to flow is offered, since
blood flowing from the aortic isthmus to the descending aorta can still bypass the
coarctation by flowing through the ampulla. However, once the ductus is completely constricted and the ampulla disappears obstruction to flow may occur

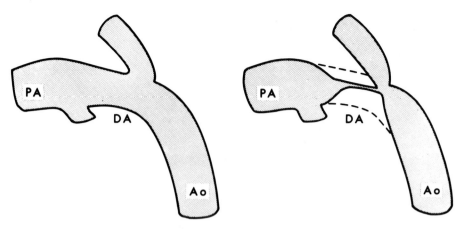

Fig. 25. Diagrammatic representation of the role of the ductus arteriosus in producing aortic obstruction in juxtaductal coarctation of the aorta. Left panel shows the vessels in the fetus with the ductus arteriosus widely patent. Right panel shows identical major vessel pattern in the newborn with the ductus arteriosus constricted. PA, main pulmonary trunk; DA, ductus arteriosus; and Ao, descending aorta.

(Fig. 25). We suggest that this may explain the sudden occurrence of left ventricular failure in infants with juxtaductal coarctation of the aorta, since in some instances complete ductal constriction may occur rapidly. Support for this hypothesis comes from experimental studies we have performed.

We simulated surgically juxtaductal coarctation in fetal lambs by invaginating the posterolateral wall of the aorta to produce a shelf similar to that found in patients. Immediately following birth, no pressure difference was present between the ascending and descending aorta. However, following the administration of oxygen and acetylcholine to constrict the ductus arteriosus, we were able to produce a systolic pressure difference of about 30 mm Hg.

SUMMARY

The normal fetal circulation and distribution of cardiac output in the fetus have been described. The manner in which various congenital heart malformations may influence the course of the fetal circulation and thereby alter the development of various vascular structures is presented. The clinical features of congenital heart disease are markedly influenced by the circulatory changes occurring at and after birth. Since fetal development of the ductus arteriosus and the pulmonary circulation may be abnormal in the presence of congenital heart malformations, their postnatal response may not be normal. Furthermore, since progressive maturation of the pulmonary arterioles and ductus arteriosus occurs during advancing gestation, in premature infants after birth these structures may not show the degree of responsiveness usually seen in the full-term infant. Experimental work on the effects of induced cardiac anomalies on the development of the fetal circulation should be encouraged to increase our understanding of the relationships between congenital heart disease and the cardiovascular adaptation following birth.

REFERENCES

1. Barcroft, J.: Researches on Prenatal Life. Oxford, Blackwell, 1946.

2. Barclay, A. E., Franklin, K. J., and Prichard, M. M. L.: The Foetal Circulation and Cardiovascular System, and the Changes That They Undergo at Birth. Oxford, Blackwell, 1944.

3. Dawes, G. S.: Foetal and Neonatal Physiology. Chicago, Year Book, 1968.

4. Dawes, G. S., Mott, J. C., and Widdicombe, J. G.: The foetal circulation in the lamb. J. Physiol. (London) 126:563, 1954.

5. Assali, N. S., Kirschbaum, T. M., and Dilts, P. V., Jr.: Effects of hyperbaric oxygen on uteroplacental and fetal circulation. Circ. Res. 22:573, 1968.

6. Rudolph, A. M., and Heymann, M. A.: The circulation of the fetus in utero: Methods for studying distribution of blood flow, cardiac output and organ blood flow. Circ. Res. 21:163, 1967.

7. Rudolph, A. M., and Heymann, M.A.: Validation of the antipyrine method for measuring fetal umbilical blood flow. Circ. Res. 21: 185, 1967.

8. Rudolph, A. M., and Heymann, M. A.: Circulatory changes with growth in the fetal lamb. Circ. Res. 26:298, 1970.

9. Behrman, R. E., Lees, M. H., Peterson, E. N., DeLannoy, C. W., and Seeds, A. E.: Distribution of the circulation in the normal and asphyxiated fetal primate. Amer. J. Obstet. Gynec. 108:956, 1970.

10. Rudolph, A. M., Heymann, M. A., Teramo, K. A. W., Barrett, C. T., and Raiha, N. C. R.: Studies on the circulation of the previable human fetus. Pediat. Res. 5:452, 1971.

11. McNamara, D. G.: Coartation—Course and prognosis in infancy and childhood. In Kidd, B. S. L., and Keith, J. D. (Eds.): The Natural History and Progress in Treatment of Congenital Heart Defects. Springfield, Ill., Charles C. Thomas, 1971.

12. Reynolds, S. R. M.: Fetal and neonatal pulmonary vasculature in guinea pigs in relation to hemodynamic changes at birth. Amer. J. Anat. 98:97, 1956.

13. Dawes, G. S., Mott, J. C., Widdicombe, J. G., and Wyatt, D. G.: Changes in the lungs of newborn lamb. J. Physiol. (London) 121:141, 1953.

14. Dawes, G. S., and Mott, J. C.: The vascular tone of the foetal lung. J. Physiol. (London) 169:10, 1963.

15. Cook, C. D., Drinker, P. A., Jacobson, N. H., Levison, H., and Strang, L. B.: Control of pulmonary blood flow in foetal and newly born lamb. J. Physiol. (London) 169:10, 1963.

16. Lauer, R. M., Evans, J. A., Aoki, H., and Kittle, C. F.: Factors controlling pulmonary vascular resistance in fetal lambs. J. Pediat. 67:568, 1965.

17. Cassin, S., Dawes, G. S., Mott, J. C., Ross, B. B., and Strang, L. B.: The vascular resistance of the foetal and newly ventilated lung of the lamb. J. Physiol. (London) 171:61, 1964.

18. Rudolph, A. M., and Yuan, S.: Response of the pulmonary vasculature to hypoxia and H^+ ion concentration changes. J. Clin. Invest. 45:399, 1966.

19. Colebatch, H. J. H., Dawes, G. S., Goodwin, J. W., and Nadeau, R. A.: The nervous control of the circulation in the foetal and newly expanded lungs of the lamb. J. Physiol. (London) 178:544, 1965.

20. Campbell, A. G. M., Cockburn, F., Dawes, G. F., and Milligan, J. E.: Pulmonary vasoconstriction in asphyxia during cross-circulation between twin foetal lambs. J. Physiol. (London) 192:111, 1967.

21. Barrett, C. T., Heymann, M. A., and Rudolph, A. M.: Alpha and beta adrenergic function in fetal sheep. Amer. J. Obstet. Gynec. 112:1114, 1972.

22. Campbell, A. G. M., Dawes, G. S., Fishman, A. P., Hyman, A. I., and Perks, A. M.: Release of a bradykinin-like pulmonary vasodilator substance in foetal and newborn lambs. J. Physiol. (London) 195:83, 1968.

23. Naeye, R. L.: Arterial changes during the perinatal period. Arch. Path. (Chicago) 71:121, 1961.

24. Lloyd, T. C., Jr.: Hypoxic pulmonary vasoconstriction: Role of perivascular tissue. J. Appl. Physiol. 25:560, 1968.

25. Heymann, M. A., Rudolph, A. M., Nies, A. S., and Melmon, K. L.: Bradykinin production associated with oxygenation of the fetal lamb. Circ. Res. 25:521, 1969.

26. Phillips, C. E., Jr., DeWeese, J. A., Manning, J. A., and Mahoney, E. B.: Maturation of small pulmonary arteries in puppies. Circ. Res. 8:1268, 1960.

27. Rudolph, A. M.: The changes in the circulation after birth: Their importance in congenital heart disease. Circulation 41:343, 1970.

28. Arias-Stella, J., and Saldaña, M.: The muscular pulmonary arteries in people native to high altitude. Med. Thorac. 19:292, 1962.

29. Sime, F., Banchero, N., Peñaloza, D.,

Gamboa, R., Cruz, J., and Marticorena, E.: Pulmonary hypertension in children born and living at high altitudes. Amer. J. Cardiol. 11: 150, 1963.

30. Naeye, R. L., and Letts, H. W.: The effects of prolonged neonatal hypoxemia on the pulmonary vascular bed and heart. Pediatrics 30:902, 1962.

31. Danilowicz, D., Rudolph, A. M., Hoffman, J. I. E., and Heymann, M. A.: Physiologic pressure differences between main and branch pulmonary arteries in infants. Circulation. 45:410, 1972.

32. Kennedy, J. A., and Clark, S. L.: Observations on the physiological reactions of the ductus arteriosus. Amer. J. Physiol. 136:140, 1942.

33. Born, G. V. R., Dawes, G. S., Mott, J. C., and Rennick, B. R.: The constriction of the ductus arteriosus caused by oxygen and by asphyxia in newborn lambs. J. Physiol. (London) 132:304, 1956.

34. Assali, N. S., Morris, J. A., Smith, R. W., and Manson, W. A.: Studies on ductus arteriosus circulation. Circ. Res. 13:478, 1963.

35. Kovalcik, V.: Response of the isolated ductus arteriosus to oxygen and anoxia. J. Physiol. (London) 169:185, 1963.

36. McMurphy, D. M., Heymann, M. A., Rudolph, A. M., and Melmon, K. L.: Developmental changes in constriction of the ductus arteriosus: Responses to oxygen and vasoactive substances in the isolated ductus arteriosus of the fetal lamb. Pediat. Res. 6:231, 1972.

37. McMurphy, D. M., and Boreus, L. O.: Studies on the pharmacology of the perfused human fetal ductus arteriosus. Amer. J. Obstet. Gynec. 109:937, 1971.

38. Oberhansli-Weiss, I., Heymann, M. A., Rudolph, A. M., and Melmon, K. L.: The pattern and mechanisms of response of the ductus arteriosus and umbilical artery to oxygen. Pediat. Res. In press.

39. Rudolph, A. M., Heymann, M. A., and Spitznas, U.: Hemodynamic considerations in the development of narrowing of the aorta. Amer. J. Cardiol., in press.

40. Roberts, W. C., Morrow, M. G., and Braunwald, E.: Complete interruption of the aortic arch. Circulation 26:39, 1962.

41. Naeye, R. L.: Transposition of the great arteries and prenatal growth. Arch. Path. (Chicago) 82:412, 1966.

42. Rudolph, A. M., Scarpelli, E. M., Golinko, R. J., and Gootman, N.: Hemodynamic basis for clinical manifestations of patent ductus arteriosus. Amer. Heart J. 68:447, 1964.

43. Hoffman, J. I. E., and Rudolph, A. M.: The natural history of ventricular septal defects in infancy. Amer. J. Cardiol. 16:162, 1965.

44. Wagenvoort, C. A.: The pulmonary arteries in infants with ventricular septal defects. Med. Thorac. 19:162, 1962.

45. Peñaloza, D., Sime, F., Banchero, N., Gamboa, R., Cruz, J., and Marticorena, E.: Pulmonary hypertension in healthy men born and living at high altitudes. Amer. J. Cardiol. 2:150, 1963.

46. Vogel, J. H. K., McNamara, D. G., and Blount, S. G., Jr.: Role of hypoxia in determining pulmonary vascular resistance in infants with ventricular septal defects. Amer. J. Cardiol. 20:346, 1967.

47. Kitterman, J. A., Edmunds, L. H., Jr., Gregory, G. A., Heymann, M. A., Tooley, W. H., and Rudolph, A. M.: Patent ductus arteriosus in premature infants: Incidence, relation to pulmonary disease and management. Submitted for publication.

48. Wilcken, D. E. L., Charlier, A. A., Hoffman, J. I. E., and Guz, A.: Effects of alterations in aortic impedance on the performance of the ventricles. Circ. Res. 14:283, 1964.

49. Douglas, J. E., Rembert, J. C., Sealy, W. C., and Greenfield, J. C.: Factors affecting shunting in experimental atrial septal defects in dogs. Circ. Res. 24:492, 1969.

50. Danilowicz, D., Rudolph, A. M., and Hoffman, J. I. E.: Delayed closure of the ductus arteriosus in premature infants. Pediatrics 37: 74, 1966.

51. Gregory, G. A., Kitterman, J. A., Phibbs, R. H., Tooley, W. H., and Hamilton, W. K.: Treatment of the idiopathic respiratory-distress syndrome with continuous positive airway pressure. New Eng. J. Med. 284:1333, 1971.

52. Peñaloza, D., Arias-Stella, J., Sime, F., Recavarren, S., and Marticorena, E.: The heart and pulmonary circulation in children at high altitudes. Pediatrics 34:568, 1964.

53. Edwards, J. E., Christensen, N. A., Clagett, O. T., and McDonald, J. R.: Pathologic considerations in coarctation of the aorta. Proc. Mayo Clin. 23:324, 1948.

Pathogenesis of Congenital Atrioventricular Block

Maurice Lev

CONGENITAL ATRIOVENTRICULAR (AV) BLOCK, as strictly de-fined, is that which is known to be present at birth. However, in a broad sense, since it may not be discovered at birth, any AV block that is detected early in life, in which there is no evidence of myocarditis, trauma, or other etiologic agent, and in which no previous examination has revealed sinus rhythm, or in which other congenital malformations of the heart or other organs are coexistent, may be termed congenital heart block. This broader definition may thus include some cases of acquired AV block in a congenitally malformed heart.

The pathology of congenital AV block has been reviewed in the past by Lev.[1-8] Such blocks are either isolated (present in an otherwise normally formed heart), or they may be associated with other cardiac abnormalities. It would appear that the isolated type is more common.[9-17]

ORIGINS OF CONGENITAL AV BLOCK

There are at present three known pathogenetic mechanisms for the creation of congenital AV block: (1) lack of communication between the atrial musculature and the more peripheral part of the conduction system;[18] (2) interruption of the AV bundle (bundle of His);[19] and (3) pathologic changes in an aberrant conduction system.[20]

Lack of Communication Between Atrial Musculature and the More Peripheral Conduction System (Fig. 1)

In these cases, the musculature of the atrial septum in its peripheral portion is deficient and there is diminished or no connection between the atria and the AV node. The AV node may be normally developed but shows no such connection, or the node may be deficient, absent, or abnormal in shape. Where it is absent, there is no connection between the atrial musculature and the penetrating portion of the bundle of His. In an occasional case, not only is the node absent, but the penetrating portion of the AV bundle is also absent, and only the branching portion may be present, giving off the bundle branches.

From the Congenital Heart Disease Research and Training Center, Hektoen Institute for Medical Research; the Departments of Pathology, Northwestern University Medical School; the University of Chicago School of Medicine; the Abraham Lincoln School of Medicine, University of Illinois; The Chicago Medical School, University of Health Sciences; and Loyola University, Stritch School of Medicine, Chicago, Ill.

Supported by Grant HE 07605-09 from the National Institutes of Health, National Heart and Lung Institute, Bethesda, Md.

Maurice Lev, M.D.: *Director, Congenital Heart Disease Research and Training Center, Hektoen Institute for Medical Research; Professor of Pathology, Northwestern University Medical School; Professorial Lecturer, University of Chicago School of Medicine; Lecturer in Pathology, Abraham Lincoln School of Medicine, University of Illinois; Lecturer in Pathology, The Chicago Medical School, University of Health Sciences; Lecturer, Department of Pathology, Loyola University, Stritch School of Medicine; and Career Investigator and Educator, Chicago Heart Association, Chicago, Ill.*

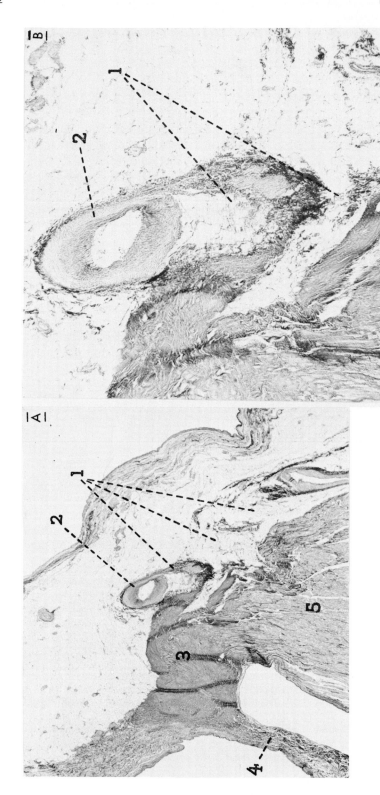

Fig. 1. Lack of communication between the atria and the more peripheral conduction system. Weigert-van Gieson stain. (A) × 15; (B) × 48; 1, region of AV node; 2, branch of ramus septi fibrosi; 3, central fibrous body; 4, mitral valve; and 5, ventricular musculature. (By permission.[4])

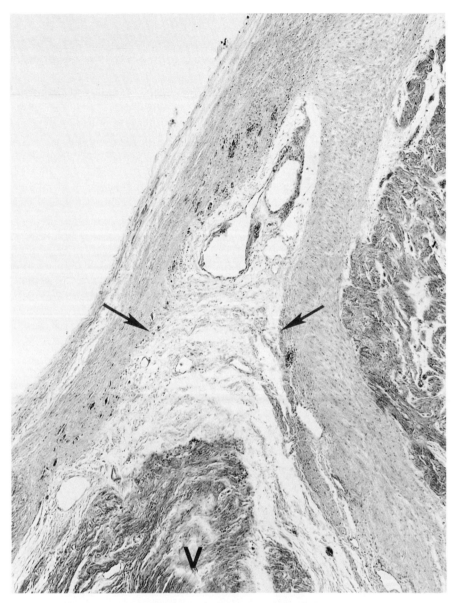

Fig. 2.   Interruption of the penetrating portion of the bundle of His, which is replaced by space and loose connective tissue. Hematoxylin-eosin stain. × 50. Arrows point to region of penetrating portion of AV bundle. V, ventricular muscle. (By permission.[19])

These cases have been seen in otherwise normally developed hearts,[3, 21–24] or are associated with fibroelastosis,[18] fibroelastosis with patent ductus,[18] fibroelastosis with fetal (preductile) coarctation,[18] patent foramen primum,[25] atrial septal defect of the fossa ovalis (secundum) type,[26] and complete transposition with common ventricle.[27]

Interruption of the A V Bundle (Bundle of His) (Fig. 2)

In these cases, the atrial connections to the AV node are intact. However, there is interruption in the penetrating portion of the AV bundle. The branching portion of the AV bundle may be present or absent. The bundle branches, in their beginning, may be intact, or defective. However, a portion of one or both bundle branches are connected to the ventricular myocardium.

This type has been found to be associated with otherwise normally developed hearts,[25,28] or associated with single ventricle with transposition and pulmonary atresia,[29] isolated mixed levocardia with atrial inversion,[30] persistent ostium primum,[31] cor triloculare biventriculare,[32] ventricular septal defect,[33] fibroelastosis,[34] adult (postductal) type of coarctation with fibroelastosis,[19] atrial septal defect of the fossa ovalis type,[19] aneurysm of the pars membranacea,[35,37] and aneurysm of the aortic sinus of Valsalva.[35]

Pathologic Changes in an Aberrant Conduction System

In the case of Lev, Fielding, and Zaeske[20] (Figs. 3–5), which was a case of mixed levocardia with ventricular inversion (corrected transposition), ventricular septal defect, and fetal coarctation, the usually formed peripheral conduction

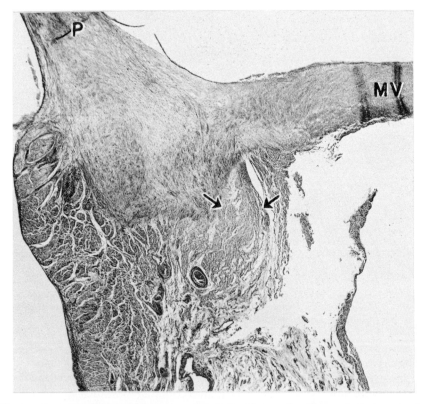

Fig. 3. Abnormal conduction system in a case of mixed levocardia with ventricular inversion (corrected transposition) with fetal coarctation and ventricular septal defect. Normally situated AV node. Weigert-van Gieson stain. × 27. P, pars membranacea, and MV, annulus of mitral valve. Arrows point to node. (By permission.[20])

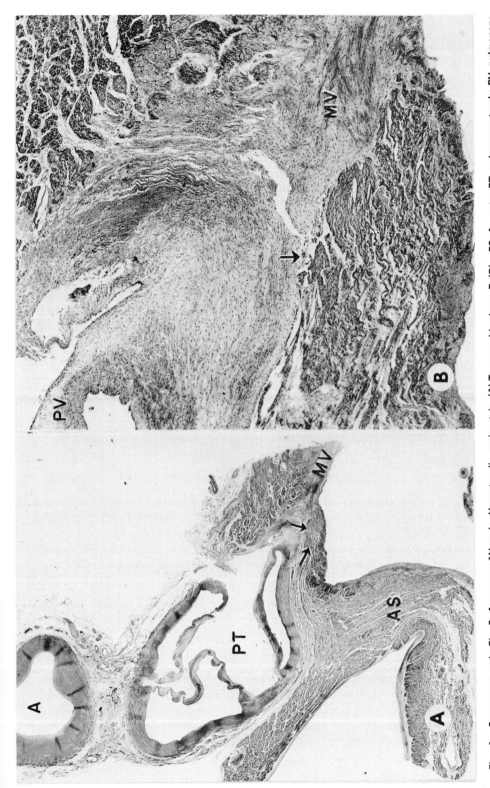

Fig. 4. Same case as in Fig. 3. Accessory AV node. Hematoxylin-eosin stain. (A) Topographic view x 7, (B) x 50. A, aorta; PT, pulmonary trunk; PV, pulmonary valve; AS, atrial septum; and MV, mitral annulus (right-sided). Arrows point to node. (By permission.[20])

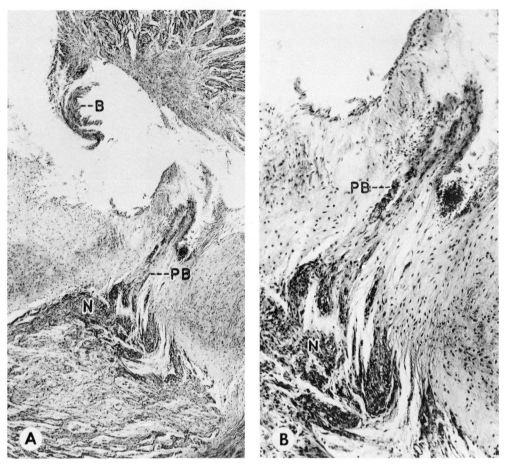

Fig. 5.   Same case as in Figs. 3 and 4. Accessory AV node and accessory AV bundle penetrating mitral (right-sided) annulus. Hematoxylin-eosin stain. (A) x 65, (B) x 135. Note the scar in
the AV node and the hemorrhage and fibrosis of the AV bundle. N, accessory node; PB, Accessory
bundle penetrating annulus; and B, bundle reaching the roof of the morphologic left (right-sided)
ventricle. (By permission.[20])

system consisted of an AV node. This was not connected to the usually positioned
AV bundle and bundle branches, which were absent. Instead, an accessory conduction system was present with an accessory AV node, lying anteriorly in the
right AV groove, adjacent to the pulmonary artery, and well connected to the
atria. This node formed an aberrant AV bundle, which penetrated the right AV
groove, and continued on the superior surface of the ventricular septal defect.
It gave off the bundle branches in reverse formation. Fibrosis and hemorrhage in
the accessory penetrating bundle had produced the block.

    There is still a group of anomalies, which have been described as being asso-
ciated with atrioventricular block, for which conduction system studies have not
been done as yet. These are hypoplasia of the aortic tract complex (hypoplastic
left heart syndrome),[38,39] tetralogy of Fallot,[40] complete transposition with tricuspid stenosis or atresia,[41–43] pulmonary atresia with tricuspid stenosis without transposition (pulmonary atresia with intact ventricular septum[45]), muscu-

lar subaortic stenosis,[46] Marfan's disease,[47-49] patent ductus arteriosus with double aortic arch,[50] and congenital absence of the left epicardium.[51] It is possible that blocks associated with these anomalies may reveal new pathogenetic mechanisms.

Acquired (nonsurgical) heart block in congenital heart disease,[52-54] when it occurs associated with atrial or ventricular septal defects, may be due to hemodynamic stresses, with fibrosis or necrosis of the AV bundle. Such a case was studied by Lev, Paul, and Cassels[26] in a heart with atrial septal defect of the fossa ovalis type. Necrosis and hemorrhage were found in the normally formed penetrating portion of the AV bundle. Some blocks, so acquired, may not be permanent, and operative closure of the defect may relieve the block.[55] It is also possible in corrected transposition to acquire AV block without ventricular septal defect. This may be due to the prolonged course of the AV bundle in this anomaly.

Familial AV Block[18,56-60]

Congenital AV block may be familial, or it may occur in families in which other members have the Wolff-Parkinson-White Syndrome.

THEORETICAL CONSIDERATIONS OF EMBRYOLOGIC FAULT IN CONGENITAL AV BLOCK

Congenital AV block may obviously be due to an abnormality in the formation of the conduction system, or an abnormality in the formation of the structures related to the conduction system. Therefore, it is necessary to consider the embryologic development of the AV node, bundle and bundle branches, and of the central fibrous body (trigonum fibrosum dexter) and the pars membranacea.

Embryologic Development of the AV Node, Bundle and Bundle Branches

Originally, Retzer[61] thought that the AV node and bundle developed from the sinus venosus. Mackenzie[62] likewise believed the AV node to be derived from the sinus venosus, while the AV bundle arose from the atrial canal. Koch[63] and Aschoff[64] thought that only the posterior part of the AV node arose from the sinus while the anterior part of the node and the bundle were derived from the atrial canal. Patten[65] suggested that the AV node is developed from the myocardium of the left sinus horn.

Most authors[66,67,68,69,70] believe, however, that the AV node and bundle in the mammal originates from the atrial canal musculature. They originate from the posterior part of this canal, which lies behind the posterior endocardial cushion at a time when the musculature of this canal is still unbroken. According to Sanabria,[68] the primordia of these structures appear before the inferior septum has joined the posterior endocardial cushion, and before the endocardial cushions have fused. The proliferation of the primordial tissue of the canal to form the AV node and bundle, occurs under the general influence of the stimulus for muscular proliferation and septation produced by the alignment of the septum primum and the septum inferior with the endocardial cushions and their fusion. These processes are the concomitants of the shift of the auricular canal to the right and the ventral deviation of the bulbus. During this phase there is atrophy of the anterior part of the atrial canal musculature and with the subsequent development of valves there is atrophy of the lateral walls. There is a difference of opinion as to whether both the AV node and bundle originate in situ,[68,70] or whether the bundle originates from a proliferation of AV nodal tissue.[69] There is also a difference of opinion as to whether the bundle branches originated in situ from the ventricular trabeculae[68,70] or whether they originate from a proliferation of the tissue of the bundle of His.[69] The left originates before the right.

In man,[69] the AV node and bundle originates at 8–10 mm. By 13 mm, the left bundle branch has developed considerably and the right first makes its appearance. At 16.5 mm, the left bundle branch is completely developed, and at about 22–25 mm the right bundle branch is traced to the moderator band. Histologic differentiation of these structures is a continuing process up to birth.

Embryologic Development of the Central Fibrous Body and Pars Membranacea

The central fibrous body is normally formed by the union of the anterior and posterior endocardial cushions, later re-enforced by a fibrous extension from the aorta, during the second phase of the development of the heart. This phase concerns itself with the absorption of the bulbus, and the reorientation of the atrial canal to the bulbus. The details of this phase were originally described by Pernkopf and Wirtinger[71] and recently confirmed by Asami.[72] During this process, the aortic conus comes to lie in the groove between the developing mitral and tricuspid orifices and valves as the endocardial cushions fuse. At the end of this process, the bulbar musculature is still present at the aortic base posteriorly. However, this eventually becomes fibrosed, thus contributing to the formation of the central fibrous body.

The distal and right extension of the central fibrous body is the pars membranacea. This consists of an atrioventricular portion, and ventriculo-ventricular portion. Many versions of the formation of the pars membranacea have been given.[66,73–76] This structure is probably formed by the endocardial cushions, with or without participation by the bulbar cushions.

Possible Embryologic Fault in Congenital AV Block

In lack of communication between the atria and the AV node, an inviting hypothesis is that in the process of formation of the central fibrous body, and the obliteration of the posterior portion of the aortic part of the bulbus, the atrial connections are also obliterated, and in some cases further damage is done to the AV node and bundle and even the beginning of the bundle branches. Thus, we may be dealing with an abnormality in the aortic extension of the central fibrous body. In interruption of the AV bundle we may be dealing with abnormalities in the mitral or tricuspid extensions of the central fibrous body or of the pars membranacea. An alternate explanation of the latter would be that there was lack of union between the developing AV node and the AV bundle. This would lead one to assume that these structures originally develop separately.

Where the conduction system is abnormally formed with aberrant communications, as in the case of Lev, Fielding, and Zaeske,[20] we may postulate that the musculature behind the anterior endocardial cushion is stimulated to form a conduction system from the atrial canal, rather than that behind the posterior cushion.

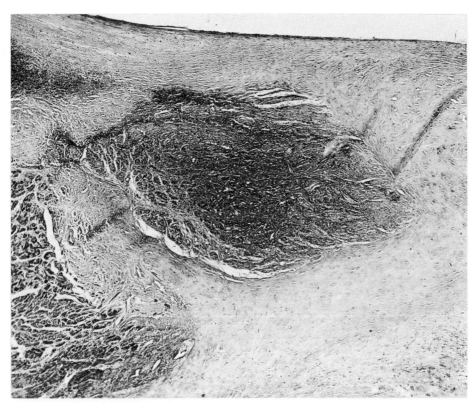

Fig. 6.   Replacement of penetrating portion of AV bundle by hemorrhage, due to surgery. He-matoxylin-eosin stain. × 40. (By permission.[80])

ATRIOVENTRICULAR BLOCK PRODUCED BY SURGERY IN CONGENITAL HEART DISEASE

This has been studied by Reemstma, Delgado, and Creech,[77] Lenègre and Blondeau,[78] Titus, Daugherty, and Edwards,[79] Lev, et al.[80] and Hudson.[35] Block has been obtained by operative procedures on VSD, ASD of the primum type, tetralogy of Fallot, common AV orifice, corrected transposition, and calcified bicuspid aortic valve.[35,81–84] The pathologic change leading to block is usually produced by surgical severance, hemorrhage, necrosis or inflammation of the penetrating portion of the AV bundle, or of the beginning of the branching portion (Fig. 6). Some blocks are temporary, due to edema or hemorrhage. Some patients with surgical AV block may resume sinus rhythm as long as 2 yr later.

HORIZONS

More work remains to be done on the conduction system in congenital AV block associated with congenital malformations. This is especially needed in atrioventricular block with atrial or ventricular inversion (corrected transposition).[14,85–88]

REFERENCES

1. Lev, M.: Anatomic basis for atrioventricular block (Symposium on Cardiac Arrhythmias). Amer. J. Med. 37:742, 1964.

2. — : The normal anatomy of the conduction system in man and its pathology in atrioventricular block. Ann. N. Y. Acad. Sci. 111:817, 1964.

3. — : The anatomy and pathology of the conduction system in the human heart. Hebrew Med. J. 1:262, 1962.

4. — , Benjamin, J. E., and White, P. D.: A histopathologic study of the conduction system in a case of complete heart block of 42 years' duration. Amer. Heart J. 55:198, 1958.

5. — : The pathology of complete atrioventricular block. Progr. Cardiovasc. Dis. 6:317, 1964.

6. — : The conduction system in congenital heart disease. Amer. J. Cardiol. 21:619, 1968.

7. — : The anatomic basis for disturbances in conduction and cardiac arrhythmias. Progr. Cardiovasc. Dis. 2:360, 1960.

8. — : The architecture of the conduction system in congenital heart disease: I. Common atrioventricular orifice. Arch. Path. (Chicago) 65:174, 1958.

9. Moss, A. J., Adams, F. H., and O'Loughlin, B. J.: Congenital malformation of the cardiac conduction system. J. Dis. Child. 97:72, 1959.

10. Richter, I.: Kompletter Herzblock im Kindesalter. Mschr. Kinderheilk. 107:326, 1959.

11. Moss, A. J.: Congenital complete atrioventricular block; clinical features, hemodynamic findings, and physical working capacity. J. Lancet 81:542, 1961.

12. Landtman, B., Linder, E., Hjelt, L., and Tuuteri, L.: Congenital complete heart block. A clinical study of 27 cases. Ann. Paediat. Fenn. 10:99, 1964.

13. Moreau, P., Gerbaux, A., and Lenègre, J.: L'étiologie des blocs auriculo-ventriculaires. Arch. Mal. Coeur. 56:609, 1963.

14. Nakamura, F. F., and Nadas, A. S.: Complete heart block in infants and children. New Eng. J. Med. 270:1261, 1964.

15. Jouve, A., Géraud, R., Torresani, J., Arnoux, M., and Moliner, A.: Les blocs auriculo-ventriculaires isolés présumés congénitaux. Arch. Mal. Coeur. 59:1770, 1961.

16. Kangos, J. J., Griffiths, S. P., and Blumenthal, S.: Congenital complete heart block: a classification and experience with 18 patients. Amer. J. Cardiol. 20:632, 1967.

17. Swiderski, J.: Trwaly Blok przedsion-Kowo-Komorowy serca II i III stopnia u dzieci. Pediat. Pol. 43:15, 1968.

18. Lev, M., Silverman, J., Fitzmaurice, F. M., Paul, M. H., Cassels, D. E., and Miller, R. A.: Lack of connection between the atria and the more peripheral conduction system in congential atrioventricular block. Amer. J. Cardiol. 27:481, 1971.

19. — , Cuadros, H., and Paul, M. H.: Interruption of the atrioventricular bundle with congenital atrioventricular block. Circulation 43: 703, 1971.

20. — , Fielding, R. T., and Zaeske, D.: Mixed levocardia with ventricular inversion (corrected transposition) with complete atrioventricular block; a histopathologic study of the conduction system. Amer. J. Cardiol. 12:875, 1963.

21. Smithells, R. W., and Outon, E. B.: Congenital heart block. Arch. Dis. Child. 34:223, 1959.

22. Latta, H., and Crittenden, I. H.: Acquired lesions of the conduction system in familial congenital heart block. Lab. Invest. 13:214, 1964.

23. Sotello-Avila, C., Rosenberg, H. S., and McNamara, D. G.: Congenital heart block due to a lesion in the conduction system. Pediatrics 45:640, 1970.

24. Lenègre, J., and Gay, J.: Un cas de bloc auriculo-ventriculaire complet-solitaire-probablement congènital par destruction du noeud de Tawara. Arch. Mal. Coeur. 63:740, 1970.

25. Wallgren, A., and Winblad, S.: Congenital heart block. Acta Paediat. 20:175, 1938.

26. Lev, M., Paul, M. H., and Cassels, D. E.: Complete atrioventricular block associated with atrial septal defect of the fossa ovalis (secundum) type. A histopathologic study of the conduction system. Amer. J. Cardiol. 19:266, 1967.

27. Linder, E., Landtman, B., Tuuteri, L., and Hjelt, L.: Congenital complete heart block. II. Histology of the conduction system. Ann. Paediat. Fenn. 11:11, 1965.

28. Monnett, P., and Perrin, A.: Bloc auriculo-ventriculaire congénital sous la dépendance d'une interruption du système Hisien vérifieé par coupes sériées et sans anomalie macroscopique cardiaque. Arch. Franc. Pédiat. 15:1357, 1958.

29. Wilson, J. G., and Grant, R. T.: A case of congenital malformation of the heart in an infant associated with partial heart block. Heart 12:295, 1925–26.

30. Yater, W. M.: Congenital heart block. Review of the literature; report of a case with incomplete heterotaxy; the electrocardiogram in dextrocardia. Amer. J. Dis. Child. 38:112, 1929.

31. —, Lyon, J. A., and McNabb, P. E.: Congenital heart block. Review and report of the second case of complete heart block studied by serial sections through the conduction system. JAMA 100:1831, 1933.

32. —, Leaman, W. G., and Cornell, V. H.: Congenital heart block; report of the third case of complete heart block studied by serial sections through the conduction system. JAMA 102:1660, 1934.

33. Huntingford, P. J.: The aetiology and significance of congenital heart block. (The report of a case studied by serial section of the heart.) J. Obstet. Gynaec. Brit. Comm. 67:259, 1960.

34. Mottu, T., Kapanci, Y., Varonier, H., Bernhardt, E., and Thelin, F.: Bloc auriculo-ventriculaire complet associé à une fibroélastose de l'endocarde. Cardiologia 46:180, 1965.

35. Hudson, R. E. B.: Surgical pathology of the conduction system of the heart. Brit. Heart J. 29:646, 1967.

36. Cohn, A. E., and Lewis, T.: Auricular fibrillation and complete heartblock. A description of a case of Adams-Stokes Syndrome, including the postmortem examination. Heart 4:15, 1912–13.

37. Harris, A., Davies, M., Redwood, D., Leatham, A., and Siddons, H.: Aetiology of chronic heart block. A clinico-pathological correlation in 65 cases. Brit. Heart J. 31:206, 1969.

38. Donoso, E., Braunwald, E., Jick, S., and Grishman, A.: Congenital heart block. Amer. J. Med. 20:869, 1956.

39. Bernard, R., Gérard, R., and Gras, A.: Les hypoplasies congénitales de l'aorte (a propos d'une observation avec bloc auriculo-ventriculaire associé chez un nourrisson de 18 mois). Arch. Franc. Pediat. 17:921, 1960.

40. Bernreiter, M., and O'Connell, F.: Congenital heart block. Report of a case. JAMA 150:792, 1952.

41. Dickson, R. W., and Jones, J. P.: Congenital heart block in an infant with associated multiple congenital cardiac malformations. Amer. J. Dis. Child. 75:81, 1948.

42. Aitchison, J. D., Duthie, R. J., and Young, J. S.: Palpable venous pulsations in a case of transposition of both arterial trunks and complete heart block. Brit. Heart J. 17:63, 1955.

43. Wyss, S., and Töndury, G.: Zum Kongenitalen Totalen Atrioventrikular-Block. Z. Kreislaufforsch 52:478, 1963.

44. Belobradek, Z., Herout, V., and Jurkovic, V.: Isolated tricuspid insufficiency combined with Adams-Stokes syndrome. Acta Cardiol. 14:486, 1959.

45. Hoekenga, M. T.: Complete heart block in an infant associated with multiple congenital cardiac malformations. Amer. J. Dis. Child. 69:231, 1945.

46. Gilgenkrantz, J. M., Cherrier, F., Petitier, H., Dodinot, B., Houplon, M., and Legoux, J.: Cardiomyopathie obstructive du ventricule gauche avec bloc auriculo-ventriculaire complet; considerations therapeutiques. Arch. Mal. Coeur. 61:439, 1968.

47. Bawa, Y. S., Gupta, P. D., and Goel, B. G.: Complete heart block in Marfan's syndrome. Brit. Heart J. 26:148, 1964.

48. Moretti, G. F., Staeffen, J., Bertrand, E., and Broustet, A.: Bloc auriculo-ventriculaire complet dans le syndrome de Marfan. Presse Med. 72:605, 1964.

49. Chopra, K. L., Krishnan, S., and Joseph, P. P.: Intermittent bundle branch block and complete heart block in Marfan's syndrome. Indian Heart J. 22:53, 1970.

50. Jennings, G. H.: Two contrasted cases of complete heart block observed over many years. Brit. Heart J. 33:50, 1971.

51. Varriale, P., Rossi, P., and Grace, W. J.: Congenital absence of the left pericardium and complete heart block. Dis. Chest 52:405, 1967.

52. Yater, W. M., Barrier, C. W., and McNabb, P. E.: Acquired heart block with Adams-Stokes attacks dependent upon a congenital anomaly (persistent ostium primum); report of case with detailed histopathologic study. Ann. Intern. Med. 7:1263, 1934.

53. Rogers, H. M., and Rudolph, C. C.: Congenital ventricular septal defect with acquired complete heart block. Amer. Heart J. 41:770, 1951.

54. Berman, D. A., and Adicoff, A.: Corrected transposition of the great arteries causing complete heart block in an adult. Amer. J. Cardiol. 24:125, 1969.

55. Conklin, E. F., Giustrar, F. X., Ditolla, E. M., Rappaport, I., Mistretta, C., and Gregory, J. J.: Secundum atrial septal defect with complete heart block and Adams-Stokes attacks. New York J. Med. 70:1080, 1970.

56. Wendkos, M. H., and Study, R. S.: Familial congenital complete A-V heart block. Amer. Heart J. 34:138, 1947.

57. Crittenden, I. H., Latta, H., and Ticinovich, D. A.: Familial congenital heart block. Amer. J. Dis. Child. 108:104, 1964.

58. Kahler, R. L., Braunwald, E., Plauth, W. H., and Morrow, A. G.: Familial congenital heart disease; familial occurrence of atrial septal defect with A-V conduction abnormalities; supraventricular aortic and pulmonic stenosis and ventricular septal defect. Amer. J. Med. 40:384, 1966.

59. Tsagaris, T. J., Bustamante, R. A., and Friesendorff, R. A.: Familial heart disease. Dis. Chest 52:153, 1967.

60. Rodriguez-Coronel, A., Isenberg, J. I., and Bliss, H. A.: Supernormal conductivity of the A-V node with anomalous A-V excitation in a patient with hereditary A-V block. Acta Cardiol. 23:179, 1968.

61. Retzer, R.: Ueber die muskulöse Verbindung zwischen Vorhof und Ventrikel des Säugetierherzens. Arch. Anat. Physiol. Anat. Abteilung Heft. 1:1904.

62. Mackenzie, I.: The excitatory and connecting muscular system of the heart. (A study in comparative anatomy.) In proceedings of 17th Internat. Congress Med., London, Section 1. Anatomy and Embryology. London, H. Frowde, 1913, Part 1, p. 121.

63. Koch, W.: Ueber die Bedeutung der Reizbiedungsstellen (kardiomotorischen Zentren) des rechten Vorhofes beim Säugetierherzen. Arch. Ges. Physiol. 151:279, 1913.

64. Aschoff, L.: Bericht über die Verhandlungen der XIV. Tagung der Deutschen pathologischen Gesellschaft in Erlangen vom 4.—6. April 1910. Zbl. Allg. Path. 21:433, 1910.

65. Patten, B. M.: The development of the sinoventricular conduction system. Univ. Mich. Med. Bull. 22:1, 1956.

66. Mall, F. P.: On the development of the human heart. Amer. J. Anat. 13:249, 1912.

67. Tandler, J.: Anatomie des Herzens. Jena, 1913, G. Fischer.

68. Sanabria, T.: Recherches sur la différenciation du tissu nodal et connecteur du coeur des mammifères. Arch. Biol. 47:2, 1936.

69. Walls, E. W.: The development of the specialized conducting tissue of the human heart. J. Anat. 81:93, 1947.

70. Field, E. J.: The development of the conducting system in the heart of sheep. Brit. Heart J. 13:129, 1951.

71. Pernkopf, E., and Wirtinger, W.: Die Transposition der Herzostien-ein Versuch der Erklärung dieser Erschinung. Z. Anat. Entwicklungsgesch. 100:563, 1933.

72. Asami, I.: Beitrag zur Entwicklung des Kammerseptums im menschlichen Herzen mit besonderer Berücksichtigung der sogenannten Bulbus drehung Z. Anat. Entwicklungsgesch. 128:1, 1969.

73. Tandler, J.: In Keibel, F., and Mall, F. P. (Eds.): Manual of Human Embryology, Vol. II. Philadelphia, J. P. Lippincott, 1912.

74. Frazer, J. E.: The formation of the pars membranacea septi. J. Anat. 51:19, 1917.

75. Odgers, P. N. B.: The development of the pars membranacea septi of the human heart. J. Anat. 72:247, 1937-8.

76. Hamilton, W. J., Boyd, J. D., and Mossman, H. W.: Human Embryology. Cambridge, England, W. Heffer & Sons, 1945.

77. Reemtsma, K., Delgado, J. P., and Creech, Jr., O.: Heart block following intracardiac surgery: localization of conduction tissue injury. J. Thorac. Cardiovasc. Surg. 39:688, 1960.

78. Visioli, O., Baragan, J., and Lenègre, J.: Disorders of post operative conduction in the surgery of congenital septal defects. Anatomo-electrical study. Atti. Soc. Ital. Cardiol. 2:169, 1962.

79. Titus, J. L., Daugherty, G. W., Kirklin, J. W., and Edwards, J. E.: Lesions of the atrioventricular conduction system after repair of ventricular septal defect. Relation to heart block. Circulation 28:82, 1963.

80. Lev, M., Fell, E. H., Arcilla, R., and Weinberg, M. H.: Surgical injury to the conduction system in ventricular septal defect. Amer. J. Cardiol. 14:464, 1964.

81. Sayed, H. M.: Complete heart block following open heart surgery. J. Cardiovasc. Surg. 6:426, 1965.

82. Hurwitz, R. A., Riemenschneider, T. A., and Moss, A. J.: Chronic postoperative heart block in children. Amer. J. Cardiol. 21:185, 1968.

83. Smith, T. W., McFarland, J. C., Buckley, M. J., and Austen, W. G.: Late recovery of conduction following surgically induced atrioventricular block. Ann. Thorac. Surg. 9:372, 1970.

84. Averill, K. H., Vogel, J. H. K., Pryor, R., and Blount, Jr., S. G.: Complete heart block following intracardiac surgery; reversion to normal sinus rhythm after twenty-five months. Amer. J. Cardiol. 14:556, 1964.

85. Walker, W. J., Cooley, D. A., McNamara, G. M., and Moser, R. H.: Corrected transposition of the great vessels, atrioventricular heart block and ventricular septal defect. A clinical triad. Circulation 17:249, 1958.

86. Wright, F. S., Adams, Jr., P., and Anderson, R. C.: Congenital atrioventricular dissociation due to complete or advanced atrioventricular heart block. J. Dis. Child. 98:72, 1959.

87. Siggers, D. C., and Deuchar, D. C.: Long-term use of implanted pacemakers in the control of complete heart block. Guy Hosp. Rep. 119:323, 1970.

88. Jausseran, J. M., Amichot, J. L., Serafini, V., Torresani, J., and Jouve, A.: Bloc auriculoventriculaire complet et transposition corrigée des gros vaisseaux. Marseille Med. 107:305, 1970.

Recognition and Management of Cardiologic Problems in the Newborn Infant

Norman S. Talner and A. G. M. Campbell

T HE MORTALITY FROM CONGENITAL HEART DISEASE is highest during the first few mo of life with one-quarter to one-third of all infants born with cardiac defects expiring before the age of 1 mo, most within the first wk.[1] On the basis of these data, it becomes readily apparent that any program designed to increase the salvage of critically ill infants with cardiac disorders must rest on a foundation of prompt recognition, safe and rapid transport to an infant cardiac center, accurate physiologic and anatomic diagnosis, and appropriate medical or surgical management. This portion of the symposium on neonatal heart disease will be primarily concerned with the presentation of a broad, systematic appraisal of the infant suspected of having a cardiologic problem. As such, it will consider the two major high-risk situations—the cyanotic infant with a large right-to-left shunt, and the infant thought to be in congestive heart failure. Each may exist singly or be present in combination. Cyanosis and congestive heart failure will be analyzed with special reference to the underlying pathophysiology, stressing clinical and laboratory methods that will permit delineation of the specific nature of the problem and lead to a rational approach to management and potential salvage.

FUNCTIONAL BASIS FOR HYPOXIA IN THE NEWBORN

Central to the theme of the infant with cyanosis or congestive heart failure is the presence of tissue hypoxia. This may be defined as a state in which a diminished rate of oxygen utilization by mitochondria exists in relation to the tissue oxygen requirements. Tissue hypoxia can arise as the result of any defect(s) in oxygen transport that may take place at the pulmonary, circulatory, or tissue level. (Fig. 1). As outlined by Duc,[3] hypoxia can be associated with a low oxygen content in arterial blood (hypoxemia) or with a normal oxygen content (normoxemia). Furthermore, hypoxemia can occur either with a diminished arterial oxygen tension or with a low oxygen content without a decrease in oxygen tension. When the partial pressure of oxygen in arterial blood is reduced, the most commonly encountered clinical problem, this may be caused by hypoventi-

From the Department of Pediatrics, Yale University School of Medicine, and the Yale-New Haven Medical Center, New Haven, Conn.

Some of the patients were studied in the Children's Clinical Research Center, supported by Grant RR-00125 from the General Clinical Research Centers Program of the Division of Research Resources, National Institutes of Health.

Norman S. Talner, M.D.: Director, Pediatric Cardiology, Yale-New Haven Medical Center, and Professor of Pediatrics, Yale University School of Medicine, New Haven, Conn.; recipient of Career Development Award HD-18438 from the National Institutes of Health, USPHS. A. G. M. Campbell, M. B., M.R.C.P. (Edin.): Director, Newborn Services, Yale-New Haven Medical Center, and Associate Professor of Pediatrics, Yale University School of Medicine, New Haven, Conn.

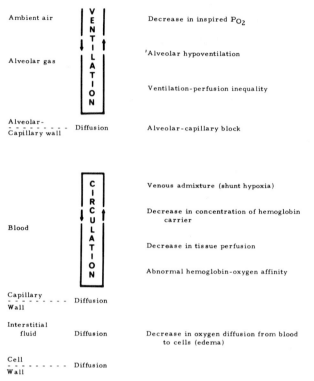

Fig. 1. Pathophysiologic basis for hypoxia. (Modified after Dejours.[2])

lation, right-to-left intracardiac or intrapulmonary shunting, ventilation-perfusion inequality, or a diffusion defect.[4]

When hypoxia is seen with a low oxygen content in the face of a normal oxygen tension, the basic problem relates to the amount of oxygen container (hemoglobin) available. Since the total hemoglobin pool is limited as in anemia, the amount of oxygen transported to the tissues is low, despite attempts at compensation achieved by an increase in cardiac output. The correction of this defect requires replacement of the hemoglobin stores, which will increase oxygen-carrying capacity.

A significant decrease in systemic blood flow can limit oxygen supply to the tissues, despite a normal or near-normal oxygen content and oxygen tension. This can be observed in septic shock or with congestive heart failure associated with impaired systemic perfusion. Therapy under these circumstances requires augmentation of the blood flow to the peripheral tissues.

Abnormalities of hemoglobin-oxygen binding can also produce tissue hypoxia with normal oxygen tensions and content as well as blood flow. The presence of fetal hemoglobin in the newborn could possibly interfere with oxygen transport because of the high affinity of fetal hemoglobin for oxygen, which limits the amount available to the tissues. However, other mechanisms that will increase oxygen delivery to the tissues do exist, and they will be considered later.

In assessing cyanosis in the newborn, it must be stressed that blueness is only recognized when at least 5 g/100 ml of reduced or abnormal hemoglobin is present in capillary blood. Therefore, with the high hemoglobin content in the newborn, less arterial unsaturation is required to reach the critical level of reduced hemoglobin. The presence of fetal hemoglobin with increased oxygen affinity allows for cyanosis to become evident only with a significant decrease in arterial oxygen tension. For example, as cited by Lees,[5] with normal pH levels at 37° C, cyanosis can be recognized at an arterial saturation of approximately 80% with an oxygen tension about 50 mm Hg, if adult hemoglobin predominates. If fetal hemoglobin is the major oxygen carrier, however, cyanosis will only be observed at a Pa_{O_2} of 40 mm Hg, due to the leftward shift in the oxygen dissociation curve. On the other hand, if the infant is anemic, blueness may not be noted even with a severe decrease in oxygen saturation.

CLINICAL BASIS FOR HYPOXIA IN THE NEWBORN

When hypoxia associated with a decreased arterial oxygen tension or oxygen content, compromised systemic blood flow, or abnormal oxygen-hemoglobin affinity is approached from the clinical standpoint, consideration must be given to the possible involvement of four major organ systems (heart, lungs, central nervous system, and hemopoietic), each of which will now be discussed.

Cardiac Basis for Hypoxia

Many cardiac malformations are associated with a decrease in arterial oxygen tension with or without accompanying congestive heart failure. When cardiac failure is not present, hypoxemia usually arises from a right-to-left shunt as a consequence of obstruction to pulmonary blood flow, the switching of the major arterial streams (transposition of the great arteries), or, rarely, the anomalous connection of a systemic venous channel to the left heart. To these may be added abnormalities in ventilation-blood flow relationships and hypoventilation when congestive heart failure complicates the hypoxic state.

The common cardiac lesions associated with hypoxemia without necessarily congestive heart failure in the newborn are transposition of the great arteries, tricuspid and pulmonary atresia, valvar pulmonic stenosis, severe tetralogy of Fallot, and Ebstein's malformation of the tricuspid valve.

When the various causes of cardiac failure are analyzed in terms of their basic hemodynamic abnormality, they could be categorized in the following fashion: (1) *volume-pressure loading* of the myocardium, as would be seen with large volume left-to-right shunts, arteriovenous fistulae, total anomalous pulmonary venous return without pulmonary venous obstruction (examples of volume loading), or left or right ventricular outflow obstruction, coarctation, anomalous pulmonary venous return with pulmonary venous obstruction (examples of pressure loading); (2) *primary depression of contractile element function* that may arise from inflammatory disease of the myocardium, hypoxemia and acidemia, electrolyte abnormalities such as hypocalcemia and hypokalemia, hypoglycemia, and coronary occlusive disease; and (3) *arrhythmias* with heart rates in excess of 220/min or less than 40/min.

Although cardiac malformations can usually be tolerated without difficulty in utero, the circulatory adjustments that mark the transition from intra- to extrauterine existence exert a profound influence on the clinical picture of infants born with a congenital or acquired cardiac disorder. We propose to illustrate how alterations in the fetal-flow pathways and pulmonary vasculature operate as the major determinants of the clinical picture of cardiac disease in the newborn by delaying the appearance of clinical difficulty, altering the underlying hemodynamic state so that the presentation is atypical, or accelerating the manifestations of a cardiac problem.

Ductus Arteriosus: The ductus arteriosus is the principal determinant of the clinical picture in a number of pathologic states encountered during the newborn period. Notably in the hypoplastic left-heart syndrome, signs of low systemic perfusion appear when ductal constriction occurs. These infants may tolerate their severe defect for 1 to 2 days, while the ductus remains widely patent. The systemic vascular bed is apparently adequately perfused in retrograde fashion from the pulmonary artery with blood of low oxygen tension. When the ductus constricts, pulses diminish, and a severe metabolic acidemia develops. With low systemic perfusion, it is noteworthy that the systemic arterial oxygen tension rises, reflecting an increase in the pulmonary-to-systemic blood flow ratio. These metabolic alterations in an infant with aortic atresia are shown in Fig. 2. Thus, with the hypoplastic left-heart picture, the fetal pathway —the ductus arteriosus—is the major limiting factor in allowing short-term survival. Left-to-right shunting through an incompetent foramen ovale and the lowered resistance in the pulmonary vascular bed following delivery are obviously also of considerable import.

The ductus arteriosus can also modify the clinical picture in infants with obstruction to pulmonary venous return in association with anomalous pulmonary venous connection. With the ductus open, the obstructed pulmonary circuit can to some extent be unloaded via this channel into the systemic circulation. This serves to delay clinical signs of systemic and pulmonary venous congestion, and to mask the underlying pathology. A right-sided angiocardiogram will reveal flow via fetal pathways, and only on close scrutiny may the anomalous pulmonary venous pathway be recognized. Combined umbilical artery and umbilical venous catheterization in a newborn with tachypnea and a reticular-granular pattern in the lung field should provide help when the anomalous pulmonary venous connection is below the diaphragm. The P_{O_2} in the umbilical venous blood sampled at the level of the inferior vena cava will then exceed that in the umbilical artery, due to the insertion of the pulmonary venous trunk into the portal circuit or ductus venosus (Fig. 3).

The ductus arteriosus provides the only avenue for lung blood flow in infants with pulmonary atresia. In this condition, the size of the ductal left-to-right

	pH	P_{CO_2} mm Hg	P_{O_2} mm Hg	Lactate mM/L
PDA open	7.31	32	34	3
PDA const.	7.04	18	55	12

Fig. 2. Metabolic alterations observed in infant with aortic atresia prior to and following constriction of the ductus arteriosus.

	pH	P_{O_2} mm Hg	P_{CO_2} mm Hg
Umb. Art.	7.28	35	43
Umb. Vein	7.29	42	40

Fig. 3. Simultaneous blood-gas and pH samples obtained from the umbilical artery and vein in infant with anomalous pulmonary venous connection to portal vein. Note that umbilical venous P_{O_2} exceeds that in umbilical artery.

shunt is usually small as borne out by the extremely low levels of arterial oxygen tension. Rudolph has raised the possibility that the ductus is underdeveloped in these infants because, in fetal life, it only carried 8%–10% of left ventricular output rather than most of the right ventricular flow, as would occur in the normal fetal state.[6]

It is also pertinent to point out that closure of the ductus arteriosus can be delayed in any condition occurring in a newborn deficient in oxygenation at the pulmonary level. The diagnosis of persistence of the fetal pathways, therefore, requires definition as to the specific cause for continued patency of a fetal flow pattern (asphyxia, pulmonary disease, hypoglycemia, high blood viscosity, etc.).

Ductus Venosus: The role of the ductus venosus in possibly providing a low-resistance bypass in infants with anomalous pulmonary venous connection into the portal system has been reported by Rudolph.[6] Signs of clinical difficulty may be delayed if the ductus venosus remains open postnatally. When this pathway is obliterated, pulmonary venous blood must now pass through the high-impedance hepatic circuit and increased pulmonary venous obstruction results.

Foramen Ovale: The third fetal pathway, the foramen ovale, occupies a central role in the clinical problems associated with certain cardiac malformations. In lesions producing elevation of left atrial pressure, such as obstructive disease of the left heart, large volume left-to-right communications at the ventricular and pulmonary artery level, and endomyocardial disease, flow from left to right at the atrial level through an incompetent foramen ovale has been observed. Abolition of the left atrial hypertension may be followed by a disappearance of the atrial shunt. Left-to-right atrial shunting through a foramen ovale may serve to maintain low pulmonary venous pressures and possibly prevent pulmonary edema. At the same time, however, left ventricular filling pressures are diminished, and this may compromise systemic perfusion.

In conditions where there is severe obstruction to right ventricular outflow, an elevated right atrial pressure will permit a right-to-left atrial shunt. This flow pathway provides the only means for survival in infants with pulmonary atresia and intact ventricular septum, as well as in tricuspid atresia.

The foramen ovale is usually the principal pathway for systemic and pulmonary venous blood to reach the systemic circulation in patients with total anomalous pulmonary venous connection. On the other hand, a left-to-right atrial communication exists as the only pathway for admixture of pulmonary and systemic venous blood in mitral and aortic atresia.

The patency of the foramen ovale is important to the survival of infants with transposition of the great arteries and intact ventricular septum. What little admixture of the pulmonary and systemic circuits that does take place occurs at the atrial and pulmonary artery levels. The postnatal fall in pulmonary vascular resistance permits aortic-to-pulmonary shunting across the ductus arteriosus. The foramen ovale provides for a left-to-right atrial flow pattern. Creation of a large atrial communication in this situation to increase systemic oxygenation is mandatory.

Pulmonary Vascular Bed: The pulmonary vasculature occupies the key role in the timing of symptomatology in infants with large communications at the ventricular or pulmonary artery levels. Signs of congestive heart failure typically become manifest between 1 and 3 mo of age. This relates to the delayed postnatal fall in pulmonary vascular resistance with cardiac failure developing if this decrease is relatively rapid. In infants born at high altitude, the pulmonary vasoconstricting effects of the reduced atmospheric oxygen tensions limit left-to-right shunting and make cardiac failure less likely.[7] A few term, newborn infants have been observed to develop signs of severe cardiac failure within a few days of birth and in whom cardiac catheterization and angiocardiographic studies indicated that the basic problem was a large ventricular septal defect or patent ductus arteriosus. The early onset of failure in these infants is related to an abrupt fall in pulmonary vascular resistance immediately after birth caused by an abnormally rapid regression of vascular smooth muscle or deficiency in the amount of smooth muscle present. The latter defect has also been cited by Danilowicz et al.[8] as the reason for the early onset of cardiac failure in the premature infant with a patent ductus arteriosus.

Congestive Heart Failure in the Fetus: During the past few years, newborns have been observed with classic signs of congestive heart failure that were apparent during the first few hr of life. This raised the possibility that cardiac failure existed in utero. When the various conditions that could produce signs of decompensation at birth were reviewed, they could be classified into three broad categories. The first group consisted of volume loading of the ventricle(s) as a consequence of massive tricuspid regurgitation, pulmonary valve insufficiency, a large systemic arteriovenous fistula, or anemia. The second category comprised those infants with antenatal closure of the foramen ovale or ductus arteriosus with problems related to volume and pressure loading. The final group had as its hemodynamic common denominator depression of contractile element function arising from neonatal asphyxia, hypoglycemia, hypocalcemia, myocardial inflammatory disease, coronary artery disorders, or adrenal insufficiency.

(1) Volume loading (tricuspid regurgitation): Four newborn infants with tricuspid insuffiency have been investigated where the clinical picture of massive cardiomegaly with cyanosis and systemic venous congestion was noted during the first few hours of life.[9] On auscultation, each had a pansystolic murmur along the lower right sternal margin. The liver, which was strikingly enlarged, appeared to pulsate with ventricular systole. An electrocardiogram revealed evidence of right atrial and right ventricular enlargement. On heart catheterization, right atrial mean pressure and right ventricular systolic and end-diastolic pressures were elevated. The right atrial pressure pulse was dominated by the V wave with a rapid *y* descent, and was thought compatible with tricuspid regurgitation. Right ventricular angiography demonstrated massive tricuspid

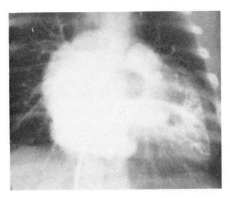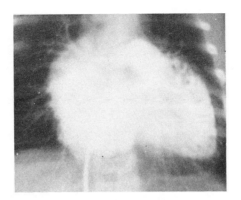

Fig. 4. Right ventricular angiogram in a 12-hr-old infant with massive tricuspid regurgitation through a normally inserted tricuspid valve. Right-to-left shunting at atrial level can also be noted.

insufficiency (Fig. 4) and, in addition, a right-to-left shunt was present at the atrial level accounting for the presence of hypoxemia. One of these patients had the typical displacement of the tricuspid valve seen with the Ebstein malformation, while the other three had a normally inserted tricuspid valve with a dilated ring.

The severity of tricuspid insufficiency in the immediate newborn period relates to the high pulmonary vascular resistance present in utero with systemic pressures in the right ventricle. Similar clinical problems have been associated with congenital absence of the pulmonary valve and can be explained in like fashion.[9] The postnatal course of these infants with tricuspid regurgitation is of interest in terms of natural history. While two infants with severe cardiac failure died, two others have survived. Their clinical state improved dramatically over a 3-day period. The level of oxygen saturation rose from the range of 50%–95% and heart size diminished considerably (Fig. 5). One infant now has no clinical or laboratory evidence of tricuspid insufficiency, while the other has only minimal signs of regurgitation. Similar experiences have been reported by others.[10]

Systemic arteriovenous fistulae: All of the infants with large systemic arteriovenous fistulae (cerebral, hepatic) show signs of congestive heart failure at or soon after birth. With this malformation, the large low-resistance runoff through the fistula competes in utero with the other low-resistance circuit—the placenta. A high output state in the fetus develops. This serves to maintain pulmonary artery pressures at systemic levels postnatally with elevation of the pulmonary vascular resistance to a point that permits right-to-left shunting through the ductus arteriosus and/or foramen ovale (Fig. 6). We have observed this phenomenon on two occasions. In one instance, ligation of a hepatic artery feeding an arteriovenous malformation was followed by a precipitous fall in pulmonary vascular resistance and massive left-to-right shunting through an enlarged ductus arteriosus.

The systemic vascular bed participates in the circulatory adjustments to a large arteriovenous fistula. Coarctation-like physical findings have been reported by Deverall[11] and Walker[12] and are ascribed to regional redistribution of cardiac output. Most of the systemic flow is diverted through the fistula with

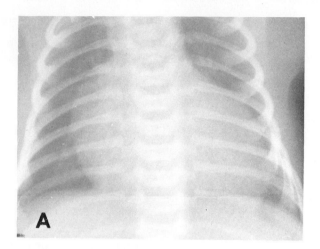

Fig. 5. Chest roentgeno-
grams obtained at a few hr of
age (A) and 3 days of age (B) in
infant with tricuspid insufficiency. Note striking decrease
in cardiac size, secondary to
diminution in magnitude of
regurgitation.

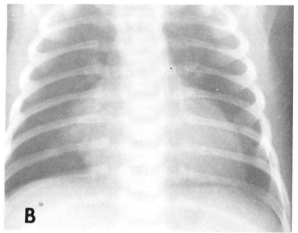

distal systemic flow maintained in right-to-left fashion through the ductus arteriosus. Spontaneous closure of the ductus after birth may then be followed by
signs of reduction in systemic perfusion.

Anemia: High output congestive heart failure with volume overload in
utero can also occur with severe anemia as in hemolytic disease or the twin-
transfusion or maternal-fetal transfusion syndromes.

(2) Volume and pressure loading (premature closure of the foramen ovale):
Premature closure of the foramen ovale results in volume loading of the right-
heart chambers in the fetus with the potential for underdevelopment of the
left heart. At birth, with the presumed fall in pulmonary vascular resistance,
flow through the pulmonary circuit increases. The left side cannot accommo-
date this sudden increment in blood volume leading to signs of pulmonary congestion, right ventricular failure, and death. In three instances, this circulatory
abnormality resulted in stillbirth with anasarca and hydramnios.[13]

Premature closure of the ductus arteriosus: Closure of the ductus arteriosus
in utero has been described by Arcilla et al.[14] This author reported a newborn
who had tricuspid insufficiency and severe heart failure at birth that disap-

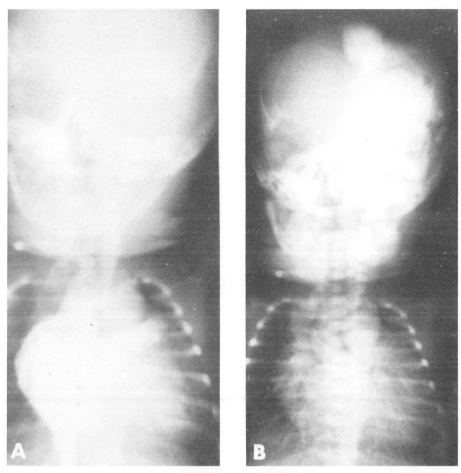

Fig. 6.   Right-to-left shunting via the foramen ovale (A) in infant with a large cerebral arteriovenous fistula (B).

peared the next day. Hemodynamic studies at 4 hr of age revealed a large cone-shaped ductus arteriosus arising from the pulmonary artery but terminating blindly at its aortic end. In the fetus, ductal occlusion with a high pulmonary vascular resistance should strikingly raise the outflow impedance imposed on the right ventricle. Fetal survival would be possible if increased shunting via the foramen ovale took place. Perinatal problems could arise, however, if this atrial connection was small. Following delivery, the right-heart-pressure over-load should diminish as pulmonary vascular resistance diminishes.

(3) Myocardial dysfunction: Myocardial function may also be depressed by the biochemical changes associated with neonatal asphyxia. The combina-tion of acidemia and hypoxemia has been shown to impair cardiac performance in the newborn lamb by Downing et al.[15] Correction of these metabolic altera-tions with alkali, glucose, and artificial ventilation can often reverse the signs of cardiac failure. This has been documented by Burnard and James[16] and con-firmed in our laboratory.

More obscure causes of myocardial dysfunction at birth include infants with hypoglycemia, hypocalcemia, obstruction to coronary blood flow, and loss of adrenal function. Their clinical state is characterized by low systemic perfusion and respiratory distress, and probably represents the end results of severe metabolic alterations operating singly or in combination to impair the performance of the newborn myocardium. Two infants with anterolateral myocardial infarction at birth have been observed by our group. One of these expired and postmortem examination revealed hemorrhagic infarction of the left ventricle secondary to a thrombus in the anterior descending left coronary artery. A second infant with electrocardiographic and enzyme evidence of infarction has survived and is clinically well.

Two additional patients with adrenal gland pathology presented with cardiac failure at birth. The mechanism for this is probably the myocardial depressant effects of increased potassium ion concentration as suggested by Sommerville et al.[17]

It should be pointed out that in those instances where hemodynamic studies were performed in infants with an apparent metabolic etiology for cardiac failure, left-to-right atrial shunting and right-to-left ductal flow were observed. Thus, the fetal flow pathways can remain patent in the newborn period with acquired cardiac disorders as well as with congenital defects.

Pulmonary Basis for Hypoxia

The hypoxemia that arises from obstructive disease of the airway or primary lung problems is on the basis of alveolar hypoventilation, unevenness of ventilation in relation to blood flow, or intrapulmonary right-to-left shunting. These functional changes can exist singly or be present in combination. The cyanosis associated with pulmonary disorders can usually be abolished by the administration of 100% oxygen, but not when the major physiologic problem relates to fixed intrapulmonary right-to-left shunting as is sometimes observed in the respiratory distress syndrome. Elevation of carbon dioxide tension commonly accompanies the cyanosis of pulmonary disease and, in fact, a tension over 60 mm Hg should immediately suggest a primary lung problem. The acidemia observed with pulmonary disease, however, frequently represents a combination of metabolic and respiratory components.

It should be kept in mind when assessing the infant suspected of having a cardiopulmonary problem that hypoxemia and acidemia on any basis can result in persistence of an elevation of pulmonary vascular resistance,[18] with flow from right-to-left via fetal flow circuits. Severe hypoxemia and acidemia can also depress myocardial function so that pulmonary factors, while primary, can be accompanied by signs of myocardial and circulatory insufficiency.

Central Nervous System and Hypoxia

When cyanosis is observed with central nervous system disease, it is a manifestation of alveolar hypoventilation. This may be on an intermittent basis, with periodic respirations or apneic spells, or can be persistent. Again, a high pulmonary vascular resistance can be expected due to hypoxemia and acidemia as has been described with primary pulmonary disease. Myocardial depression can also occur secondary to the effects of hypoxemia and acidemia.

Hematologic Basis for Hypoxia

Severe anemia as would result from hemolytic disease or hemorrhage will limit oxygen transport to the tissues by decreasing the amount of oxygen carrier available. Several infants have also been observed who were cyanotic, and who had abnormally high hemoglobin concentrations secondary to a large placental transfusion from the mother or twin.[19] These plethoric infants showed signs of congestive heart failure and were found to be shunting via fetal pathways. It is postulated that an elevated pulmonary vascular resistance is maintained by the combined increased viscosity and blood volume.

The rare infant with an abnormal hemoglobin, such as methemoglobin, may be alarmingly blue but without significant distress in the newborn period. If the percentage of abnormal hemoglobin is more than 50%, respiratory symptoms usually develop. The underlying problem is the presence of an oxygen carrier with a limited affinity for oxygen, even though arterial oxygen tension may be normal. Determination of oxygen saturation that is derived from the oxygen tension, pH, and temperature will be falsely high, and the defect must be demonstrated by measuring the oxygen saturation by spectrophotometry.

ADAPTATION OF THE NEWBORN INFANT TO HYPOXIA

The newborn infant adapts to hypoxia with the same fundamental compensatory mechanisms available to the adult. These include increased adrenergic activity, respiratory alterations, and modulation of oxygen transport that is dependent on shifts in hemoglobin-oxygen affinity and an increased red blood cell production.

As the arterial oxygen tension falls or congestive heart failure is apparent, sympathoadrenal function is stimulated, which results in an increase in heart rate and maintenance of the contractile state (beta-receptor function) and a regional redistribution of cardiac output, i.e., renal and skin vasoconstriction (alpha-receptor function). This serves to maintain perfusion of the more vital areas, such as the brain and myocardium at the expense of regions of less import, i.e., the skin and kidneys. Catecholamine metabolites are increased in the urine of hypoxic infants and those in congestive heart failure.[20] Peripheral vasoconstriction has been shown to be present in neonatal asphyxial states and congestive heart failure.[21,22]

Respiratory adaptation to hypoxia occurs via stimulation of peripheral (P_{O_2}) and medullary chemoreceptors (pH, P_{CO_2}). The result is a hyperventilatory response with a decrease in P_{CO_2} and a rise in pH. In infants who are hypoxemic with either obstruction to pulmonary blood flow or transposition of the great arteries, sampling of pulmonary venous blood demonstrates the presence of a respiratory alkalosis (see Fig. 9B). This represents an attempt at respiratory compensation for the metabolic acidemia that accompanies the hypoxic state.[23] When pulmonary congestion occurs as a consequence of high pressures and/or flows in the pulmonary circuit, an increase in respiratory frequency takes place due to activation of vagal pathways.[24] Accumulation of fluid in the pulmonary interstitial space apparently initiates this respiratory alteration which serves to preserve gas exchange in the presence of pulmonary edema. As fluid invades the alveolar spaces, however, a fall in Pa_{O_2} occurs early, and in the more severe stages a rise in carbon dioxide tension is noted as well.

The delivery of oxygen to the tissues can be influenced by shifts in hemoglobin-oxygen affinity. This has been related to temperature, pH, P_{CO_2}, and the intrinsic nature of the hemoglobin and red cell content of 2, 3-diphosphoglycerate (DPG) and ATP. Fetal hemoglobin has a high affinity for oxygen with a shift in the equilibrium curve to the left. An increase in hydrogen ion concentration, carbon dioxide tension, body temperature, as well as 2, 3-DPG and ATP, shifts the equilibrium curve to the right. The oxygen-hemoglobin equilibrium curve can be expressed by its P50 value, the whole blood oxygen tension at which hemoglobin is 50% saturated at pH 7.4 and temperature 37° C. This value is approximately 27 mm Hg in the adult, while it is in the order of 20 mm Hg in the term infant and, therefore, to the left.

The differences in oxygen affinity between adult and fetal red blood cells have been explained on the basis that the affinity of 2, 3-DPG for hemoglobin F is considerably less than it is for hemoglobin A.[25,26] Orzalesi and Hay have also shown that other factors influence the position of the oxygen-hemoglobin dissociation curve in the newborn infant.[27] The content of adult versus fetal hemoglobin as well as red blood cell content of 2, 3-DPG all serve to set the level of P50. These investigators also demonstrated that the oxygen affinity of fetal blood decreases during gestation. This is dependent on the relative proportion of adult versus fetal hemoglobin at any level of red cell 2, 3-DPG.

Since the final step in oxygen transport is the movement of oxygen from the blood to the tissues, shifts of hemoglobin-oxygen equilibrium are of importance in the maintenance of tissue oxygenation and organ function. A leftward shift in the curve would place the infant at a physiologic disadvantage from impaired inability to unload oxygen, and augmentation of cardiac output to meet tissue demands is required. On the other hand, a rightward shift, which facilitates the release of oxygen at a relatively higher partial pressure, appears to be clinically advantageous in any hypoxic state. In this regard, Miller et al. have demonstrated increased 2, 3-DPG levels and P50 values in infants with congestive heart failure and severe hypoxemia.[28]

An increase in red blood cell mass serves as the long-term accommodation to hypoxemia (right-to-left shunting, high altitude). Compensatory polycythemia appears related to the release of erythropoietin from the kidneys, although the precise metabolic pathway has not as yet been elucidated.[29]

DIAGNOSTIC APPROACH TO THE HIGH-RISK INFANT

Having established the physiologic determinants of the high-risk clinical situation in the newborn, an approach to diagnosis can be formulated, which should lead to specific delineation of the problem. These consist of (1) patterns of respiration, (2) cardiac check list, (3) chest roentgenogram, (4) electrocardiogram, (5) hemoglobin and hematocrit, (6) blood-gas determinations and pH, including the response to 100% oxygen, (7) metabolic studies, (8) methemoglobin determinations, and (9) cardiac catheterization and angiocardiography. Each of these will be considered in detail and, in addition, two relatively new noninvasive methods for assessing cardiac abnormalities in the newborn—the echocardiogram and radionuclear angiogram—will be briefly discussed.

Respiratory Patterns

Careful observation of the infant's respiratory pattern with regard to frequency, depth, grunting, retractions, and flaring of the alae nasi often provides valuable physiologic information as to the nature of the underlying condition. The normal respiratory rate of the sleeping infant is less than 50/min with no significant evidence of intercostal activity. The various respiratory patterns encountered and their functional significance are shown in Table 1.

Cardiac Check List

Although the physical findings in the infant with heart disease may contribute only in a limited way to a precise anatomic definition of the problem, there are several important clues to be derived from the physical examination.

Heart Rate: A rate in excess of 200/min should raise the suspicion of a tachyarrhythmia, while a heart rate less than 40/min could indicate complete heart block. Tachycardia secondary to hypoxemia with or without congestive heart failure is to be expected as a result of increased autonomic activity.

Peripheral Arterial Pulsations: Weakly palpable arterial pulses with lowered blood pressure in association with mottled extremities are commonly observed when systemic perfusion is compromised. A discrepancy between the brachial and femoral pulses should always raise the possibility of coarctation. Bounding arterial pulsations are found in high output states such as arteriovenous fistula, aortic runoffs into the pulmonary circuit, hyperthyroidism, or severe anemia.

Table 1. Respiratory Patterns in the High-Risk Newborn Infant

Response	Pattern	Physiologic Significance	Clinical Correlate
Hyperpnea	Frequency ↑ Tidal volume ↑	Hyperventilation mediated via hypoxic stimulation of chemoreceptors and hydrogen ion stimulation of medullary centers	Obstruction to pulmonary blood flow Transposition of great arteries
Tachypnea	Frequency ↑ Tidal volume ↓	Adjustment to fluid accumulation in pulmonary interstitial spaces associated with ↓ in lung compliance	Volume loading pulmonary circuit Pulmonary venous obstruction Obstructive lesions of left heart
Grunting [30]	Prolonged expiratory phase under positive pressure	Serves to ↓ pulmonary capillary & venous distension & lessen transudation Improves alveolar ventilation Opens atelectatic alveoli	Pulmonary parenchymal disease Hyaline membrane disease Transient tachypnea Left heart failure (late)
Periodic breathing	Variation in frequency and tidal volume Apneic spells	Damage to respiratory centers	Central nervous system disease

Triple or Quadruple Rhythm: Auscultation of an S_3 and S_4 should raise the suspicion of Ebstein's malformation of the tricuspid valve.

Single S_2:   If splitting of the second heart sound cannot be appreciated, absence of a semilunar valve should be considered. However, synchronous closure of both the pulmonary and aortic valves, as occurs with transposition of the great arteries, will allow the examiner to hear only a single heart sound, where in actuality two semilunar valves exist. Clearly audible splitting of S_2, however, may be a useful clinical finding in certain situations (volume loading at the atrial level).

Cardiac Murmurs: A search for intracranial or hepatic bruits should be carried out in any infant with cardiac failure. Pansystolic murmurs along the left sternal border may be heard with interventricular communications and tricuspid regurgitation. Basal, systolic, ejection murmurs are often heard with obstructive lesions of the right and left heart. However, it must be emphasized that classic auscultatory findings may be absent or atypical in many lesions presenting in the newborn period. Murmurs can be heard with pulmonary and metabolic problems and can be absent in the presence of serious cardiac malformations.

Hepatic Enlargement: Hepatomegaly is the cardinal sign of systemic venous congestion in the newborn. Neck vein distension and peripheral edema are only rarely observed. Systemic venous congestion usually follows in the wake of signs of left-sided congestive heart failure but is the only manifestation when there is right-heart obstruction. Systolic pulsation of the liver accompanies right ventricular failure and has been seen with massive tricuspid atresia-stenosis complexes or obstructive lesions of the right ventricle.

Sweating: Excessive perspiration has been noted with infants with congestive heart failure.[31] This is further evidence of increased activity of the autonomic nervous system.

Feeding Problems: The infant with cardiac failure frequently tires with feedings. This is the infantile equivalent of dyspnea on exertion. Failure to thrive is observed with congestive heart failure and severe hypoxemia. Hypermetabolism, noted in infants with cardiac failure, reflects the increased oxygen demands consequent to enhanced autonomic activity and the loads imposed on cardiorespiratory performance.[32] A weight gain which is out of proportion to the caloric intake is indicative of fluid retention accompanying cardiac failure.

Chest Roentgenogram

A high-quality film of the chest is mandatory in the evaluation of any infant suspected of having a cardiopulmonary disorder. Information can be obtained as to the size and shape of the heart and status of the pulmonary vascular bed. Cardiac enlargement strongly suggests an underlying cardiac disorder. However, metabolic and airway problems can be associated with cardiomegaly. In addition, the presence of pulmonary parenchymal disease, diaphragmatic hernia, pneumothorax, pneumomediastinum, all important causes of respiratory distress, can be confirmed or excluded by the radiologic examination. The position of the abdominal viscera may suggest more complex cardiac malformations and, therefore, provide valuable information prior to proceeding with diagnostic studies.

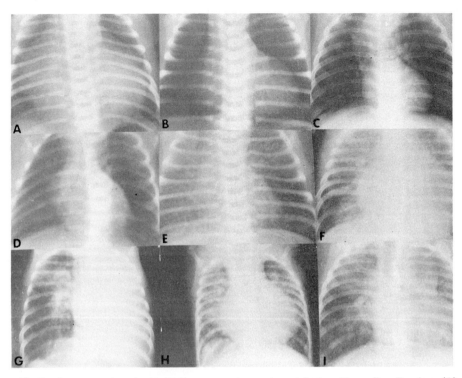

Fig. 7. Representative chest roentgenograms in newborn infants with cardiac disorders. (A) Massive cardiomegaly demonstrated at 6 hr of age in infant with tricuspid regurgitation. (B) Striking diminution in pulmonary vascular markings in association with cardiac enlargement (valvar pulmonic stenosis with intact ventricular septum). (C) Decrease in pulmonary vascular markings, right aortic arch in infant with severe tetralogy of Fallot. (D) Egg-shaped cardiac contour without cardiomegaly and normal pulmonary blood flow in patient (aged 2 days) with transposition of the great arteries. (E) Normal-sized heart with reticular-granular lung pattern seen with obstruction to pulmonary venous return. (F) Prominent pulmonary venous markings with cardiac enlargement in newborn with aortic atresia. (G) Increase in pulmonary blood flow, cardiac enlargement, and left lower lobe atelectasis seen in an infant with a large ventricular septal defect. (H) Prominent pulmonary arterial and venous pattern and cardiac enlargement in patient with patent ductus arteriosus. (I) Cardiomegaly, increased pulmonary blood flow and prominent shadow in left upper lung field seen in newborn with anomalous pulmonary venous connection to left superior vena cava (no evidence of pulmonary venous obstruction).

Several examples of the type of data that can be obtained from the routine roentgen examination of the chest are shown in Fig. 7. In our institution, we employ high-quality magnification films of the chest that permit very precise differentiation of vascular and parenchymal patterns of the lung as shown in Fig. 8.[33]

Electrocardiogram

The electrocardiogram is usually of limited help in the evaluation of the critically ill infant because, in the transition from the fetal to neonatal circulation, sufficient time may not elapse to manifest selective ventricular hypertrophy. Furthermore, respiratory problems can be associated with some degree of ventricular hypertrophy. Under certain circumstances, the electrocardiogram may be of considerable help. Left ventricular hypertrophy accompanies right-heart bypass situations such as tricuspid and pulmonary atresia. It can even exist with

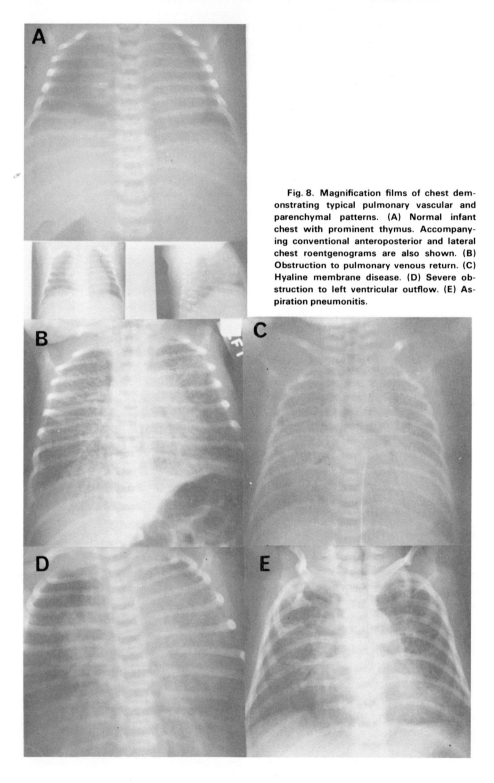

Fig. 8. Magnification films of chest demonstrating typical pulmonary vascular and parenchymal patterns. (A) Normal infant chest with prominent thymus. Accompanying conventional anteroposterior and lateral chest roentgenograms are also shown. (B) Obstruction to pulmonary venous return. (C) Hyaline membrane disease. (D) Severe obstruction to left ventricular outflow. (E) Aspiration pneumonitis.

valvar pulmonary stenosis if the right ventricular chamber is small, although right ventricular hypertrophy is more common. Fortunately, the frontal electrical axis permits a reasonable means for differentiation. Left axis deviation favors tricuspid atresia, while a normal axis can be seen with pulmonary atresia and right axis deviation occurs with pulmonary stenosis. Right ventricular hypertrophy is the electrocardiographic pattern with right ventricular obstruction as observed in patients with severe tetralogy of Fallot or pulmonic stenosis with an intact ventricular septum. Peaked P waves indicating right atrial enlargement are characteristic of practically all lesions with right ventricular obstruction or bypass. In Ebstein's malformation, prominent P waves, increased P-R interval, right ventricular conduction delay, and, on occasion, Wolff-Parkinson-White syndrome Type B may be present.

A counterclockwise frontal loop with right ventricular hypertrophy or combined hypertrophy suggests an endocardial cushion defect or double outlet right ventricle syndrome. Abnormal initial QRS forces are often associated with common ventricle or ventricular inversion.

The electrocardiogram is useful also in the detection of electrolyte abnormalities such as hyper- and hypokalemia and hypocalcemia, as well as cardiac arrhythmias.

Hemoglobin and Hematocrit

Newborn infants can be cyanotic from abnormally high hemoglobin concentrations (hematocrit > 70%). Heart size may be increased and tachypnea is often present. If distress is marked, phlebotomy can improve the clinical state. Severe anemia, on the other hand, is also accompanied by signs of congestive heart failure and transfusion with packed cells, or exchange transfusion is required. Routine determination of the hemoglobin and hematocrit should allow for the early detection of the fundamental problem producing circulatory difficulty.

Blood-Gas Determinations and pH

Confirmation of the presence of central cyanosis (arterial hypoxemia) requires the determination of arterial oxygen tensions. To further aid in the delineation of cardiopulmonary disorders, the carbon dioxide tension and pH of arterial blood should also be estimated. While the infant is breathing room air, the sample should be obtained from a catheter inserted into an umbilical artery, from a puncture of the right radial, brachial, or temporal artery, or from a warmed heel. Ultramicro methods (requiring 0.1–0.2 ml) must be available to minimize loss of significant amounts of blood. It should also be stressed that right-to-left shunting via the ductus arteriosus exists in many cardiac and lung disorders and, therefore, a sample obtained from the heel or umbilical artery reflects the Pa_{O_2} of blood in the descending aorta, and not necessarily that of blood perfusing the central nervous system.

The blood-gas and pH data taken in conjunction with clinical and radiologic information should permit accurate appraisal of the basic physiologic abnormalities. Our group has reported on certain patterns of blood-gas and pH alterations seen in association with varying hemodynamic states (Fig. 9).[34,35] Volume-load-

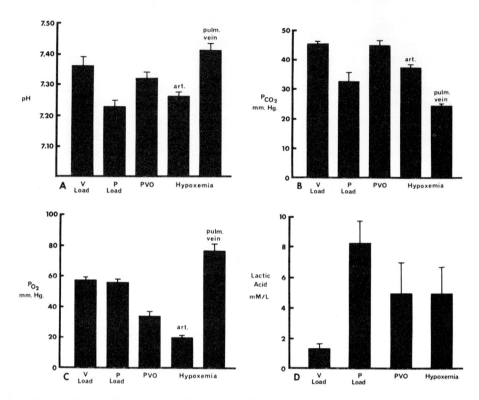

Fig. 9. (A) pH, (B) carbon dioxide tensions, (C) oxygen tensions, and (D) lactic acid levels encountered in high-risk infants with volume loading (V load), pressure loading (P load), pulmonary venous obstruction (PVO), and severe hypoxemia.

ing situations with severe pulmonary venous congestion have a slight decrease in predicted Pa_{O_2} due to intrapulmonary right-to-left shunting and ventilation-perfusion abnormalities. This is accompanied by a mild respiratory acidemia as would be expected in the presence of pulmonary edema. With mild congestive heart failure, however, a respiratory alkalosis has been observed. When severe pulmonary venous obstruction exists in association with some anomalies of the pulmonary venous connection, a respiratory acidemia is again present. There is more significant lowering of arterial oxygen tension in this group because of obligatory right-to-left atrial shunting.

With severe left-heart obstruction (critical aortic stenosis, aortic atresia) and a high pulmonary-to-systemic blood flow ratio, oxygen tension is only slightly decreased. The metabolic acidemia arises from impaired tissue perfusion.

When the arterial oxygen tension is extremely low (< 30 mm Hg), as would be encountered in obstruction to pulmonary blood flow or transposition of the great arteries with limited mixing, a metabolic acidemia also develops as a consequence of increased anaerobic metabolism. Under these circumstances, systemic blood flow is augmented but, despite this, the amount of oxygen delivered is insufficient to meet tissue demands.

The response to 100% oxygen administration is a useful guide in the assessment of abnormalities in cardiopulmonary function. If cyanosis is on the basis of right-to-left shunting, then only a trivial rise (< 8–10 mm Hg) in oxygen tension is to be expected following the administration of the enriched oxygen mixture for 10–15 min, a time sufficient to wash out nitrogen. Unfortunately, this will not distinguish between intrapulmonary or intracardiac shunting. A significant rise in Pa_{O_2} (> 30 mm Hg) points to a ventilation-perfusion problem or hypoventilation. An elevated P_{CO_2} favors the latter, while normal or decreased P_{CO_2} occurs in the former. Patients with congestive heart failure may have large increases in Pa_{O_2} with 100% oxygen as the pulmonary factors related to impaired oxygenation are corrected. To be kept in mind is the fact that a high oxygen mixture and restoration of pH to normal will lower the pulmonary vascular resistance and, therefore, alter shunting via fetal flow pathways.

Metabolic Studies

Glucose: Severe hypoglycemia in the newborn period occurs in infants of low birth weight or in those of diabetic mothers.[36] We have observed cardiomegaly and signs of cardiac failure in many of these infants. In a few, the clinical signs of tricuspid insufficiency were apparent. Following correction of hypoglycemia, the cardiac and respiratory findings disappeared. Benzing has reported on hypoglycemia as a complication of congestive heart failure in infants with congenital cardiac defects.[37] These data indicated that blood glucose levels should be monitored in any infant with cardiorespiratory distress and, if found to be low, corrected in order to provide suitable substrate for metabolism.

Calcium: In the circumstances where hypoglycemia has been encountered (the severely stressed infant), hypocalcemia may coexist. Since calcium is essential in the excitation-coupling phenomenon of cardiac muscle function, this metabolic defect must be corrected. The QT interval of the electrocardiogram serves as a useful guide to the presence of hypocalcemia.

Methemoglobin Determinations

Rarely a newborn infant is cyanotic because of the presence of an abnormal hemoglobin, such as methemoglobin with a decreased affinity for oxygen. These infants develop severe distress if the per cent of abnormal hemoglobin is more than 50%. Administration of 100% oxygen will not alter the arterial oxygen saturation, and blood withdrawn from a peripheral artery will not become oxygenated on exposure to room air, although the arterial oxygen tension is normal. Absorption spectroscopy will confirm the diagnosis, and methylene blue may be required to treat the condition.

Cardiac Catheterization and Angiocardiography

By the above approach to diagnosis, infants can usually be selected who require cardiac catheterization and selective angiography. Under some circumstances where the situation is unclear, studies are performed to clarify the underlying state and lead to proper management. Accepting the premise that no infant is too ill to be investigated if the information so derived will aid treatment, attention to certain details are required if the studies are to be performed with the least possible risk (< 6% mortality).[38]

Optimal definitive diagnosis and cardiac care can only be carried out in an infant cardiac center. This requires the commitment of a trained, experienced professional and technical staff, as well as facilities with around-the-clock diagnostic and therapeutic capabilities.

At our center approximately 50 of these high-risk infants under 1 mo of age are evaluated each year. None of these receives sedation or general anesthesia. The infant's body temperature is monitored continuously and maintained in the neutral range using a servo-controlled heating device. Blood gases, pH, and glucose levels are frequently checked throughout the course of the study.

The femoral or saphenous veins are selected for catheter insertion and the largest venous channel chosen (common femoral vein), if a balloon septostomy is being considered. Soft No. 4–5 catheters (Elecath, NIH type) are used, and an umbilical artery catheter is placed in the descending aorta during the first few days of life for monitoring systemic pressure and blood-gas tensions and pH.

Pressures are measured through a transducer (Statham 23 DB) and recorded on a multichannel unit (Electronics for Medicine) with a direct-writing attachment. A tachometer is utilized for assessing changes in heart rate. In our catheterization unit, facilities are available for both biplane cine and cut-film angiograms with video circuitry used for instant replay of contrast injections. At least 15 min are allowed to lapse between injections to minimize the hazards of hyperosmolar solutions.

Oxygen saturations are determined using a reflection oximeter (American Optical) that requires 0.2 cc samples. Acid-base status is checked with an Astrup unit. If respiratory failure exists ($P_{CO_2} > 55$ to 60 mm Hg), intubation and controlled positive pressure ventilation are utilized.

The pediatric cardiovascular surgeon is in attendance during the study so that, if indicated, the infant can be moved directly from the catheterization laboratory to the operating room.

With special attention to heart rate, blood pressure, ventilation, temperature control, hypoglycemia, and acid-base equilibrium, control of cardiac failure in the high-risk infant can be successfully managed through diagnostic studies aimed at precisely defining the nature of this suspected cardiac problem.

Echocardiogram and Radionuclear Angiogram

Two additional methods have become available which should be of value in the precatheterization assessment of infants with cardiopulmonary disorders.

Echocardiography represents a noninvasive method that may permit delineation of certain cardiac defects without risk to the infant.[39] The principle of the method involves the analysis of reflected ultrasound waves ($> 20,000$/cps). These waves, when traversing a homogenous medium such as fluid, travel in a straight line but they are reflected on impact with an interface between two media of differing densities. In nonhomogenous tissues, these waves are returned as echoes wherever they strike zones of variable acoustic impedance. Since the ultrasound waves have a relatively constant transit time through most soft tissues, measurement of the transducer-interface distance can be performed. The echocardiogram is capable of identifying the right and left ventricular cavity, the ventricular septum, positions and motions of both atrioventricular values, as well as the mitral semilunar valve relationship. As such, it has been shown to be a useful method in such conditions as the hypoplastic left- or right-heart syndrome, double outlet right ventricle, single ventricle, and transposition of the great arteries.

Wesselhoeft et al. have reported on a screening procedure designed to rule out significant cardiac malformations as the cause of cyanosis in a critically ill infant.[40] The technique, which involves the use of intravenous nuclear angiography (technetium), has the advantage of safety and ease of performance. The studies are carried out using a gamma camera with a multiple hole collimator. Although revealing far less anatomic detail than standard contrast angiography, the information derived was adequate to eliminate infants without primary cardiac problems from consideration for cardiac catheterization. It was also of aid in planning cardiac catheterization and thus facilitated the diagnostic study.

MEDICAL MANAGEMENT OF THE INFANT WITH CARDIAC DISEASE

Hypoxemia

If the underlying cardiac problem is severe hypoxemia from obstruction to pulmonary blood flow, then the obvious requirement is an immediate surgical procedure to improve the level of oxygenation. In proceeding to the operating room, the infant should be kept at 37° C, receive 10% glucose to prevent hypoglycemia, and be given increments of sodium bicarbonate to correct metabolic acidemia. If ventilation is inadequate, it should be controlled by endotracheal intubation and a respirator.

For the infant with transposition of the great arteries with limited mixing of the pulmonary venous, and systemic venous blood, balloon septostomy using the Rashkind technique is performed at the time of diagnostic catheterization.[41] The preferred catheter is a double-lumen 6.5 French inserted into the common femoral vein. This requires an incision made above the inguinal crease. The catheter is manipulated into the left atrium and pulmonary vein. Once the catheter location in the left atrium is verified, the balloon is inflated with 2–3 ml of contrast material and rapidly pulled across the atrial septum with an abrupt tug. If palliation is successful, a rise in arterial P_{O_2} should occur with saturations in the range of 60–70%. This should relieve the hypoxemia and acidosis and control the signs of congestive heart failure. On occasion, the rise in oxygen saturation may be delayed for 2–3 days, but previously existent acidemia remains corrected. If a significant rise in arterial oxygen tension does not occur, then a surgical septectomy is in order.

Several other congenital cardiac lesions can also be palliated by balloon atrial septostomy. These include tricuspid and pulmonary atresia which in addition to enlarging the atrial communication requires a surgical procedure to increase pulmonary blood flow. In infants with anomalous pulmonary venous return with severe congestive heart failure, obstruction may exist at the level of the foramen ovale. Under these circumstances, a balloon atrial septostomy may allow for control of cardiac failure and permit the infant to grow to a time when surgical correction can be carried out at relatively low risk.

Congestive Heart Failure

The treatment of the infant with congestive heart failure must take into consideration the underlying physiologic disturbance. Therapy is directed towards achieving an increase in the contractility of the myocardium, augmentation of peripheral perfusion, and a decrease in pulmonary and systemic venous congestion. It should be stressed that with certain conditions medical management cannot adequately control the effects imposed by the hemodynamic load, particularly when there is severe obstruction to left or right ventricular outflow. Under these circumstances, surgical intervention is required to remove the pressure load on the myocardium.

The pharmacologic armamentarium consists primarily of digitalis glycosides and certain diuretic agents aided by various supportive measures.

Digitalis Glycosides: The cardiac glycosides remain the principal therapeutic agents in the management of congestive heart failure in the infant. Digoxin is the most widely used preparation, although some centers have achieved considerable success with digitoxin. The aim with digitalis is to produce clinical improvement (decrease in heart rate, respiratory frequency, heart size, and hepatic enlargement) without accompanying signs of toxicity.

Guidelines for the use of digoxin in infants are shown in Table 2. This program is used for premature or term infants in moderate-to-severe cardiac failure. For the patient with minimal signs of cardiac failure consisting of slight cardiac enlargement, tachycardia, and tachypnea, we have begun treatment with a maintenance digoxin dose of 0.02 mg/kg of body weight in divided doses every 12 hr, which will achieve full digitalization over a period of 5–7 days. For the more seriously ill infant, loading doses as outlined are needed.

The choice of the intravenous, intramuscular, or oral route of administration will be dependent on the severity of the clinical picture. When there is compromise of peripheral perfusion, as in the hypoplastic left-heart syndrome, intravenous medication is required. Otherwise, we utilize either the intramuscular or the oral route with the choice dictated by whether the patient is able to manage feedings.

Special precautions should be taken with premature infants whose tolerance to glycosides is less than in the term infant, possibly related to diminished renal clearance of the medication. Similar recommendations hold for the infant with inflammatory disease of the myocardium where the sensitivity of the cardiac muscle to glycoside is definitely increased. Under these conditions, we advise half

Table 2. Suggested Digitalis Dosages for Infants with Congestive Heart Failure

Agent	Dosage Form		Loading Dosage	Maintenance Proportion of TDD[*]
	Oral	Parenteral		

Digoxin	Elixir 0.05 mg/ml	0.1 mg/ml	Prematures
			  0.035 mg/kg i.m.
			Term
			  Oral: 0.05–0.07 mg/kg
			  Parenteral: 75% of oral dose
			Loading dose provided over
			24 hr period as $\frac{1}{2}, \frac{1}{4}, \frac{1}{8}, \frac{1}{8}$
				$\frac{1}{4}-\frac{1}{3}$ given in two divided doses in 24 hr

[*] TDD, total digitalizing dose.
[*] By Permission.[35]

the estimated dose of digoxin and monitor the electrocardiogram continuously throughout therapy.

During the postoperative period, heightened sensitivity to digitalis is present so that it is sometimes necessary to use lower dosages and work up gradually to higher levels as needed. It has also been shown in the experimental animal that changes in pH, P_{CO_2}, and P_{O_2} alter the responsiveness to cardiac glycosides. Halloran et al. have demonstrated in the dog that an elevated P_{CO_2} increases the amount of digitalis required to produce toxicity.[42] The availability of laboratory methods for estimating digoxin concentrations in the blood will perhaps afford a better means for controlling therapy and avoiding toxicity.

Infants with supraventricular arrhythmias without apparent underlying heart disease or with the Wolff-Parkinson-White syndrome are managed with digoxin. If there is cardiac disease present, we choose to perform cardioversion, and this usually has achieved prompt restoration of a sinus mechanism.

The duration of digitalis therapy varies but the need for medication is rarely present after the first year of life except with endomyocardial disease.

Isoproterenol: For the management of acute congestive heart failure in which there has been an unsatisfactory response to cardiac glycosides, beta-receptor stimulation with isoproterenol has been instituted. A circulatory support solution consisting of 20 ml of 7.5% sodium bicarbonate and 30 ml of 20% glucose is mixed in a 50 ml syringe into which sufficient isoproterenol is added to deliver 0.1 to 0.2 μg/kg/min by an infusion pump. Glucose is used because of the problems associated with hypoglycemia, while the sodium bicarbonate is required to neutralize the effects of metabolic acidemia.

Diuretic Therapy: Diuretics occupy a prominent role in the management of congestive heart failure. There are several classes of agents available that are capable of selectively interfering with transport mechanisms related to renal tubular reabsorption and, in this fashion, promote natriuresis and diuresis.

The newer diuretic preparations, furosemide and ethacrynic acid, have replaced organic mercurials in the acute management of cardiac failure. These potent diuretic drugs interfere with diluting mechanisms in the distal cortical tubules and block sodium transport in the loop of Henle or ascending limb.

The dosages of the various diuretic agents are shown in Table 3. For acute,

Table 3. Diuretic Agents

Preparation	Dosage and Route of Administration	
Potent natriuretics		
1. Ethacrynic acid	i.v.	1 mg/kg/dose
	Oral	2–3 mg/kg/day
2. Furosemide	i.v.	1 mg/kg/dose
	Oral	2–3 mg/kg/day
Thiazide		
1. Chlorothiazide	Oral	20–40 mg/kg/day
2. Hydrochlorothiazide	Oral	2–5 mg/kg/day
Aldosterone antagonists		
1. Spironolactone	Oral	1–2 mg/kg/day

Intermittent therapy is recommended on a long-term basis to prevent electrolyte complications. By permission.[35]

severe cardiac failure, we have used ethacrynic acid or furosemide by the intravenous route with a diuretic response generally noted in 1–2 hr. For maintenance therapy, we shift to the oral preparations of these medications given on
an intermittent basis, usually every other day. When peripheral edema with secondary aldosteronism is present, we add an aldosterone antagonist to the program. Thiazide diuretics have also been utilized in the management of moderately severe congestive heart failure in place of furosemide or ethacrynic acid.
It should be stressed that use of potent diuretics requires frequent checking of the
serum electrolyte concentrations.

Other Supportive Measures

Position: Newborn infants with congestive heart failure should be managed
in an incubator providing a neutral thermal environment—that temperature at
which the overall metabolic and circulatory needs are minimal. Environmental
temperature within the incubator can be optimally controlled using a skin
thermistor servo control device, which allows the incubator temperature to be
adjusted automatically to keep a skin temperature of $36°–37°C$. These infants
should be placed on a $20°–30°$ incline to permit pooling of blood in the dependent areas of the body, and thereby decrease the work of breathing.

Oxygen: Humidified oxygen is often necessary to overcome the impaired
oxygenation occasioned by the presence of pulmonary edema. Forty to fifty per
cent oxygen is all that is usually required, and higher concentrations should be
avoided to minimize damage to the respiratory mucosa. The level of arterial
oxygen tension must be monitored in the premature infant.

Rotating Tourniquets: In pulmonary edema, three tourniquets may be
rotated every 10–15 min, leaving one extremity free at all times. The blood pressure should be maintained between systolic and diastolic levels. This will enforce
entrapment of blood in the periphery and ease the load on the compromised myocardium and pulmonary circulation.

Artificial Ventilation: In infants with severe pulmonary edema and accompanying respiratory failure ($P_{CO_2} > 60$ mm Hg), ventilatory support is indicated
with nasoendotracheal intubation and use of a volume-controlled respirator.
This has been accomplished in a few infants with large volume left-to-right shunts
in severe cardiac failure and has allowed us to proceed with diagnostic studies
and palliative surgery under conditions in which blood-gas tensions and pH
values more closely approximate normal.

Sedation: Situations in which the infant with pulmonary edema is extremely
restless have been encountered that required the judicious use of morphine sulfate in subcutaneous doses of 0.05 mg/kg. These infants must be watched very
carefully, and blood gases must be monitored for signs of respiratory failure
when this approach is instituted.

Diet: In most instances, cardiac failure can be controlled by the use of
digitalis and diuretic agents without the need for severe sodium restriction. We
try to avoid intravenous therapy in infants with cardiac failure and will begin
gavage feeding with a simulated breast milk formula as needed. This type of
formula provides a low solute and protein load.

In evaluating management, one should always keep in mind that the underlying hemodynamic situation may not be improved by an aggressive medical thera-peutic program and that surgery may become mandatory.

In those conditions where there are large volume loads, such as ventricular septal defect or patent ductus arteriosus, banding of the pulmonary artery or ligation of the ductus arteriosus may be indicated. Control of cardiorespiratory failure prior to surgical intervention is advisable, but this cannot always be ob-tained. It is also important to manage infections before undertaking surgery. In the face of critical obstructive lesions (pulmonary or aortic stenosis), one may have to go immediately to surgery once the diagnosis has been established.

Controversy continues to exist around the approach to the infant with coarcta-tion of the aorta. Infants with simple coarctation can usually be managed medically, but if a response to medical treatment is unsatisfactory, surgical in-tervention is required. In infants with the combination of coarctation and large shunt lesions, resection of the coarctation plus banding of the pulmonary artery is necessary.

REGIONAL INFANT CARDIAC PROGRAM

In an attempt to achieve more optimal management of the critically ill infant with heart disease, a regional program involving 11 New England hospitals has been developed to provide definitive care for infants suspected of having cardiac problems.[44] The major purposes of this program are to increase case finding, to encourage early referral, and to improve transportation, diagnosis, and treat-ment. A brief review of some aspects of this program in the light of our experi-ence at the Yale-New Haven Hospital will serve as an illustration of our ap-proach to improved diagnosis and management.

Case Identification

As part of the Regional Infant Cardiac Program and of several ongoing pro-grams of postgraduate education in Connecticut, numerous seminars, workshops, lectures, and demonstrations have been held on the care of the critically ill infant. These have focused not only on congenital heart disease but also on the many other problems of the newborn infant that require early identification and rapid, safe transportation to a more appropriately staffed and equipped regional center. Cardiorespiratory difficulty in the first few days or wk of life was by far the most frequent reason for referral in 1970 and 1971 (Table 4). The early identification of the infant with serious congenital heart disease has been particularly stressed. For maximum impact, cyanosis and tachypnea, two cardinal, suspicious signs in early infancy, have been given special emphasis. Community physicians and nurses have been encouraged to act early, even if the infant should later be shown

Table 4. Relative Incidence of Cardiorespiratory Problems of the Newborn Period in a Regional Referral Service During 1970 and 1971

Referring Diagnosis	1970	1971	Total	%
Congenital heart disease	55	51	106	24
Other respiratory distress	90	98	188	43
All other problems	74	70	144	33
Totals	219	219	438	100

to have some pulmonary or metabolic cause for his distress. These infants may be just as critically ill and in need of the special services available at the referral center and, as previously indicated, may be extremely difficult to differentiate from infants with a serious heart defect. As experience has grown, so has the ability to define a primary pulmonary or metabolic cause for the hypoxemia and congestive heart failure from a congenital cardiac defect. In 1970, of 13 infants who were suspected to have congenital heart disease but later shown to have normal hearts, eight were catheterized. In 1971, using an approach as outlined above more extensively, only two out of nine who presented in a similar manner were catheterized. It should be pointed out that all infants referred to the cardiac center on suspicion of congenital heart disease are supported by the regional program for certain expenses, such as transportation and parental visiting, irrespective of the eventual diagnosis.

The relative incidence of the various types of congenital heart disease that leads to the onset of serious symptoms and signs in the newborn period, as experienced at our medical center in 1970 and 1971, are shown in Table 5. It has been estimated that congenital heart defects of sufficient severity to cause difficulty for the infant in the neonatal period will occur at a rate of approximately 2/1000 births. From Table 6, it can be seen that while the expected number of serious defects is being identified in those infants delivered at the Yale-New Haven Hospital (22/9504 or 2.3/1000), there are still some infants born in this

Table 5. Relative Incidence and Mortality of Different Diagnostic Groups of Infants Presenting with Signs and Symptoms of Heart Disease at Yale-New Haven Medical Center During 1970 and 1971

	Born Y-NHH	Referred from Region	Total	Neonatal Mortality Per Cent
"Hypoplastic" left heart syndrome	3	13	16	93.8
Transposition of great arteries	2	13	15	33.3
"R.H. bypass" syndrome (e.g., pulmonary and tricuspid atresia)	0	13	13	53.8
PDA (with CHF in premature infants)	5	8	13	0.0
Other L–R shunts (e.g., VSD, ECD)	1	16	17	11.7
Coarctation of aorta syndrome	1	8	9	44.4
Complex or multiple abnormalities	3	9	12	50.0
Miscellaneous	7	8	15	14.4
Total congenital heart disease	22	88	110	37.3
CHF "secondary myocardial dysfunction," etc.	4	18	22	9.1
Total	26	106	132	32.6

Table 6. Estimated Accuracy of Identification of Serious Congenital Heart Disease in Newborn Period During 1970 and 1971

1970 and 1971	Yale-New Haven Hospital	Region Served
Total Births (2-yr period)	9504	56,000 (approx.)
Potential Serious CHD (2/1000)	19	112 (approx.)
Actual CHD	22	88
Unrecognized	0	24 (approx.)

region who die without transfer to the referral center. With about 28,000 births (excluding the Yale-New Haven Hospital), the potential number of infants with serious congenital heart disease is over 50/yr. Our present referral average of 44/yr suggests that possibly 10–20 infants each year continue to be denied definitive diagnosis and treatment.

Information and Communication

In conjunction with the educational programs outlined above, virtually all Connecticut hospitals with newborn nurseries (33) have been visited individually by one of us and have been included in regional workshops. We feel that such personal contacts with regional physicians and nurses have been important in improving communication between the community hospitals and the medical center and vice versa. Apart from disseminating information about the regional program and its aims throughout the community, such contacts have also led to earlier use of telephone consultations for advice and quicker referral before deterioration in the infant's condition makes further diagnosis or treatment impossible. The installation of direct telephone lines to the Newborn Special Care Nursery has removed one minor but irritating difficulty in communication for the referring physicians.

Transportation

There is little merit in advocating early identification and referral of infants in cardiorespiratory distress, if it is difficult or impossible for the practicing physician to arrange for speedy and safe transportation to the referral center. The type of ambulance transportation available in many communities is quite unsuited to the special needs of newborn infants and will merely impose additional, unacceptable hazards to the baby. Such difficulties over transportation are often the basis for a decision to retain the infant in the community hospital for "further observation." Any such delay in definitive diagnosis and treatment for severely hypoxic infants is usually fatal.

At the Yale-New Haven Hospital each year, over 200 infants are admitted to the Newborn Special Care Nursery from regional hospitals. About 20%–25% of this total are infants suspected of having congenital heart disease (Table 4). We were greatly concerned about infants arriving in a variety of conveyances with serious hypothermia, severe acidosis, hypoglycemia, obstructed airways, and other preventable complications of unskilled supervision with inadequate equipment and facilities. The purchase of a transport incubator by referring hospitals will help prevent hypothermia in ambulances, but this is only one small part of the problem of transporting sick infants. We believe that the major requirement of any safe system is the presence throughout the journey of experienced and skilled supervision. The actual mode of transport, whether it be ambulance, private car, or helicopter, seems to us to be of secondary importance. The use of a helicopter of other form of transport may clearly be dictated by regional, geographic, and climatic conditions, but, in Connecticut, an ambulance is adequate for almost all circumstances.

Because of these concerns, a transportation service for the special care nursery was developed using two cooperating, local, ambulance companies in rotation.

When a community physician decides that transfer of an infant to the medical center is indicated, he can request help with transportation at the time of his initial telephone call. An ambulance is dispatched within 15–30 min to the community hospital, accompanied always by a pediatrician and occasionally by both a nurse and a pediatrician from the special care nursery. A transport incubator (Air Shields, Inc. or Ohio Medical Products), which is kept in readiness at all times, and other essential items of equipment for observation and emergency care are taken on each call. All equipment is stored, maintained, and cleaned between calls by the special care nursery staff. Much of the equipment was obtained through a grant from the Maternal and Child Health Section of the Connecticut State Department of Health.

The presence of a physician (usually an intern or resident in pediatrics but can be any available, experienced person on the staff of the special care nursery) is the most important feature of this method of transportation. Any extra time spent on the double journey from the medical center to the community hospital and back is more than compensated by the advantage of his presence in the ambulance. He can play a crucial role in the management of the infant from the moment of his arrival at the community hospital until return to the center. For example, before leaving the community hospital, he can initiate and maintain correction of acidosis or hypoglycemia by insertion of an umbilical catheter or intravenous infusion and thus better prepare the infant for transfer. He can support respiration by suction, intubation, and artificial ventilation, and be immediately available for a large variety of emergency procedures during the ambulance journey. Since the service was initiated, in about 10% of the calls the accompanying physician has been required to utilize such emergency measures as intubation, cardiac massage, and aspiration of a pneumothorax, and over this period no infant has died during transfer, and several have survived because of such intervention. These infants have generally arrived at the medical center in a better state of oxygenation, acid-base balance, and with a normal body temperature. It is difficult to make exact comparisons between this group of infants and that transferred by community ambulances, as the majority of referring physicians now utilize this service (Table 7). However, we have noticed a reduced mortality among infants with congenital heart disease who were transferred to the medical center, by this method.

Two other positive features of this transportation service are worth mentioning. First, the presence of a physician removes the need (if any ever exists) for the excessive and dangerous speed usually associated with an emergency ambulance journey. It is now more appropriate for the vehicle to be driven smoothly and evenly so that the physician's observation and monitoring of the infant is facili-

Table 7. Utilization of Ambulance Transportation Service From its Initiation in September 1970 until December 1971 (16 mo)

Diagnosis	Yale Ambulance		Local Ambulances		Total
	Infants	%	Infants	%	
CHD	43	71.7	17	28.3	60
Other conditions	129	64.5	71	35.5	200
Total	172	66.2	88	33.8	260

tated. In this regard, a portable cardiac monitor with a visual trace (oscilloscope) is much more useful than one with a purely audible signal, which is often not heard above the engine noise. If an emergency should arise, it is important that the ambulance be stopped until the physician can react to the emergency by carrying out whatever resuscitative procedure is indicated. Second, as the infant's mother in the first few days of life is usually confined to the community hospital, she will be unable to visit the medical center. To have a chance to meet the doctor and nurse from the special care nursery, who will be caring for her baby, relieves much of the distress and anxiety occasioned by the infant's transfer. In addition to obtaining important items of history, the doctor or nurse can explain the special care nursery and its staff, features, and policies to the mother in a way that will prepare her for the first visit to see her baby. They can also outline the likely course of management during the early hours of admission. If special problems are present involving family, finances, or social circumstances, the unit's full-time social worker can be notified in advance and participate at an early stage in the management of the sick infant and his family.

Initial evaluation of this program to date indicates that approximately 60% of infants can be saved with this aggressive approach based on early case finding, safe transportation, and prompt diagnosis and treatment.

CONCLUSION

The systematic approach to the infant suspected of having a life-threatening cardiac problem requires an appreciation of normal neonatal cardiopulmonary adaptation and the physiologic basis for hypoxia. Hypoxemia and congestive heart failure in the newborn have been considered in relation to the operation of fundamental, physiologic mechanisms and the role in which fetal circulatory pathways and the pulmonary vasculature act as major determinants of the clinical expression of cardiac disease.

The cardiac, respiratory, central nervous system, and hematologic bases for hypoxia have been discussed and an organized approach to clinical and laboratory evaluation presented. The medical management of life-threatening cardiac problems has been outlined and placed in the context of an ongoing regional infant cardiac program. Initial evaluation of this endeavor indicates that the salvage of upwards of 60% of these infants can be achieved by stressing early case finding, ease of communication between community hospitals and infant cardiac center, safe transportation, precise diagnosis, and appropriate medical and surgical treatment.

REFERENCES

1. Keith, J. D.: Congestive heart failure. Review article. Pediatrics 18:491, 1956.

2. Dejours, P.: Applied physiology, I. Hypoxia, cyanosis, hypercapnia and asphyxia. *In* Respiration. New York, Oxford University Press, 1966, p. 202.

3. Duc, G.: Assessment of hypoxia in the newborn. Suggestions for a practical approach. Pediatrics 48:469, 1971.

4. Finley, T. N., Swenson, E. W., and Comroe, J. H., Jr.: The cause of arterial hypoxemia at rest in patients with "alveolar-capillary block syndrome." J. Clin. Invest. 41:618, 1962.

5. Lees, M. H.: Cyanosis of the newborn infant. Recognition and clinical evaluation. J. Pediat. 77:484, 1970.

6. Rudolph, A. M.: The changes in the cir-

culation after birth. Their importance in congenital heart disease. Circulation 41:343, 1970.

7. Vogel, J. H. K., McNamara, D. G., and Blount, S. G., Jr.: Role of hypoxia in determining pulmonary vascular resistance in infants with ventricular septal defects. Amer. J. Cardiol. 20:346, 1967.

8. Danilowicz D., Rudolph, A. M., and Hoffman, J. I. E.: Delayed closure of the ductus arteriosus in premature infants. Pediatrics 37:74, 1966.

9. Reisman, M., Hipona, F. A., Bloor, C. M., and Talner, N.S.: Congenital tricuspid insufficiency. A cause of massive cardiomegaly and heart failure in the neonate. J. Pediat. 66:869, 1965.

10. Schiebler, G. L., Van Mierop, L. H. S., and Krovetz, L. J.: Diseases of the tricuspid valve. In Moss, A. J., and Adams, F. H. (Eds.): Heart Disease in Infants, Children and Adolescents. Baltimore, William & Wilkins, 1968, Chap. 23, Part 2.

11. Deverall, P. B., Taylor, J. F. N., Sturrock, G. S., and Aberdeen, E.: Coarctation-like physiology with cerebral arteriovenous fistula. Pediatrics 44:1024, 1969.

12. Walker, W. J., Mullins, C. E., and Knovick, G. C.: Cyanosis, cardiomegaly, and weak pulses. A manifestation of massive congenital systemic arteriovenous fistula. Circulation 29:777, 1964.

13. Lev, M., Arcilla, R., Rimoldi, H. J. A., Licata, R. H., and Gasul, B. M.: Premature narrowing or closure of the foramen ovale. Amer. Heart J. 65:638, 1963.

14. Arcilla, R. A., Thilenius, O. G., and Ranniger, K.: Congestive heart failure from suspected ductal closure in utero. J. Pediat. 75:74, 1969.

15. Downing, S. E., Talner, N. S., and Gardner, T. H.: Influences of arterial oxygen tension and pH on cardiac function in the newborn lamb. Amer. J. Physiol. 211:1203, 1966.

16. Burnard, E. D., and James, L. S.: Failure of the heart after undue asphyxia at birth. Pediatrics 28:545, 1961.

17. Sommerville, R. J., Nora, J. J., Clayton, G. W., and McNamara, D. G.: Adrenal insufficiency mimicking heart disease in infancy. Pediatrics 42:691, 1968.

18. Rudolph, A. M., and Yuan, S.: Response of the pulmonary vasculature to hypoxia and hydrogen ion concentration changes. J. Clin. Invest. 45:399, 1966.

19. Gatti, R. A., Muster, A. J., Cole, R. B., and Paul, M. H.: Neonatal polycythemia with transient cyanosis and cardiorespiratory abnormalities. J. Pediat. 69:1063, 1966.

20. Lees, M. H.: Catecholamine metabolite excretion of infants with heart failure. J. Pediat. 69:259, 1966.

21. Celander, O.: Studies of the peripheral circulation. In Cassels, D. E. (Ed.): The Heart and Circulation in the Newborn and Infant. New York, Grune & Stratton, 1966, p. 98.

22. Talner, N. S.: Pathophysiology of cardiac failure in the newborn. In Adams, F. H., Swan, H. J. C., and Hall, V. E. (Eds.): Pathophysiology of Congenital Heart Disease. Los Angeles, University of California Press, 1970, p. 126.

23. Gootman, N. L., Scarpelli, E. M., and Rudolph, A. M.: Metabolic acidosis in children with severe cyanotic congenital heart disease. Pediatrics 31:251, 1963.

24. Churchill, E. D., and Cope, O.: The rapid shallow breathing resulting from pulmonary congestion and edema. J. Exp. Med. 49:531, 1929.

25. Bauer, C., Ludwig, I., and Ludwig, M.: Different effects of 2, 3-diphosphoglycerate and adenosine triphosphate on the oxygen affinity of adult and foetal human haemoglobin. Life Sci. 7:1339, Part I, 1968.

26. Tyuma, I., and Shimizu, K.: Effect of organic phosphates on the difference in oxygen affinity between fetal and adult hemoglobin. Fed. Proc. 29:1112, 1970.

27. Orzalesi, M. M., and Hay, W. W.: The regulation of oxygen affinity of fetal blood. I. In vitro experiments and results in normal infants. Pediatrics 48:857, 1971.

28. Miller, W. W., Oski, F. A., and Delivoria-Papadopoulos, M.: Increased oxygen release in hypoxemia and heart failure. Pediat. Res. 4:444, 1970.

29. Jacobson, L. O., Goldwasser, E., Fried, W., and Plzak, L.: Role of the kidney in erythropoiesis. Nature (London) 179:633, 1957.

30. Knelson, J. H., Kowatt, W. F., and DeMuth, G. R.: The physiologic significance of grunting respiration. Pediatrics 44:393, 1969.

31. Morgan, C. L., and Nadas, A. S.: Sweating and congestive heart failure. New Eng. J. Med. 268:580, 1963.

32. Lees, M. H., Bristow, J. D., Griswold, H. E., and Olmsted, R. W.: Relative hypermetabolism in infants with congenital heart disease and undernutrition. Pediatrics 36:183, 1965.

33. Ablow, R. C., Greenspan, R. H., and Gluck, L.: Advantages of the direct magnification technic in the newborn chest. Radiology 92:745, 1969.

34. Talner, N. S.: Biochemical and clinical studies of congestive heart failure in the newborn. Proc. Ass. Europ. Paediat. Cardiol. 6:15, 1970.

35. — : Congestive heart failure in the infant. A functional approach. Pediat. Clin. N. Amer. 18:1011, 1971.

36. Amatayakul, O., Cumming, G. R., and Haworth, J. C.: Association of hypoglycaemia with cardiac enlargement and heart failure in newborn infants. Arch. Dis. Child. 45:717, 1970.

37. Benzing, G., III, Schubert, W., Hug, G., and Kaplan, S.: Simultaneous hypoglycemia and acute congestive heart failure. Circulation 40:209, 1969.

38. Braunwald, E., and Swan, H. J. C.: Cooperative study on cardiac catheterization. Circulation 37 (Suppl. 3): 17, 1968.

39. Chesler, E., Joffe, H. S., Beck, W., and Schrire, V.: Echocardiography in the diagnosis of congenital heart disease. Pediat. Clin. N. Amer. 18:1163, 1971.

40. Wesselhoeft, H., Hurley, P. J., Wagner, H. N., Jr., and Rowe, R. D.: Nuclear angiography in the diagnosis of congenital heart disease in infants. Circulation 45:77, 1972.

41. Rashkind, W. J., and Miller, W. W.: Creation of an atrial septal defect without thoracotomy. A palliative approach to complete transposition of the great artieries. JAMA 196:991, 1966.

42. Halloran, K. H., Schimpff, S. C., Nicolas, J. G., and Talner, N. S.: Digitalis tolerance in young puppies. Pediatrics 46:730, 1970.

43. Laragh, J. H.: The proper use of newer diuretics: Diagnosis and treatment. Ann. Intern. Med. 67:3, 1967.

44. New England Infant Cardiac Program. New Eng. J. Med. 281:800, 1969.

Hemodynamic Investigation of Congenital Heart Disease in Infancy and Childhood

Thomas P. Graham, Jr. and Jay M. Jarmakani

HEMODYNAMIC EVALUATION of the patient with congenital heart disease can involve a number of different approaches for attempting to define anatomic and physiologic responses to the congenital lesion. The measurements generally made are those to determine blood flow, pressure, chamber dimensions and volumes. With the use of these basic variables and their derivatives, information relative to vascular resistance, valve or shunt orifice sizes, myocardial distensibility, and basic muscle mechanics can be obtained.

The basic variables and their derivatives, pressure (P) and dP/dt, volume (V) and dV/dt, and flow (Q), which is equal to dV/dt, can be influenced importantly by four major determinants of myocardial performance. These determinants are illustrated schematically in Fig. 1.

The first determinant to be considered has been labeled preload, and it can be estimated by the measurement of end-diastolic volume (EDV). With an increase in preload such as would be produced by an increase in venous return during intravenous fluid therapy, there is an increase in ejection fraction (EF), cardiac output (CO), and peak dP/dt. These changes are all manifestations of the Frank-Starling mechanism, whereby the heart responds to an increase in ventricular filling with an increase in the rate and extent of ventricular emptying.

The second determinant shown is afterload, and it can be considered as the force opposing myocardial fiber shortening. This variable can be estimated by aortic pressure under normal conditions, and an increase in systemic vascular resistance will constitute an increase in afterload. With the increase in afterload, EDV and dP/dt normally increase. The EF, however, usually decreases, and CO may decrease or remain unchanged depending on the relative changes in EDV and EF.[1]

The third determinant considered is contractile state, which can be defined as the rate and force of contraction from a given preload. An increase in contractile state per se is associated with an increase in dP/dt, EF, and CO from a decreased or unchanged EDV.[1] Contractile element velocity at zero load (V_{max}) has been used as an indicator of contractile state.

The fourth determinant is heart rate. An increase in heart rate can produce a decrease in EDV as the diastolic filling period is curtailed. An increase in the

From the Department of Pediatrics, Division of Pediatric Cardiology, Duke University Medical Center, Durham, N.C.

Supported in part by USPHS Grants HE-11307, and HE-10179, and Grant RCDA HE-38557 from the National Heart Institute.

Thomas P. Graham, Jr., M.D.: Associate Professor of Pediatrics, and Director, Division of Pediatric Cardiology, Vanderbilt University Medical Center, Nashville, Tenn. Jay M. Jarmakani, M.D.: Assistant Professor of Pediatrics, Division of Pediatric Cardiology, Duke University Medical Center, Durham, N.C.

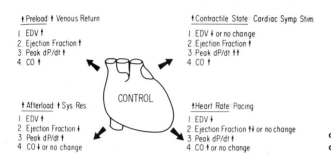

Fig. 1. Schematic diagram of the four major determinants of myocardial performance.

frequency of contraction also produces a variable increase in contractile state, which is dependent on the level of contractile state prior to the rate increase and the frequency range over which heart rate is altered. Because of the simultaneous decrease in preload and increase in contractile state, the overall effects on EF, CO, and dP/dt are variable. In general, EF decreases slightly, CO decreases or remains unchanged, and dP/dt increases.[1]

In most clinical situations, there are no isolated alterations of one of these determinants without simultaneous changes in the others. Therefore, a knowledge of the effects of all four determinants is of obvious importance in the assessment of a patient's hemodynamic data.

The objectives of the remainder of this manuscript will be to describe current techniques for measurements of blood flow, chamber volume, pressure, and myocardial muscle function with particular reference to their application in the infant and child with congenital heart disease.

BLOOD FLOW DETERMINATIONS

The estimation of systemic and pulmonary blood flow, as well as the delineation of abnormal circulatory pathways, are functions of major importance in any investigation of congenital heart disease. The four general methods that have been used for these determinations are discussed below.

Fick Method with Oxygen Sampling

The Fick method has been the mainstay of cardiac catheterization estimations of pulmonary and systemic flow. The formulas used have been presented and discussed in detail by Bing et al.[2]

(1)   Systemic flow (liters/min) $= Qs = \dfrac{\dot{V}O_2(cc/min)}{(Ao\ O_2 - MVBO_2)\ vol/100\ ml} \times 0.1$

VO_2 = total body oxygen consumption, $Ao\ O_2$ = aortic O_2 content, and $MVBO_2$ = mixed venous blood O_2 content.

(2)   Pulmonary flow $= Qp = \dfrac{\dot{V}O_2\ (cc/min)}{(PVO_2 - PAO_2)\ vol/100\ ml} \times 0.1$

PV = pulmonary vein O_2 content and PA = pulmonary artery O_2 content.

In the presence of shunts, a further determination, effective pulmonary flow (Qep), is calculated. Qep can be defined as the volume of systemic venous return which reaches the pulmonary alveoli.

(3)   Effective pulmonary flow $= Qep = \dfrac{\dot{V}O_2\ (cc/min)}{(PVO_2 - MVBO_2)\ vol/100\ ml} \times 0.1$
      (liters/min)

(4)   Left to right shunt (liters/min) = Qp − Qep

(5)   Right to left shunt = Qs − Qep

   The accuracy of these methods depends on the ability to measure accurately $\dot{V}O_2$, O_2 content of blood, and hemoglobin in situations in which O_2 saturation determinations are used and converted to O_2 content. In addition, a steady state for $\dot{V}O_2$ and A-V O_2 difference must be present during the time of sampling. Accurate measurements of $\dot{V}O_2$ are not always possible particularly in infants in whom these measurements are frequently crucial to proper management. Fortunately estimations of pulmonary to systemic flow ratios and shunts are possible using only O_2 saturations as illustrated below.

(6)   Qp/Qs = formula 2/formula 1

$$= \frac{Ao\ O_2 - MVBO_2}{PVO_2 - PAO_2} \text{ where all samples are } O_2\% \text{ saturations.}$$

(7)   % L-R shunt = formula 4/formula 2 × 100 = Qp − Qep/Qp × 100

by simplifying the equations

$$= \frac{PA - MVB \times 100}{PV - MVB}$$

$$= \% \text{ of Qp that is shunted blood}$$

(8)   % R-L shunt = formula 5/formula 1 × 100 = Qs − Qep/Qs × 100

by simplifying the equations

$$= \frac{PV - Ao}{PV - MVB} \times 100$$

$$= \% \text{ of Qs that is shunted blood}$$

   The relationship between Qp/Qs ratio and per cent left-to-right shunt is an exponential one as shown in Fig. 2. This is an important point to remember when using these equations. Thus an increase in shunt of only 8%, from 75% to 83%, is associated with an increase in Qp/Qs ratio of 50%, from 4/1 to 6/1. Calculations of shunts < 25% are probably within the limits of error for this method. Likewise shunts above 80% are probably best expressed simply as > 80% with Qp/Qs > 5/1.

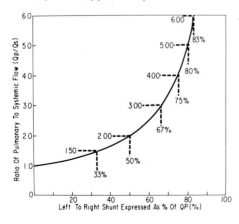

Fig. 2.   Exponential relationship between Qp/Qs ratio and per cent left-to-right shunt.

Indicator Dilution

Indicator dilution techniques, usually employing indiocyanine green, are extremely valuable for cardiac output quantitation, delineation of abnormal circulatory pathways, and estimation of left to right as well as right to left shunts. This subject has been dealt with extensively by the cardiovascular group at the Mayo Clinic[3] and will only be briefly outlined here.

Left-to-Right Shunts: (% QP) = C(p + BT)/Cp = C(p + 2BT)/Cp where Cp = peak concentration of indicator and C(p + BT) = concentration of indicator at time of peak concentration plus one buildup time, and C(p + 2BT) = concentration of indicator at time of peak concentration plus two buildup times.[3]

Regression equations derived from comparing these ratios with oxygen-estimated shunts are used for converting the ratios to %Qp.[3]

Right-to-Left Shunts: (% Qs) = (BT″ × MC″)/(BT″ × MC″ + 0.46 MCT × MC′) where BT″ = buildup time for initial abnormally early portion of curve, MC″ = maximal concentration for initial abnormally early portion of curve, MCT = time from injection to maximal concentration of second peak of curve, MC′ = maximal concentration of second peak.

This equation is used for quantitation of right to left shunts by comparing the ratio of the early-appearing first peak of the curve representing shunted blood with the second peak representing blood traversing the lungs.[3] This technique is extremely valuable for detection and quantitation of right to left shunts.

Special Techniques: Selective injection of indicator to detect location of shunts is another valuable technique which has been described in detail elsewhere.[3] In addition, simultaneous sampling of indicator from two withdrawal sites has been used for quantification of pulmonary blood flow in the presence of left to right shunting.[3]

Cardiac Output (CO): This use has been the largest single application of indicator dilution curves. By use of a sterilized cuvette, blood can be reinfused and multiple curves performed for repeated estimations of CO during exercise or pharmacologic interventions.

Hugenholtz et al.[4,5] have employed a fiberoptic catheter system for rapid determinations of CO during exercise and isoproterenol infusion. This technique requires arterial sampling of indicator in the ascending aorta and is a valuable adjunct to tests of overall cardiovascular function during imposed stressful conditions.

Radionuclides: These have been used in several different ways for detection and quantitation of shunts, and for estimation of cardiac output.

The krypton index has been used for detection and quantitation of left to right shunts.[6] This method involves the inhalation of ^{85}Kr with the recording of the subsequent washout of indicator. This method is sensitive for the detection of small shunts and relatively simple to perform. It does, however, require patient cooperation.

One of the most practical and useful radionuclide methods for use in infants and small children has been developed by Spach et al.[7] This method uses ^{131}I-sodium iodohippurate as the indicator, which is injected into the central circulation and thus can be used in infants and young children. The dose is quite small, 15 μCi–45 μCi maximum/injection, and with rapid renal excretion the biologic half life is quite short. This technique utilizes external probes and thus blood sampling is not required. Detection and quantitation of left to right shunts and detection of right to left shunts can be performed quite rapidly. Three to four injections can be performed before background activity becomes a significant problem.

One example of the practical usefulness of this procedure to detect abnormal circulatory pathways is shown in Fig. 3. Injections have been made sequentially into first the right ventricle (RV), and then the left ventricle (LV) in an infant with transposition of the great arteries (TGA). Probes are positioned to detect activity over the heart and over the head. The LV injection (Panel B) is distinctly abnormal with the heart curve showing a break on the downslope with delayed washout of activity consistent with continued recirculation through the heart and lungs. The head curve shows a very slow, delayed appearance of activity indicating considerable delay in LV to cerebral circulation. The RV curves (Panel A) unequivocally confirm the diagnosis of TGA. The heart curve shows a much smaller break on the downslope than the LV curve, and the RV head curve shows almost immediate activity following injection, indicating a direct circulatory pathway from RV to cerebral circulation. Thus, with only two injections of radionuclide taking less than 1 min and without blood sampling, TGA can be diagnosed even in the smallest infant without affecting hemodynamics.

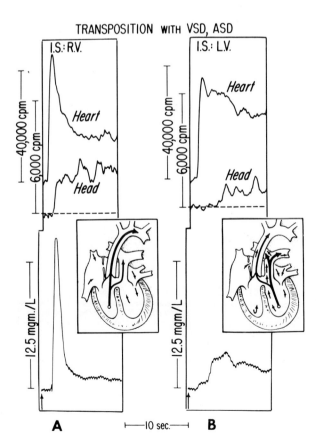

Fig. 3. Use of radionuclide injections in right ventricle (A) and left ventricle (B) for diagnosis of transposition of the great vessels. External probes over head and heart are used to detect radioactivity. Indicator dilution curves with cardiogreen are shown in lower panels for comparison. (By permission.[7])

The diagnostic combination of curves for total anomalous pulmonary venous connection is shown in Fig. 4. The first injection is into the right ventricle (Panel A), and the head curve shows a very delayed appearance of activity consistent with prolonged pulmonary recirculation. The heart curves show an early break on the downslope consistent with a large left to right shunt. The right atrial injection (Panel B) shows a similar heart curve, but the head curve shows early activity consistent with a large right to left shunt. This combination of curves, then, is diagnostic of total anomalous pulmonary venous connection, and again the diagnosis can be made without requiring blood sampling and without disturbing systemic and pulmonary hemodynamics.

A final use of radionuclides has been in imaging of the central circulation using a scintillation camera. In this technique a large detector is placed over the patient's chest and following intravenous ^{99m}Tc radioactivity can be detected traversing the central circulation in a manner analogous to a venous angiogram. A representative study from a normal patient is shown in Fig. 5. This method has been used to detect systemic venous abnormalities, intracardiac defects, and right to left shunts.[8-10] In addition, it may be useful in estimation of ventricular volume,[11] as well as in quantitation of left to right shunts by measuring activity vs. time over a preset "window," which can be placed over pulmonary artery or lung. This technique is safe, does not disturb circulatory hemodynamics, and is associated with low radiation exposure.

Flowmeters

Electromagnetic flowmeters have now been miniaturized and incorporated into cardiac catheters for detection of velocity of blood flow. By integration of

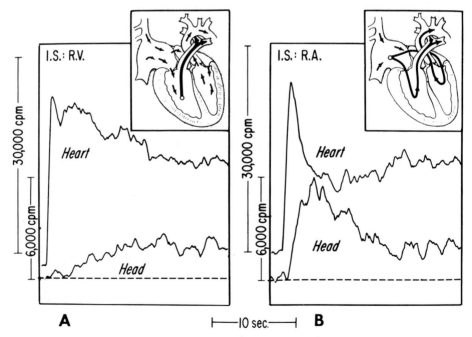

Fig. 4. Use of radionuclide injections in right ventricle (A) and right atrium (B) for diagnosis of total anomalous pulmonary venous connection. (By permission.[7])

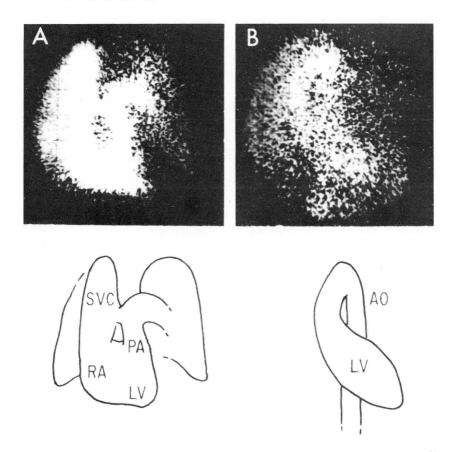

Fig. 5. Scintillation camera imaging of the central circulation following intravenous [99m] Tc.
(A) Right heart phase; (B) left heart phase.

the velocity-time signal, blood flow can be determined. This catheter can be manipulated into aorta as well as pulmonary artery for instantaneous measurements of blood flow both before and after exercise or pharmocologic interventions and should prove a useful adjunct to current techniques.

A somewhat specialized method for blood flow determinations during cardiac catheterization has been developed by Greenfield et al.[12] using the instantaneous pressure gradient technique. This method has been useful to detect alterations in systemic flow with varying hemodynamic interventions.

The fourth general method of blood flow determination, those derived from LV volume determinations, are discussed below.

LEFT HEART VOLUME DETERMINATIONS

The determination of ventricular and atrial volumes can aid considerably in evaluating myocardial pumping characteristic in congenital heart disease. The work of Dodge et al.[13] has been instrumental in developing accurate methodology for this approach in adults with acquired heart disease. Miller and Swan[14] and Hugenholtz et al.[15] first applied these techniques to congenital heart disease.

Methodology

Biplane cineangiocardiography at 60 frames/sec is usually required to accurately detect end-diastole and end-systole in infants and young children with rapid heart rates. Anteroposterior (AP) and lateral (LAT) views are employed, and the first cine of the catheterization is normally used for volume estimation. Left heart volumes frequently can be derived from the levogram phase of pulmonary artery cines or from left atrial (LA) or left ventricular (LV) cines. The electrocardiogram, left ventricular or aortic pressure when feasible, and cine exposure signals are recorded on photographic paper during the ciné. A calibrated wire grid of 625 1 cm × 1 cm squares is filmed at the completion of the study at the position the patient's heart occupied in order to correct projected images for x-ray magnification. Peripheral field distortion of the images usually can be avoided by keeping the left heart in the center of the radiographic field.

The area-length method assuming an ellipsoid of revolution reference figure has been adopted most widely for left heart volume estimation. There is an excellent correlation between calculated volumes and known volumes of postmortem hearts using this method.[13,16] The simplified form of the equation for calculating LV or LA volumes is: $V = 0.849$ (Aap) • (Alat)/shortest LL, where V = calculated volume, Aap = area of the LV or LA in the AP view, Alat = area in the LAT view, and LL = the shortest of the two measured longest lengths, whether in the AP or LAT view.

All methods for LV volume estimation consistently overestimate volume, probably because of the trabeculations and papillary muscles that are included in the volume estimation. Therefore, a regression equation derived from postmortem studies is required to correct the calculated volume. Different regression equations have been derived for large (> 15 ml) vs. small volumes as follows: for $V \geq 15$ ml, $V' = 0.732\ V$ and for $V > 15$ ml, $V' = 0.974\ V - 3.1$ with V' = corrected or regressed volume and V = calculated volume.[17] A regression equation is not required for LA volume estimation.

An estimate of LV wall mass also can be derived from AP and lateral angiocardiograms.[18] In this method the LV lateral wall thickness is measured at end-diastole at a point midway between the aortic valve and the apex in the AP view. This wall thickness, h, is then added to the major semiaxis (LL/2) and the two minor semiaxes to calculate muscle volume plus end-diastolic volume (EDV). By subtracting LVEDV from this total volume, muscle volume is derived and multiplied by the specific gravity of heart muscle (1.050) to derive muscle mass (LVM). For children this value is corrected by a regression equation derived from postmortem data.[16] Additional details of these methods have been described previously.[16,17]

The following data normally are derived for each patient studied:

(1) LVEDV (left ventricular end-diastolic volume); (2) LVESV (LV end-systolic volume); (3) LVSV (LV stroke volume = LVEDV - LVESV); (4) LVEF (LV ejection fraction = LVSV/LVEF); (5) LVSO (LV systolic output = LVSV × heart rate); (6) LVM (LV wall mass); and (7) LAMax (left atrial maximal volume).

Normal values have been derived for these variables from 56 patients with normal left hearts who have undergone routine diagnostic cardiac catheterization. From these data multiple regression equations have been derived relating volume variables to height, weight, and age for use in prediction of normal values.[17] A given patient's observed volume/predicted volume × 100 can then be expressed as a per cent of normal and related to upper and lower normal limits. These normal values, and an example of the use of the predicted values, are shown in Table 1.

The most striking feature of the normal data has been the decreased normalized size of the left ventricle and left atrium in infants vs. older children.[16, 17] This difference has been observed repeatedly and is most likely related to the more rapid heart rate of the infant group (142 ± 14 vs. 99 ± 15 for the older group, $p < 0.001$) with a relative curtailment of late diastolic filling. In addition, there is experimental evidence that left ventricular distensibility of puppies is decreased in the neonatal period as compared with adult values,[19] and thus the possibility of altered ventricular distensibility in infants might be considered as a factor in explaining the differing volumes.

Table 1. Normal Values for Left Heart Volume Variables ($\bar{x} + $ SD)

	Age 2 Yr	Age 2 Yr
LV end-diastolic volume	42 ± 10 ml/sq m	73 ± 11 ml/sq m
Predicted volume	(V) = 2.67 (wt) – 0.43 (ht) + 9.40 (age) + 19.3	(V) = 1.38 (wt) + 0.73 (ht) – 1.94 (age) – 42.3
LV ejection fraction	0.68 ± 0.05	0.63 ± 0.05
LA maximal volume	26 ± 5 ml/sq m	38 ± 8 ml/sq m
	(V) = 1.23 (wt) – 0.07 (ht) $\pm$ 2.22 (age) + 4.1	(V) = 0.60 (wt) + 0.49 (ht) – 0.71 (age) – 34.8

	All Ages
LV systolic output	4.53 ± 0.94
Predicted output =	0.21 (wt) – 0.002 (wt)^2 + 0.003 (ht) – 0.08
LV wall mass	88 ± 12 g/sq m
Predicted mass =	2.11 (wt) + 0.16 (ht) + 7.0

	Example of Use of Predicted Variable
Patient P.F. Dx:	Wt 3.2 kg, ht 59.0 m, age 0.02 yr (6 days)
Truncus arteriosus	
Predicted LVEDV =	2.67 (3.2) – 0.43 (49) + 9.40 (0.02) + 19.3
=	8.5 – 21.1 + 0.2 + 19.3
=	6.9 ml
Observed LVEDV =	13.1/6.9 x 100 = 190% of normal

Upper and Lower Limits of Normal for Volume Variables as a Per Cent of Normal		
	($x \pm 2$ SD)	
LV end-diastolic volume	128%	74%
LV wall mass	124%	76%
LV systolic output	138%	63%
LA maximal volume	135%	65%
LV ejection fraction (as % of LVEDV)		
< 2 yr	80%	55%
> 2 yr	75%	50%

The infant also has an increased ejection fraction when compared with older children[17] (Table 1). This increase in the extent of ventricular emptying may be related to an increase in myocardial contractile state secondary to the increased heart rate per se or to an augmented sympathetic influence.

The effect of a pressure overload on LVEDV in infancy is shown in Fig. 6. Here LVEDV as a per cent of predicted normal values is plotted as a function of age for infants less than 1 yr of age with aortic stenosis (AS) or coarctation of the aorta. All seven infants with isolated AS have LVEDV values that are within the normal range. The two youngest infants with AS had severe heart failure at the time of cardiac catheterization. Despite the presence of failure, these infants had not utilized the Frank-Starling mechanism to increase output by increasing LVEDV, thus suggesting an alteration in myocardial distensibility. Both infants died shortly following the study, and neither infant had endocardial fibroelastosis. Two infants with AS plus mitral insufficiency (MI) did show increases in LVEDV indicating the influence of an added volume overload in producing LV enlargement.

Three patients are shown who had isolated coarctation, and two of these had large increases in LVEDV. Both infants were in heart failure prior to study and both have undergone successful corrective surgery. Six infants with coarctation and associated lesions causing an added LV volume overload are shown. All have increased LVEDVs. An excellent correlation of LVEDV with degree of left to right shunt or pulmonary blood flow has been demonstrated previously in patients with isolated ventricular septal defect or patent ductus arteriosus.[20]

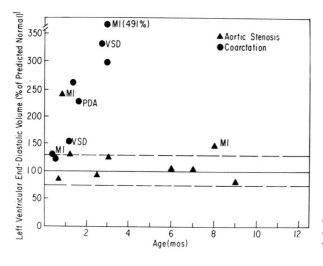

Fig. 6.   Left ventricular end-diastolic volume as a per cent of normal for infants with a left ventricular pressure overload.

In Fig. 7, mean values for LVEDV expressed as ml/sq m are shown for seven different groups of infants studied during the first year of life. Again the normal LVEDV for infants with an isolated pressure overload (AS or coarctation) is demonstrated. In marked contrast, infants with a volume overload (VSD, PDA, or systemic or coronary A-V fistula) have increases in LVEDV to over twice normal. Finally infants with myocardial disease show an average LVEDV which is over four times normal. A number of infants with myocardial disease have LVEDVs that are equal in absolute value to normal adult volumes,[16] indicating the marked utilization of the Frank-Starling mechanism to compensate for myocardial dysfunction.

In Fig. 8, LV ejection is shown for the same group of patients shown in Fig. 6. Two of the seven patients with isolated AS have depressed ejection fractions, the same patients who were in severe heart failure. An acute increase in resistance to ejection per se can cause a decreased LVEF in animals.[1] Thus a decreased ejection fraction in the presence of AS might not necessarily infer a decrease in myocardial contractile state. Older children with AS have an increased LVEF, suggesting that hypertrophy can compensate adequately for the altered resistance to ejection.[21] Thus, the ability to increase muscle mass rapidly may be an important determinant of the degree of compensation in response to a severe hemodynamic overload in infancy.

One infant with AS plus MI also shows a depressed ejection fraction and died shortly following the study. Mitral insufficiency per se can result in an increase in ejection fraction when induced acutely by providing a low resistance pathway for ejection.[22] Thus a low ejection fraction in the presence of mitral

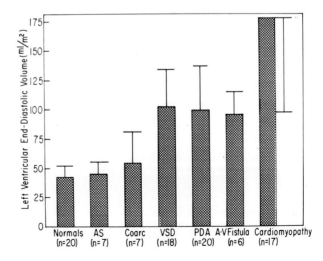

Fig. 7. Left ventricular end-diastolic volume in ml/sq m for seven different infant patient groups studied during the first yr of life.

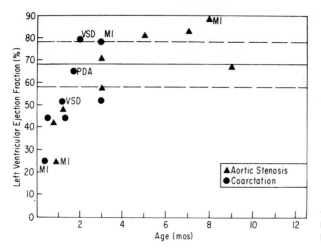

Fig. 8. Left ventricular ejection fraction for infants with a left ventricular pressure overload.

insufficiency is strongly suggestive of impaired myocardial performance. These data suggest a poor prognosis for infants with AS and a depressed ejection fraction, and thus emergency valvulotomy would appear to be indicated.

All three infants with isolated coarctation show a depressed ejection fraction, and all have survived corrective surgery. These findings substantiate that a depressed ejection fraction in the presence of an isolated pressure overload does not necessarily imply severe myocardial disease.

Left ventricular wall mass is shown in Fig. 9 for seven of the patients shown in the previous figures. Because of overlying thymus, overlying right ventricle, or poor delineation of the LV lateral wall, LV mass cannot always be determined in infants. For all the patients shown, LV hypertrophy is indicated by the increased values for estimated LV wall mass. An excellent correlation has also been found for LVM and degree of left to right shunt in LV volume overload[20] and for degree of obstruction in older patients with AS or coarctation.[21]

Left atrial maximal volume is shown in Fig. 10. Only one patient with iso-

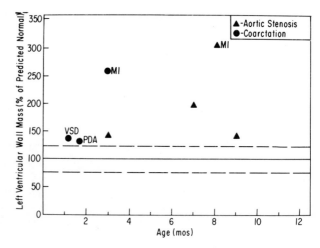

Fig. 9. Left ventricular wall mass as a per cent of normal for infants with a left ventricular pressure overload.

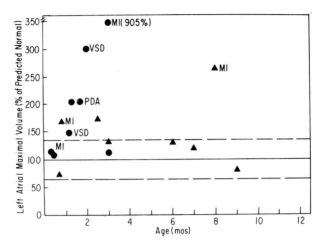

Fig. 10. Left atrial maximal volume as a per cent of normal for infants with a left ventricular pressure overload.

lated AS and one patient with isolated coarctation have increased left atrial volumes. In contrast, six of seven infants with added volume overloads have increased values for LAMax. The one infant with mitral insufficiency and normal LAMax was only 10 days old. The 3-mo-old with severe left atrial enlargement (905% of normal) had severe heart failure, which was uncontrolled following coarctation surgery and eventually required mitral valve replacement.

In Fig. 11, the use of both LA and LV volumes is shown in an infant with a patent ductus arteriosus (PDA) and an atrial defect. This infant had a large left to right shunt, but as is frequently the case with this combination the relative degree of PDA and atrial shunts was unclear. In this situation, the clearly elevated LVEDV indicated a large ductal shunt. Conversely, the small LA volume indicated a large "letoff" at the atrial level and thus a large atrial shunt. The infant had a large PDA ligated and showed moderate improvement. He continued to have symptoms of heart failure, however, and later died with an intercurrent pneumonia. At autopsy, the atrial defect was huge with only a small rim of atrial septum present. Thus the combination of

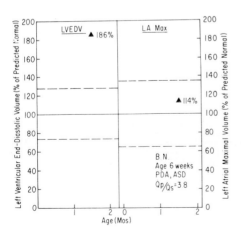

Fig. 11. Use of left ventricular and left atrial volumes to estimate size of atrial and aortic shunts in an infant with a patent ductus arteriosus and an atrial septal defect.

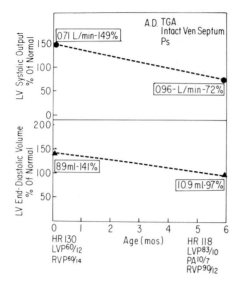

Fig. 12. Use of left ventricular volume determinations to estimate pulmonary blood flow in transposition of the great arteries.

LV and LA volumes can be quite useful in assessing the relative contributions of left to right shunting at the ventricular or aortic level versus the atrial level.

A special use of LV volume determinations which has proven clinically useful has been in patients with transposition of the great arteries (TGA). In these patients with systemic and pulmonary circuits in parallel instead of in series, Fick and indicator dilution methods for quantitation of pulmonary flow are difficult to perform and frequently unreliable. The determination of LV systolic output (LVSV × HR) by volume determinations, however, provides a reliable estimate of pulmonary flow if there is no patent ductus and bronchial flow is negligible. An example of this use is shown in Fig. 12.

A.D. was studied first at age 1 day, at which time she was noted to have equal peak right and left ventricular pressures and modest increases in LVEDV and LV output. There was no VSD or patent ductus present and thus the LVSO was equal to the pulmonary blood flow. This infant was restudied at age 6 mo because of increasing cyanosis. At this time pulmonary artery pressure was obtained, and moderately severe pulmonary stenosis was present. Both the LVEDV and LVSO had shown a decrease in terms of predicted normal values. This data then clearly indicated that a procedure only to enlarge the atrial communication would not be sufficient, but a systemic to pulmonary shunt procedure to increase pulmonary flow also was needed.

A summary of clinical uses for left heart volume variables in evaluating children with heart disease is shown in Table 2.

PRESSURE MEASUREMENTS

Pressure measured through small-diameter, fluid-filled catheters do not provide optimal frequency response for recording accurately the higher velocity components of ventricular pressure curves. By meticulous flushing to re-

Table 2. Examples of Clinical Uses of Left Heart Volume Variables

I.   Left ventricular end-diastolic volume
   1. Indicator of pulmonary blood flow: VSD, PDA, truncus, transposition, tetralogy, other complex lesions.
   2. Indicator of degree of mitral or aortic regurgitation.
   3. Indicator of degree to which Frank-Starling mechanism used for compensation: obstructive lesion, myocardial disease.
   4. Assessment of LV hypoplasia: anomalous pulmonary venous connection.
   5. Assessment of operative results.

II. Left ventricular ejection fraction
   1. Indicator of myocardial function when preload and afterload known.

III. Left ventricular systolic output
   1. Estimation of pulmonary flow in transposition.
   2. Estimation of mitral or aortic regurgitation (used with Fick output).
   3. Estimation of pulmonary flow: VSD, PDA.
   4. Estimation of cardiac output in patients without a ventricular shunt and without mitral or aortic regurgitation.

IV. Left ventricular wall mass
   1. Indicator of severity of LV pressure overload.
   2. Indicator of severity of LV volume overload.
   3. Assessment of operative result.

V.   Left atrial maximal volume
   1. Indicator of degree of mitral regurgitation.
   2. Indirect indicator of degree of pulmonary flow in patients without large atrial defects: VSD, PDA, truncus, common ventricle, other complex lesions.
   3. Indicator of size of atrial shunt in patients with atrial plus ventricular or aortic communications.

move even microbubbles, pressure recordings that are diagnostic for most purposes can be obtained. Use of No. 4F catheters in infants with very rapid heart rates, however, may result in extremely overdamped tracings that are not of diagnostic quality.

Abnormal ventricular and great vessel orientation in infants and children with congenital heart disease frequently results in difficulty in catheterization of the pulmonary artery (PA). This problem has been a common one in patients with transposition of the great arteries (TGA). Recent successful techniques for this procedure have been the coaxial catheter of Carr[23] and the substernal precutaneous puncture of Rahimtola et al.[24] In addition, with an increasing experience in catheterization of these patients, a number of clinicians have been able to enter the PA with repeated manipulation of a standard No. 5F catheter. A special technique, which is promising for achieving difficult catheter positions, is the use of the Swan-Ganz floating balloon catheter.[25] This catheter is ideal for young patients because of its size (5F) and flexibility. An example of its clinical use in a 6-mo-old infant with TGA is illustrated in Fig. 13. The catheter was inserted into the saphenous vein and advanced across an atrial communication into the left atrium. The balloon at the tip of the catheter was then inflated with CO_2, which is used to prevent injury from air embolus in case of balloon rupture. The catheter then was pushed into the left ventricle (LV) by the blood flowing across the mitral valve. By minimal manipulation, the catheter moved into the LV outflow

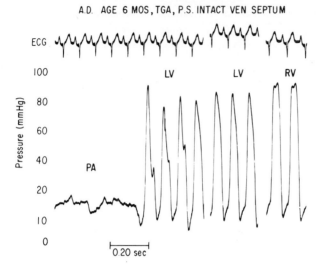

A.D. AGE 6 MOS, TGA, P.S. INTACT VEN SEPTUM

Fig. 13. Use of Swan-Ganz balloon catheter to obtain pulmonary artery pressure in transposition of the great arteries.

tract and then was pushed into the PA by the LV systolic output. The pressure tracings clearly demonstrate significant pulmonary stenosis. This information, together with the pulmonary blood flow calculated from the LV volume determinations (Fig. 12), indicated that an increase in pulmonary blood flow by means of a systemic to pulmonary shunt was needed.

The flow-directed balloon catheter also can be used for the measurement of pulmonary wedge pressure by advancing it into a small pulmonary artery and then inflating the balloon with a small amount of CO_2. It has been used extensively in adults for this purpose without the use of fluoroscopy.

High-fidelity pressure tracings can be obtained with catheter-tip micromanometers. The catheter used most extensively for this purpose has been the Statham model SF1. This catheter has an excellent frequency response but has a fairly high signal to noise ratio and some instability of baseline. It is equipped with a lumen in order to obtain accurate in vivo baseline and sensitivity by attaching the lumen to an external pressure transducer. The size (6.5F) prohibits its use in infants.

Similar high fidelity tracings can be obtained with a smaller (5F) catheter-tip micromanometer, the Statham model P866. This catheter also has some instability of baseline and is not equipped with a lumen. Therefore, in vivo baseline and sensitivity must be obtained with a separate catheter just prior to insertion of the micromanometer. An example of left ventricular pressure (P) recorded with this catheter is shown in Fig. 14. The lack of artifact in both peak pressure and early diastolic pressure is apparent in this tracing. From such data, information regarding left ventricular muscle performance can be obtained as described below.

LEFT VENTRICULAR MUSCLE FUNCTION

Attempts to characterize muscle function of the left ventricle independent of preload and afterload have centered around the application of the force-

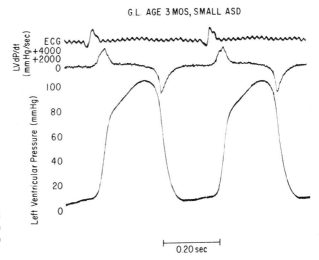

G.L. AGE 3 MOS, SMALL ASD

Fig. 14. High fidelity left ventricular pressure tracing in a 5-mo-old infant obtained with a No. 5 F micromanometer.

velocity relationship to cardiac muscle. Initial studies were performed using papillary muscle preparations,[26] and recent investigations have indicated that similar measurements can be made in the intact heart if the following assumptions are used.[27-31]

(1) Only isovolumic systole is studied since significant fiber shortening results in deviation from the basic force-velocity relationship. Thus this method of analysis excludes patients with significant ventricular shunts or mitral insufficiency.

(2) The measurement of force/unit cross-sectional area, which is equal to stress (S), can be represented by pressure (P) during isovolumic systole. Stress is approximately equal to radius (r) × P/wall thickness (h). Thus, if r and h are constants, S can be represented by P. In the calculation of velocity (below), S is present in both numerator and denominator and thus r and h cancel out.

(3) Wall thickness is assumed to be constant during isovolumic systole. Fiegl and Fry[32] found a 10% increase in h during isovolumic contraction in open chest dogs and Cothran et al.[33] reported a 6% increase in unanesthethized horses. Thus, a 5%–10% increase in h during isovolumic systole in humans may occur. It is not known whether or not this change is similar in patients with different cardiac lesions.

(4) Determinations of contractile element velocity, Vce, are performed from high fidelity pressure tracings. During isovolumic systole, Vce is directly proportional to the rate of force development (dF/dt) and inversely related to the stiffness of the functional series elastic component (dF/dl). Thus, Vce = (dP/dt)/(dF/dl) during isovolumic contraction since dP/dt can be substituted for dF/dt. The series elastic stiffness can be approximated by 28P, which has been derived from animal investigations.[26] Series elasticity has been found to remain unchanged with inotropic interventions, hypoxia, or experimental hypertrophy.[26,34-36] Thus, Vce = (dP/dt)/28P.

Both total and developed pressure (total − end-diastolic pressure) have been used in the above formulation. Current knowledge concerning muscle models is most consistent with the use of developed pressure.[34,37]

The methodology for reliable determinations of Vce requires the use of high fidelity pressure recordings (catheter-tip micromanometry) to accurately determine instantaneous values for dP/dt and P. The following description is for our current method of data collection and analysis.

High fidelity left ventricular pressure recordings are obtained prior to the first cineangiocardiogram. An electronic differentiator is used to obtain dP/dt. These data along with the electrocardiogram are recorded on photographic paper and on magnetic tape at a tape speed of 7.5 IPS. The tape is then replayed at 3.75 IPS and recorded on paper at a paper speed of 200 mm/sec. This technique yields an effective paper speed of 400 mm/sec to facilitate data analysis. Data points are then obtained each 5 msec beginning with left ventricular end-diastolic pressure and continuing until peak dP/dt. Five beats are analyzed for each patient, and data from all five beats are used to derive an average composite force-velocity, or more properly pressure-velocity curve. In using developed pressure (DP), only those data points with $DP \geq 10$ mmHg normally are used in order to avoid the early period of fractionate contraction[38] and incomplete development of the active state. Pressure and dP/dt are punched on data cards and calculations performed with a digital computer. Both first and second degree polynomial curve analysis is used to derive equations for Vce as a function of pressure. The second degree curves have demonstrated a better fit in terms of higher F and r values. The y-intercept of the derived equations is equal to Vce at zero P and thus is analogous to the maximal velocity of the unloaded muscle, Vmax. We have termed this value the Vmax index and used it to estimate myocardial contractile state. In addition, pressure-velocity curves have been derived using total pressure instead of developed pressure. These curves demonstrate an early increase in both P and Vce before the inverse relationship is established. Only that part of the curve with the inverse relationship is used for curve fitting to obtain Vmax. The maximal calculated value for Vce with this method has been termed the physiologic maximal velocity or Vpm[30] and also has been used to estimate contractile state.

Initial investigations were performed to obtain normal standards for these measurements in 20 children undergoing routine diagnostic cardiac catheterization, who had normal left hearts by routine hemodynamic measurements.[39] In addition, these patients had normal LV end-diastolic volumes,

Table 3. Normal Values for Contractile State Estimation in Children (N = 20, ages 3 to 11 yr)

		V_{max} index $(\bar{x} \pm 2\,SD)$	Upper Limit $(\bar{x} \pm 2\,SD)$	Lower Limits $(x - 2\,SD)$
Developed pressure	10 mmHg	3.33 ± 0.48	4.29	2.37
Total pressure		1.50 ± 0.39	2.27	0.72
		V_{pm} *		
Total pressure		1.30 ± 0.24	1.78	0.82

* Physiological maximal velocity = maximal calculated value for (dP/dt)/28P.

ejection fractions, systolic outputs, and LV wall masses. Normal values ± 2 SD for V_{max} index and V_{pm} are shown in Table 3. These values were derived from patients aged 3–11 yr and may not be applicable to infants as shown in Fig. 15.

In this illustration, pressure velocity curves are plotted for three patients with normal left hearts. The lowest curve is that of a patient, age 8, who is typical of the normal group. The two upper curves are from infants, ages 3 mo and 6 mo, who also have normal left hearts by the criteria described above with normal LV volumes, ejection fractions, and wall mass. Their curves and values for Vmax, however, are increased considerably above that of the normal patient and are above the upper limit of normal for Vmax index ($\bar{x}$ + 2 SD = 4.29, Table 3). These findings lend support to the previous suggestion that the higher ejection fractions in the infant's age group[17] indicate an augmented contractile state. Such an increased contractility could be due to the increased heart rate per se or may reflect an augmented sympathetic influence.

In Fig. 16, the pressure-velocity curve is shown for a 13-yr-old boy with hypertrophic subaortic stenosis and an increase in LV wall mass to 148% of normal. His pressure-velocity curve is significantly depressed from normal with the Vmax index less than the lower limit of normal ($\bar{x}$ − 2 SD = 2.37, Table 3). This depressed contractile state in the presence of hypertrophy has been shown in experimental animals[40–44] as well as in adults[45–47] with a pressure overload. Such a decrease in contractility is an inconstant finding in children with LV pressure overload.[38] This fact suggests that the factors operative in hypertrophy that affect muscle function may well be modified by age of the patient and duration of the hypertrophy.

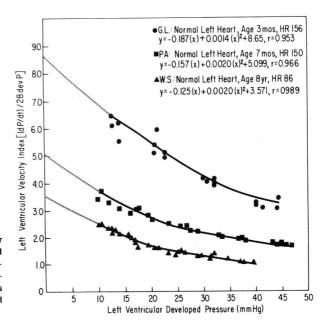

Fig. 15. Left ventricular pressure-velocity curves used to estimate myocardial contractile state. Curves in two infants have significant increases in estimated V_{max} over normal values for older children.

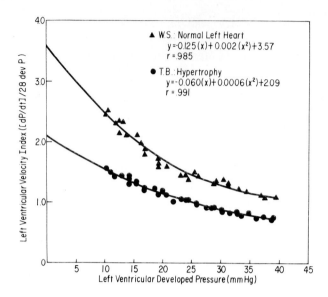

Fig. 16. Left ventricular pressure-velocity curves in a normal child compared with a depressed curve in a child with hypertrophic subaortic stenosis.

SUMMARY

Hemodynamic investigations of the infant and child with congenital heart disease encompasses accurate determinations of blood flow, pressure, ventricular and atrial volumes, and cardiac muscle function. Measurements of blood flow, pressure, and volume can provide reliable indicators of cardiac function as a pump as well as estimates of the myocardial and systemic adaptation to a congenital lesion. In addition, investigations of cardiac muscle function with the use of high fidelity pressure and dP/dt measurements can add a valuable dimension to the overall evaluation of the patient with heart disease.

ACKNOWLEDGMENT

The authors would like to thank Mrs. Martha Mason, Mrs. Barrie Scardino, Mrs. Ida Phialas, and Mrs. Costella Harris for their assistance in data processing; Miss Eugenia Cole and Miss Lucy Bullock for their help in data collection; and Mrs. Carol Lehman and Miss Wanda Taylor for their work in preparation of the manuscript.

REFERENCES

1. Tsakiris, A. G., Donald, D. E., Sturm, R. E., and Wood, E. H.: Volume, ejection fraction, and internal dimensions of left ventricle determined by biplane videometry. Fed. Proc. 28: 1358, 1969.

2. Bing, R. J., Vandam, L. D., and Gray, F. D.: Physiological studies in congenital heart disease. I. Procedures. Bull. Johns Hopkins Hosp. (Baltimore) 80:107, 1947.

3. Wood, E. H.: Diagnostic application of indicator dilution technics in quantitation of valvular regurgitation. Circ. Res. 10:531, 1962.

4. Hugenholtz, P. G., Wagner, H. R., and Ellison, R. C. Application of fiberoptic dye-dilution technic to the assessment of myocardial function. I. Description of technic and results in 100 patients with congenital or acquired heart disease. Amer. J. Cardiol. 24:79, 1969.

5. —, —, and Plauth, W. H., Jr.: Application of fiberoptic indicator dilution technic to

the assessment of myocardial function. II. The interaction of the ejection fraction and end-diastolic volume during exercise and isoproterenol infusion. Amer. J. Cardiol. 26:490, 1970.

6. Braunwald, E., Morrow, A. G., Sanders, R., Jr., and Long, R. T.: Characterization of circulatory shunts by foreign gas technics. *In* Bass, A. D., and Moe, G. K., (Eds.) Congenital Heart Disease. Washington, D.C. American Association for the Advancement of Science, 1960.

7. Spach, M. S., Canent, R. V., Jr., Boineau, J. P., White, A. W., Jr., Sanders, A. P., and Baylin, G. J.: Radioisotope dilution curves as an adjunct to cardiac catheterization. I. Left to right shunts. II. Right to left shunts. Amer. J. Cardiol. 16:165, 1965.

8. Mason, D. T., Ashburn, W. L., Harbert, J. C., Lawrence, S. C., and Eugene, B.: Rapid sequential visualization of the heart and great vessels in man using the wide-field anger scintillation camera. Circulation 39:19, 1968.

9. Graham, T. P., Jr., Goodrich, J. K., Robinson, A. E., and Harris, C. C.: Scintiangiocardiography in children. Amer. J. Cardiol. 25:387, 1970.

10. Hurley, P. J., Strauss, H. W., and Wagner, H. N., Jr.: Radionuclide angiocardiography in cyanotic congenital heart disease. Johns Hopkins Med. J. 127:46, 1970.

11. Mullins, C. B., Mason, D. T., Ashburn, W. L., and Ross, J., Jr.: Determination of ventricular volume by radioisotope angiography. Amer. J. Cardiol. 24:72, 1969.

12. Greenfield, J. C., Jr.: Pressure gradient technique. Methods Med. Res. 11:83, 1966.

13. Dodge, H. T., Sandler, H., Ballew, D. W., and Lord, J. D.: The use of biplane angiocardiography for the measurement of left ventricular volume in man. Amer. Heart J. 60:762, 1960.

14. Miller, G. A. H., and Swan, H. J. C.: Effect of chronic pressure and volume overload on left heart volume in subjects with congenital heart disease. Circulation 30:205, 1964.

15. Hugenholtz, P. G., and Wagner, H. R.: Assessment of myocardial function in congenital heart disease. *In* Adams, F. J. and Hall, V. E. (Eds.): Pathophysiology of Congenital Heart Disease. Los Angeles, University of California Press, 1970.

16. Graham, T. P., Jr., Jarmakani, M. M., Canent, R. V., Jr., Capp, M. P., and Spach, M. S.: Characterization of left heart volume and mass in normal children and in infants with myocardial disease. Circulation 38:826, 1968.

17. —, —, —, and Morrow, M. N.: Left heart volume estimation in infancy and childhood: re-evaluation of methodology and normal values. Circulation 43:895, 1971.

18. Rackley, C. E., Dodge, H. T., Coble, Y. D., Jr., and Hay, R. E.: A method for determining left ventricular mass in man. Circulation 29:666, 1964.

19. Romero, T., Friedman, W. F., and Covell, J. W.: The pressure volume relations of the fetal, newborn, and adult heart. Circulation 42 (Suppl. III):168, 1970.

20. Jarmakani, M. M., Graham, T. P., Jr., Canent, R. V., Jr., Spach, M. S., and Capp, M. P.: Effect of site of shunt on left heart volume characteristics in children with ventricular septal defect and patent ductus arteriosus. Circulation 40:411, 1969.

21. Graham, T. P., Jr., Lewis, B. W., Jarmakani, M. M., Canent, R. V., Jr., and Capp, M. P.: Left heart volume and mass quantification in children with left ventricular pressure overload. Circulation 41:203–212, 1970.

22. Urschel, C. W., Covell, J. W., Sonnenblick, E. H., Ross, J., Jr., and Braunwald, E.: Myocardial mechanics in aortic and mitral valvular regurgitation: the concept of instantaneous impedance as a determinant of the performance of the intact heart. J. Clin. Invest. 47:867, 1968.

23. Carr, I., and Wills, B.: Coaxial flow guided catheterization of the pulmonary artery in transposition of the great arteries. Lancet 2:318, 1966.

24. Rahimtoola, S. H., Ongley, P. A., and Swan, H. J. C.: Percutaneous suprasternal puncture (Radner technique) of the pulmonary artery in transposition of the great vessels. Circulation 33:242, 1966.

25. Swan, H. J. C., Ganz, W., Forrester, J., Marcus, H., Diamond, G., and Chonette, D.: Catheterization of the heart in man with use of a flow-directed balloon-tipped catheter. New Eng. J. Med. 283:447, 1970.

26. Sonnenblick, E. H.: Implications of muscle mechanics in the heart. Fed. Proc. 21: 975, 1963.

27. Taylor, R. R., Ross, J., Jr., Covell, J. W., and Sonnenblick, E. H.: A quantitative analysis of left ventricular myocardial function in the intact sedated dog. Circ. Res. 21:99, 1967.

28. Urschel, C. W., Vokonas, P. S., Hen-

derson, A. H., and Sonnenblick, E. H.: A comparison of indices of contractility derived from the isovolumic force-velocity relation. Circulation 42-III:115, 1970.

29. Mehmel, H., Krayenbuhl, H. P., and Rutishauser, W.: Peak measured velocity of shortening in the canine left ventricle. J. Appl. Physiol. 29:637, 1970.

30. Nejad, N. S., Klein, M. D., Mirsky, I., and Lown, B.: Assessment of myocardial contractility from ventricular pressure recordings. Cardiovasc. Res. 5:15, 1971.

31. Wolk, M. J., Keefe, J. F., Bing, O. H. L., Finkelstein, L. J., and Levine, H. J.: Estimation of Vmax in auxotonic systoles from the rate of relative increase of isovolumic pressure: (dP/dt)/KP. J. Clin. Invest. 50:1276, 1971.

32. Fiegl, E. O., and Fry, D. L.: Myocardial mural thickness during the cardiac cycle. Circ. Res. 14:541, 1964.

33. Cothran. L. N., Bowie, W. C., Hinds, J. E., and Hawthorne, E. W.: Left ventricular wall thickness changes in unanesthetized horses. *In* Tanz, R. D., Kavaler, F., and Roberts, J. (Eds.): Factors Influencing Myocardial Contractility. New York, Academic, 1967.

34. Parmley, W. W., and Sonnenblick, E. H.: Series elasticity in heart muscle: its relation to contractile element velocity and proposed muscle models. Circ. Res. 20:112, 1967.

35. Tyberg, J. V., Parmley, W. W., and Sonnenblick, E. H.: In vitro studies of ventricular asynchrony and regional hypoxia. Circ. Res. 25:569, 1969.

36. Parmley, W. W., Spann, J. F., J., Taylor, R. R., and Sonnenblick, E. H.: The series elasticity of cardiac muscle in hyperthyroidism, ventricular hypertrophy, and heart failure. Proc. Soc. Exp. Biol. Med. 127:606, 1968.

37. Jewell, B. R., and Blinks, J. R.: Drugs and the mechanical properties of heart muscle. Ann. Rev. Pharm. 8:113, 1968.

38. Wiggers, C. J.: The interpretation of the intraventricular pressure curve on the basis of rapidly summated fractionate contractions. Amer. J. Physiol. 80:1, 1927.

39. Graham, T. P., Jr., Jarmakani, J. M., Canent, R. V., Jr., and Anderson, P. A. W.: Evaluation of left ventricular contractile state in childhood: normal values and observations with a pressure overload. Circulation 44:1043, 1971.

40. Spann, J. F., Buccino, R. A., Sonnenblick, E. H., and Braunwald, E.: Contractile state of cardiac muscle obtained from cats with experimentally produced ventricular hypertrophy and heart failure. Circ. Res. 21:341, 1967.

41. Krayenbuhl, H. P., Pierce, E. C., II., and Agishi, T.: Left ventricular dynamics in the dog under chronic pressure load from coarctation of the aorta. Arch Kreisl auf forsch 56:25, 1968.

42. Bing, O. H. L., Matsushita, S., Fanburg, B. L., and Levine, H. J.: Mechanical properties of rat cardiac muscle during experimental hypertrophy. Circ. Res. 28:346, 1971.

43. Kaufman, R. L., Homburger, H., and Wirth, H.: Disorder in excitation-contraction coupling of cardiac muscle from cats with experimentally produced right ventricular hypertrophy. Circ. Res. 28:346, 1971.

44. Coleman, H. N., and Gunning, J. F.: Inefficient energy utilization in myocardial hypertrophy. Circulation 42-III:116, 1970.

45. Simon, H., Krayenbuehl, H. P., Rutishauser, W., and Preter, B. O.: The contractile state of the hypertrophied left ventricular myocardium in aortic stenosis. Amer. Heart J. 79:587, 1970.

46. Mason, D. T., Spann, J. F., Jr., and Zeles, R.: Comparison of the contractile state of the normal, hypertrophied, and failing heart in man. *In* Alpert, N. R. (Ed.) Cardiac Hypertrophy. New York, Academic Press, 1970.

47. Levine, H. J., McIntyre, K. M., Lipana, J. G., and Bing, O. H. L.: Force-velocity relations in failing and nonfailing hearts of subjects with aortic stenosis. Amer. J. Med. Sci. 259:79, 1970.

Perioperative Management of the Infant With Congenital Heart Disease

Welton M. Gersony and Constance J. Hayes

O VER THE PAST DECADE, rapid strides in the development of open heart surgical techniques have been translated into excellent operative results in the correction of a variety of congenital cardiac defects in older children. The cardinal challenge to the pediatrician, pediatric cardiologist, and cardiovascular surgeon has now shifted to management of the newborn with critical heart disease. Definitive or palliative surgery has become available for the great majority of these infants, but risks remain high and the salvage rate is variable.[1-4]

Optimal treatment of severe cardiac defects in the newborn may be achieved only if the primary physician recognizes the problem early, regardless of time of day or night, and promptly transfers the patient under proper environmental conditions to a central hospital where an infant cardiac program exists. The medical center, in turn, must provide on a 24-hr per day basis the highly specialized personnel, facilities, and equipment that is necessary for accurate diagnosis and successful surgical intervention. The modern "perioperative" care of a newborn infant with a severe heart defect must be considered as a unique commitment, and should not be undertaken simply as an occasional addition to a cardiac surgical program for older children and adults.

This report will outline the current approach at this institution to management of the critically ill infant with a cardiac malformation. In our experience, *unremitting attention to detail* is the single most important principle in the treatment of these seriously ill babies. Therefore, this paper will not only discuss general guidelines, but will also emphasize details of management that may often tip the delicate balance between a successful outcome and mortality.

From the Division of Pediatric Cardiology, Department of Pediatrics, College of Physicians and Surgeons, Columbia University, and Babies Hospital, Columbia Presbyterian-Medical Center, New York, N.Y.

Supported by USPHS Grant-5 T01-HE-05389-11.

Welton M. Gersony, M.D.: *Director, Division of Pediatric Cardiology, Associate Professor of Pediatrics, College of Physicians and Surgeons, Columbia University, New York, N.Y.* Constance J. Hayes, M.D.: *Assistant Professor of Clinical Pediatrics, College of Physicians and Surgeons, Columbia University, New York, N.Y.*

INITIAL MANAGEMENT

Preoperative care of the critically ill newborn with congenital heart disease, who is to require cardiac surgery, begins the moment that a serious heart lesion is suspected. Emphasis is placed on the prevention of hypothermia, hypoxia, and acidosis, and the treatment of congestive heart failure, from the time of diagnosis to the moment of operation. If travel between hospitals is necessary, it is imperative that the infant be transported by ambulance in a warm isolette accompanied by a trained nurse, and, if possible, a physician.[5] Some institutions will provide specialized vehicles that contain monitoring devices and equipment necessary for respiratory support.[6]

On admission to the medical center, the temperature is immediately measured, and the baby is placed in an incubator preheated to 33°C. This is done before a prolonged physical examination or blood sampling is carried out. Unnecessary manipulation of an exhausted, hypothermic baby is avoided as an antithetic exercise, because the result may be an excellent physical examination and a complete laboratory evaluation of an irreversibly acidotic infant, who cannot be saved. An intravenous line is established, blood gases, glucose, and electrolytes determined, and, if necessary, acidosis corrected by sodium bicarbonate administration. A portable chest x-ray is obtained, and electrocardiographic monitoring is begun after a full tracing is recorded.

Clinical diagnostic possibilities should be thoroughly evaluated. A diagnosis of heart disease made precipitately, without careful consideration of system disorders other than cardiac, can result in a sick baby with pulmonary or central nervous system disease being subjected to the additional risk of unnecessary hemodynamic study. Once a cardiac defect is strongly suspected, cardiac catheterization and angiography are carried out, with a surgical team in readiness in the event that an operation must follow immediately.

In general, catheterization should be done when a baby is in as optimal a condition as possible, *after* a clinical diagnosis of heart disease has been made, and hypothermia, hypoxia, acidosis, and congestive heart failure have been evaluated and treated. However, the procedure should be done *before* the physiologic sequelae of the cardiac defect leads to irreversible deterioration despite medical therapy. The decision as to exact timing of the cardiac catheterization may not be an easy one. Although studies on a scheduled basis are preferable whenever possible, the death during the night of a small infant with a potentially operable heart lesion who was awaiting cardiac catheterization should not occur in the modern era of aggressive management. The infant need not "prove" his ability to survive a given length of time in order to earn a place on the catheterization schedule.[3]

A key factor in the initial differential diagnosis of congenital heart disease and, hence, the timing of cardiac catheterization is the magnitude of pulmonary blood flow as determined by x-ray.[7] Medical treatment offers little or nothing to the management of marked hypoxia secondary to decreased effective pulmonary blood flow. Although initial improvement may occur after treatment of hypothermia and acidosis, the situation will only worsen with time. In some instances, a patent ductus arteriosus, which may be the only significant source of pulmonary blood flow, suddenly narrows or closes, rapidly causing terminal hypoxemia and acidosis. Since balloon septostomy or emergency surgical intervention for a palliative shunt or valvotomy may be life-saving, babies with decreased or normal pulmonary vascularity are likely to require immediate cardiac catheterization. Similarly, there are times when left ventricular obstructive disease with pulmonary congestion, (e.g. aortic stenosis, coarctation of the aorta), is present to such a severe degree that catheterization and operation may not be safely postponed, even for a few hours. On the other hand, when pulmonary vascularity is increased due to ventricular volume overload, digitalization and other anticongestive measures for 24–72 hr may improve the patient's condition considerably, and reduce the risk of cardiac catheterization and subsequent surgery. On occasion, among older babies with large left to right shunts, improvement may be so striking, that surgical intervention may not be necessary during early infancy.

CARDIAC CATHETERIZATION

The risk of cardiac catheterization is higher among seriously ill babies than older patients. The cooperative study on cardiac catheterization collected data from 16 institutions, and found a death rate of 6% among small infants as compared to a 0.44% overall mortality.[8] Varghese et al.[9] reported 19 nonsurgical deaths within the first 24 hr following hemodynamic study in 100 consecutive patients under 1 mo of age. Some degree of increased mortality may be expected for infants, but these statistics also reflect the fact that babies are often studied when in extremely poor condition, even in extremis, and that some will have cardiac lesions which are incompatible with viability. Cardiac catheterization mortality figures thus include many patients for whom death is a product of natural history, rather than a procedural complication.

The risk of hemodynamic study is dependent to a great degree on the experience and technical skill of the physician carrying out the procedure, but factors related to environmental conditions, and the cardiac catheterization team's readiness to deal with complications are also of major importance in lowering morbidity and mortality. Considerations in the management of infants during hemodynamic study are outlined below.

Analgesia

Babies are studied utilizing local anesthesia ($\frac{1}{2}$% lidocaine) without previously administered analgesics. This policy avoids further depression of already compromised cardiorespiratory function. If activity and crying become excessive, morphine sulfate will provide excellent analgesia. A low dosage range is suggested (Table 1), since even "standard" amounts of rapidly administered intravenous morphine may result in respiratory arrest. Small doses can always be repeated. Other drugs including meperidine HCL and diazepam have also been useful, and recent experiences with ketamine HCL at this institution and elsewhere have been encouraging.[10]

Blood Replacement

Warm blood, previously typed and crossmatched, should be immediately available during the cardiac catheterization of an infant. When blood loss is estimated to be 15 ml or greater in a small baby, replacement is carried out before the study is completed. Hemoglobin determinations are obtained during the subsequent 24 hr in order to reassess the need for further transfusion.

Table 1. Drugs Useful in the Management of Infants With Congenital Heart Disease

Drug	Route	Dosage	Schedule and Remarks
Digoxin (Lanoxin)	p.o.	0.06–0.075 mg/kg	Divided in 3 doses (q 6–12 hrs), more rapidly in emergency
	i.m.		2/3 of oral dose
	i.v.		
	Daily maintenance: 1/3 of digitalizing dose-divided in 2 doses		
Isoproterenol (Isuprel)	i.v.	1 mg in 100–500 ml D5W	Slow infusion
Lidocaine (Xylocaine)	i.v.	1 mg/kg/dose	Single dose over 5 min
	i.v.	30–50 μ g/kg/min	Slow infusion
Furosemide (Lasix)	i.v.	1 mg/kg/dose	For rapid diuresis, but if no effect, may
	i.m.		be repeated at higher dose level
	p.o.		
Ethacrynic acid (Edecrin)	i.v.	1 mg/kg/dose	For rapid diuresis, but if no effect, may
	p.o.		be repeated at higher dose level
Mannitol (25% solution)	i.v.	200–400 mg/kg/dose	Infusion over 1 hr
Chlorthiazide (Diuril)	p.o.	20 mg/kg/day	Divided in 2 doses; daily or every other day
Spironolactone (Aldactone)	p.o.	1.5–3 mg/kg/day	Divided in 3 doses, daily
Morphine sulfate	i.v.	0.05–0.1 mg/kg/dose	May be repeated after 1 hr
	i.m.		
Meperidine HCl	i.v.	0.5–1 mg/kg/dose	May be repeated after 1 hr
	i.m.		
Diazepam (Valium)	i.v.	0.05–0.1 mg/kg/dose	For sedation
	i.m.		
	p.o.		
Curare	i.v.	0.15–0.3 mg/kg/dose	May be repeated as necessary
Ketamine HCl	i.m.	6.5–12 mg/kg	For induction of anesthesia
	i.m.	3.25–6 mg/kg	q 1–2 hr for maintenance
Penicillin G	i.v.	100,000 U/kg/day	Divided in 4 doses (q 6 hr)
	i.m.	100,000 U/kg/day	Divided in 2 doses (q 12 hr)
Kanamycin	i.m.	12–15 mg/kg/day	Divided in 2 doses (q 12 hr)
Calcium gluconate (10% solution)	i.v.	0.5 ml/kg/dose	Administered slowly while monitoring electrocardiogram
Sodium bicarbonate	i.v.	2–3 meq/kg or base deficit x 0.3 x wt (kg)	1/2–3/4 total dose given over 1 minute, remainder over 1–2 hr. period
Arginine HCl (R-gene)	i.v.	$\frac{Cl\ deficit \times 0.2 \times wt\ (kg)}{2}$	Slow infusion over 6 hr to correct 1/2 deficit

Temperature, Oxygenation, Acid-Base

Body temperature is controlled by a transparent radiant heat canopy (Sierracin Cradle Warmer, The Sierracin Corp., Sylmar, Calif.) composed of a thin sheet of metal encased between plastic laminations, which is thermostatically controlled from a sensor on the infant's abdomen. This unit allows access to the cutdown site and may be left in place during angiography. Skin, rather than deep body temperature is utilized to adjust environmental heat, since O_2 consumption has been found to be minimal when skin temperature is maintained in the range of 36°–37°C.[11,12] Rectal temperature is also monitored, but as a reflection of the metabolic response of the infant rather than the thermal state of the environment.

Arterial blood gases are studied at regular intervals, and results indicating hypoxia, hypoventilation and/or acidosis are dealt with appropriately. Oxygen is administered when necessary via a small head box, which permits O_2 concentrations to reach the 90%–95% range in the rare event that such levels are required. Equipment for intubation and respiratory support are available in the laboratory for emergency use.

Arrhythmias

The possibility of an arrhythmia must be anticipated during the hemodynamic study. Cardiac function in a sick baby is often so compromised, that if a catastrophic arrhythmia (e.g., ventricular fibrillation) occurs, it must be terminated within seconds if the infant is to be successfully resuscitated. A DC defibrillator with small, previously lubricated paddles is turned on and adjusted before the onset of the procedure. Pacing equipment as well as pharmacologic agents utilized in the control of arrhythmias are also in readiness.

Catheterization Techniques

The hemodynamic study itself is carried out by an experienced physician, who attempts to obtain a complete diagnosis in as short a time as possible. Asepsis is carefully maintained during the procedure, but antibiotic prophylaxis has been found to be of no advantage.[13,14] Stiff catheters are avoided and extreme care is exercised in catheter manipulation, especially in areas that may be prone to perforation (e.g., left and right atrial appendage, right ventricular outflow tract, and apex of the left ventricle).

Angiocardiograms are performed through a multiple side hole catheter, which is placed in a "free" position within a chamber or vessel. Unobstructed withdrawal of blood and lack of arrhythmias with a hand injection of saline are preconditions for the pressure injection of contrast media. Diatrizoate (75% Hypaque) is utilized for angiography because of its (1) relatively high iodine content, affording good visualization of the anatomy; and (2) low viscosity, which lessens ventricular irritability and facilitates rapid administration.[15] One ml/kg/injection is administered at an optimal pressure calculated on the basis of catheter length and lumen size. Three angiocardiograms may be performed with relative safety, allowing at least 15 min between injections for the clearing of dye from the blood. Rapid administration of excessive amounts of contrast material may lead to central nervous system, cardiac, and renal complications.[16,17]

SURGERY

Within the context of the infant's disease, every therapeutic effort is made to allow him to attain optimal cardiorespiratory function prior to surgery. In extremely rare instances, an infant is taken to the operating room immediately upon admission. This is done only in situations when (1) the patient is judged to be so ill that immediate operation, even without cardiac catheterization represents his only chance of survival, and (2) the type of surgical procedure that is required is absolutely clear (e.g., systemic arterial-pulmonary shunt, pulmonary or aortic valvulotomy).

Techniques for open heart surgery in infants at this institution have been reported in detail and will be summarized here.[18] The operating room is warmed to 85° F and careful monitoring of temperature, blood pressure, blood gases and electrocardiogram are continued throughout the surgical procedure. Normothermia is maintained throughout bypass; an approach similar to that recently reported by Pierce et al.[19] Recently, successful open heart surgical procedures on small infants utilizing deep hypothermia have been described, and this technique seems extremely promising for this age group.[20-22]

Cardiopulmonary bypass is carried out using the disposable Temptrol Bubble Oxygenator (Infant Bentley Q 130 model, Bentley Laboratories, Santa Ana, Calif.) with a priming volume of 500 ml. Fresh ACD blood is prepared for pump use with heparin, calcium chloride, and tris buffer. Two and one-half percent Dextrose in $\frac{1}{2}$ strength saline is used to dilute the blood by one third of its volume. Flow rates of 200–210 ml/kg/min are employed and the stroke volume of the pump oxygenator is estabished at 7–10 ml in order to maintain a stable mean blood pressure of 40—50 mm of Hg. Perfusion is carried out through direct cannulation of the ascending aorta with a thin-walled metal cannula. The largest possible venous cannulae are employed to insure maximal unobstructed venous return. A major effort is made to minimize perfusion time, since the incidence of postoperative complications are increased when cardiopulmonary bypass is prolonged. Following termination of bypass, protamine sulfate (1.3 mg for each mg of heparin initially given), is used to restore the clotting mechanism, and freshly drawn ACD blood is slowly infused.

EARLY POSTOPERATIVE CARE

Postoperative care is initiated in an intensive care unit especially adapted for the cardiac patient (Fig. 1) with a staff attuned to the unique problems of the infant. After cardiac surgery, the infant's critical organ function must be carefully managed and his environment controlled until sufficient time has elapsed to allow the beneficial effects of improved cardiac function to become apparent. A well-trained staff of physicians and nurses must be in constant attendance to act upon monitored physiologic data and make urgent clinical decisions.

Special attention is given to several major areas of concern, which, for practicality and convenience, are discussed separately in the following sections. True separation of complications by organ systems is not possible, since functional failure in one system will cause profound physiologic and biochemical changes to ensue in another. For example, *respiratory* insufficiency will lead to hypoxia, acidosis, and hypercarbia, which in turn will compromise *cardiac* and *renal* function: neither can be managed successfully until adequate ventilation is reestablished. Clearly, it is essential that the *primary* source of each individual postoperative problem be identified and treated.

Pulmonary

Respiratory failure is probably the major postoperative complication encountered following open heart surgery among infants.[23] Cardiopulmonary bypass,

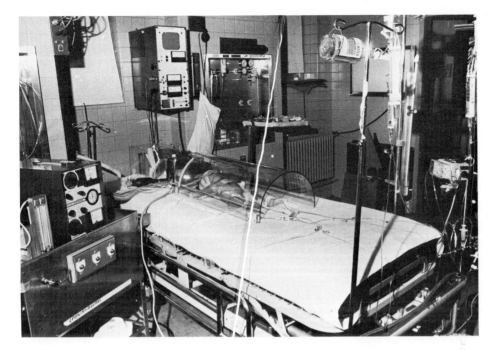

Fig. 1.   Recovery area adapted for postoper ative management of the infant with heart disease.

often carried out in the presence of chronic pulmonary congestion, results in decreased lung compliance, copious tracheobronchial secretions, atelectasis, and increased breathing efforts. In the infant left to spontaneous respirations, fatigue may rapidly ensue, and hypoventilation, acidosis, and respiratory arrest are the consequences. To cirvumvent these events, mechanical positive pressure endotracheal ventilation is instituted immediately following open heart surgery, and continued for a minimum of 1 2 hr and often up to 2 or 3 days. Initially, respirations are controlled, but an active infant, who is easily ventilated, may soon be allowed to trigger the respirator spontaneously, so that ventilation will be assisted rather than regulated. By initiating respiratory control at the onset of the postoperative period, a patent airway and adequate ventilation are assured, and emergency intubation is not required at a later time when the infant's condition may be critical. Positive pressure breathing also has the advantage of deterring pulmonary edema and maintaining vascular volume.[24] It is recognized that intubation and artificial ventilation are not without complications,[25] but for severely ill infants, the risks of initial respiratory support are more than balanced by the benefits. After closed heart surgery, vigorous babies with good air exchange and normal blood gases are not routinely placed on artificial ventilation.

   Intubation: Nasotracheal intubation is preferred for respirator care, since maximal mobility of the infant is permitted with less risk of airway displacement. Following surgery, this requires a change from the standard oral tracheal tube used in the operating room to a Portex (Portex Medical Products, Smith Industries, N. America, Ltd., Woburn, Mass.) nasotracheal tube, which is loose enough to allow a slight leak when "sigh" pressures are required.[25] A skilled physician should carry out this change-over as quickly and atraumatically as possible. Nasotracheal tubes with a 3-mm or more internal diameter are necessary in order to accept adequately sized suction catheters. Maximal stabilization of the tube is obtained by fixation to a head turban of gauze as shown in Fig. 2.[26] If the infant's condition is judged to be unusually precarious, postoperative ventilation is continued with the oral tracheal tube left in place, and nasotracheal intubation is deferred until improvement is noted. A chest x-ray is obtained soon after the onset of ventilatory support in order to observe the position of the endotracheal tube and to assess the degree of lung expansion. Tracheostomy, routinely carried out in some centers,[27] is not considered at this institution during the initial postoperative phase. Tracheostomy would be contemplated only when ventilation becomes necessary for a period exceeding 10 days.

Ventilation: A modified Bourns (Bourns, Inc. Life Systems Div., 6135 Magnolia Avenue, Riverside, Calif.) respirator is utilized for ventilatory support. This type of respirator provides relatively constant volume, positive pressure ventilation, and, when fitted with an appropriate heated humidifier, maintains inspired air at body temperature and 100% humidity.[28] Condensation within the connecting tubing is prevented by a protective sleeve of warm air encircling the inspiratory tube.[29] Initially, 100% oxygen is administered; the concentration is decreased gradually to 40%, provided that the arterial pO_2 is maintained above 60 mm. However, a "normal" pO_2 does not, in itself, guarantee

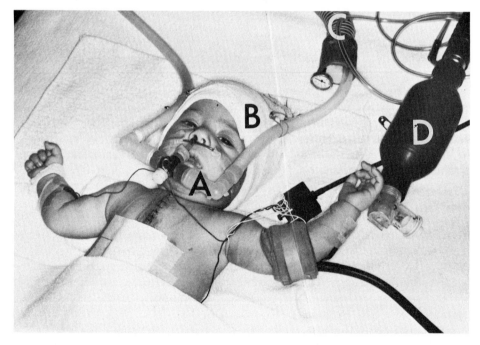

Fig. 2.   Nasotracheal intubation following open heart surgery. Nasotracheal tube is connected to the respirator via plastic elbows (A) attached to the inspiratory and expiratory tubing of the ventilator, and secured to a gauze turban (B). A sleeve of warm air (C) prevents cooling and condensation of the oxygen-air mixture. The infant inflating bag (D) is equipped with an oxygen inlet in the tail to permit close to 100% oxygen administration.

that the total amount of oxygen delivered to the tissues will be sufficient to pre-vent tissue hypoxia. Low cardiac output with poor tissue perfusion leads to in-creased lactate production, and severe acidosis will result, despite the presence of normal arterial oxygen saturation. Acidosis, in turn, may further limit oxy-genation and cardiac output by increasing pulmonary arteriolar resistance. Thus, it is important that pH be carefully monitored as well as blood gases. During the initial hours of the postoperative period, minute volume of the res-pirator is carefully adjusted, depending on pCO_2 and pH, and acidosis is cor-rected by HCO_3 administration (see Acid-Base Management), until both the pO_2 and pCO_2 are in an acceptable range, and the pH is normal (Fig. 3).

Sedation is necessary for controlled ventilation in the immediate postopera-tive period. Small intravenous doses of morphine sulfate are routinely adminis-tered, and, on occasion, curare may also be given in order to insure adequate muscle relaxation and smooth control of ventilation. Within a few hours, the infant usually requires minimal medication, and remains alert, as he adjusts to respiratory control.

Control of Secretions: Tracheobronchial aspiration under strict aseptic con-ditions is essential to the control of pulmonary secretions and maintenance of a patent airway. The infant is initially ventilated with 100% O_2, by means of a self-inflating bag (Penlon Cardiff Infant Inflating Bag, Harris Calorific Co., Medical Div., 5501 Case Avenue, Cleveland, Ohio), and if secretions are thick, 0.5 ml sterile saline, followed by 1.0 ml of air, is instilled into the nasotracheal tube. A No. 8 French catheter is quickly inserted, and tracheobronchial aspira-tion is carried out as the catheter is steadily withdrawn. The catheter used for suctioning the small infant necessarily occludes the endotracheal tube, and can be only momentarily tolerated. Therefore, suctioning, although carried out at

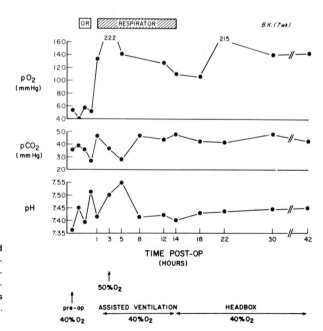

Fig. 3. Serial arterial blood gases and pH information ob-tained during the pre- and post-operative period from a 7-wk-old infant with total anomalous pulmonary venous drainage. OR: operating room.

frequent intervals, should never be prolonged. Rapid jabbing movements with the catheter in the tracheobronchial tree are avoided. This type of suctioning, as opposed to steady withdrawal, significantly drains air from the trachea and may lead to severe hypoxia. Periodic aspiration of the stomach using a small feeding tube is also carried out to allow gastric decompression and further facilitate effective ventilation.

Temperature Control

Optimal oxygenation of an infant is abetted by the maintenance of a "neutral thermal state" (skin temperature $36°-37°C$).[11,12] Despite the warm operating room and attempts to maintain normothermia during surgery, infants lose body heat after perfusion,[30] and often arrive in the intensive care unit with a subnormal temperature. Warming is immediately carried out utilizing the previously described radiant heat unit (see Cardiac Catheterization), which provides several additional advantages in the recovery room. Access to the infant is allowed at both ends of the canopy, the clear plastic affords an unobstructed view of the baby, and there is no possibility of compression of cables or drainage tubes (Fig. 1). An electric heating mattress has occasionally been necessary to warm more rapidly a markedly hypothermic infant.

Cardiovascular

Arterial and Central Venous Pressure Monitoring: A femoral arterial line is established prior to open heart surgery. This provides direct arterial pressure measurements and allows arterial sampling for blood gas determinations. Patency is maintained by intermittent irrigation with a solution containing 5% dextrose in $\frac{1}{4}$ strength normal saline to which 5 mg of heparin has been added. Later in the postoperative course, or after closed heart surgery, arterial blood pressure is monitored by the Doppler technique.[31] A second catheter, which is positioned in the inferior vena cava via the saphenous or femoral vein, is utilized for measurement of central venous pressure (CVP) and for fluid administration.

Simultaneous arterial and central venous pressure monitoring has proved to be an invaluable guide to management of the infant in the early postoperative period. Accurate knowledge of these parameters permits the early detection of hypovolemia, and the recognition of inadequate myocardial function. Changes in pressure may often be more important than actual values. Low central venous pressure associated with low arterial pressure reflects decreased intravascular volume, and suggests the need for administration of blood and/or plasma expanders. In contrast, when venous pressure remains high in the presence of arterial hypotension, poor ventricular function is likely, and inotropic agents and diuretics are indicated. The observation of pulsus alternans also signifies that myocardial function is badly compromised, and this finding may be associated with a poor prognosis. In addition, pulsus paradoxicus can easily be recognized and measured on the arterial pressure monitor. This observation strongly suggests the presence of cardiac tamponade, and if the diagnosis is established, pericardial drainage must be carried out without delay.

For most infants, central venous pressure is maintained below 10 cm, although the patient's preoperative cardiac anatomy will often necessitate adjustments.

For example: (1) The infant with total anomalous pulmonary venous drainage has a relatively small left heart, which must accept an increased blood volume postoperatively. In this situation, fluids are restricted in order to keep the central venous pressure as low as possible, consistent with an adequate cardiac output, until the left ventricle can gradually adjust without dangerous elevation of left atrial and pulmonary capillary pressure.[32] It must be emphasized, however, that central venous pressure may often not be a reliable index of left atrial pressure,[33] so that evaluation of possible left ventricular decompensation should not be dependent only upon the observation of a rising CVP, but must always be augmented by frequent auscultation of the lungs and evaluation of the chest x-ray. (2) The infant with a ventricular septal defect has a well-developed left ventricle, and postoperatively tolerates a normal central venous pressure and the more liberal administration of intravenous fluids. (3) At the opposite end of the spectrum, the patient with pulmonary atresia and a small right ventricle may require an elevated central venous pressure in order to increase right ventricular filling, and thereby improve cardiac output.

Cardiac Rate and Rhythm: The electrocardiogram is monitored continuously during the immediate postoperative period. A change in heart rate may be the first indication of a serious postsurgical complication such as hemorrhage, hypothermia, hypoventilation, or congestive heart failure. Cardiac rhythm disorders must be diagnosed quickly, since a prolonged untreated arrhythmia may add an intolerable burden to the myocardium in the critical early postoperative period. The most common arrhythmia observed among infants at this institution has been atrio-ventricular junctional rhythm. Patients with this arrhythmia will usually maintain a heart rate of greater than 80 beats per min. If slower rates are observed, intravenous isoproterenol administration may be necessary to maintain adequate cardiac output. Atrial tachyarrhythmias also occur with some frequency and cardiac glycosides may be necessary; however, in many instances, the tachycardia will be transient and no therapy is required. Multiple ventricular premature contractions or ventricular tachycardia are encountered occasionally, and if persistent, are treated with xylocaine administered by intravenous infusion. Postoperative complete heart block is treated with surgically placed pacing wires. This complication, in our experience, has not occurred among infants.

Bipolar atrial and/or ventricular wires are implanted at surgery if an arrhythmia is recognized as an intraoperative complication, or considered to be a potential postoperative problem (e.g., following a Mustard procedure for transposition of the great arteries in an infant). These wires are utilized both for diagnosis and treatment of more complicated rhythm disorders.[34]

Myocardial Performance: Causes of congestive heart failure following cardiac surgery include: (1) primary respiratory failure; (2) serious arrhythmia, (3) myocardial injury; (4) blood loss; (5) hypervolemia; and (6) significant residual hemodynamic abnormality. Specific treatment related to etiology must be carried out as indicated. Cardiac performance will gradually improve, if corrective or palliative surgery has been adequate. Isoproterenol and digoxin are the two drugs most useful in the management of low cardiac output or decompensation in the early postoperative period. The former is the first choice in the presence of arterial hypotension or bradycardia, whereas digitalis is administered for the treatment of frank congestive heart failure. For diuretic therapy in infants, the newer more potent agents, furosemide or, less often, ethacrynic acid are almost exclusively utilized in the initial hours following surgery. Later, chlorthiazide and spironolactone may be administered for a chronic diuretic regimen.

Hematologic Status

In the operating suite, at the termination of bypass, freshly drawn citrated blood is given in small increments as indicated by arterial and venous pressures, until it is estimated that normal blood volume has been restored. Later, in the recovery room, fresh whole blood is administered to replace chest tube drainage and blood samples removed for laboratory analysis. When acute blood loss has abated and the hematocrit has stabilized, Plasmanate (Plasma Protein Fraction (Human) 5%, Cutter Laboratories, Berkeley, Calif.) is substituted to replace small losses.

A coagulation profile is obtained following termination of perfusion and again upon admission to the recovery room. In our experience, protamine has adequately restored the clotting mechanism following bypass, and coagulation defects have not presented significant problems.

Acid-Base Management

Metabolic acidosis secondary to low cardiac output, renal failure, or hypovolemia must be prevented or countered promptly. An arterial pH below 7.30 may result in a cyclic decrease in cardiac output with increasing lactic acid production, and is often the forerunner of a serious arrhythmia or cardiac arrest.[23, 35] Intravenous sodium bicarbonate is utilized for correction of acidosis (Table 1). One half of the total amount is given rapidly and the remainder administered slowly over 1–2 hr. Care must be taken to avoid hyperventilation as bicarbonate stores are replaced, since the resultant alkalosis may also precipitate a cardiac arrhythmia. In addition, the frequent preoperative use of diuretics may lead to postoperative metabolic alkalosis, which may be of sufficient severity to require treatment with arginine chloride.

Renal Function and Fluid Administration

All urine is collected via an indwelling urinary catheter. Volume is measured hourly and aliquots are sampled for specific gravity as determined by refractometry.

The immature status of the infant kidney,[36, 37] often compromised by congestive heart failure and further impaired by cardiopulmonary bypass,[38] may lead to significant problems in the postoperative period. Persistent anuria or oliguria indicates the presence of either poor cardiac function, hypovolemia or acute renal failure. Blood and fluid replacement or a cardiotonic regimen will rapidly reinstitute normal urine flow in the patients with hypovolemia or cardiac failure, respectively. However, renal failure, which occurs secondary to inadequate kidney perfusion during cardiopulmonary bypass, will require more prolonged management.[39] This syndrome has been seen with decreasing frequency as bypass techniques have improved.

The concern with fluid overload as it affects cardiac function, discussed earlier, must be balanced by the necessity for sufficient fluid administration to maintain a reasonable urine volume, which in itself, is protective against acute renal failure.[40] Administration of intravenous fluids is usually adjusted within the range of 70–120 ml/kg/24 hr, depending upon the cardiac lesion and venous and arterial pressures (see Cardiovascular). Determination of serum solids by refractometry as an estimation of hydration has been reported to be useful in the calculation of fluid requirements.[41] All fluids, including those necessary to maintain patency of the monitoring lines, are included in the input measurements. Fluid balance is continuously reassessed from a cardiovascular and renal viewpoint, and adjustments are made in the rate of intravenous infusion as necessary.

Globin pigments in the peripheral blood secondary to hemolysis have been recognized as an important etiologic factor in acute renal failure following prolonged use of the pump oxygenator. Thus, the presence of hemoglobinuria is considered to be an indication for diuretic therapy in order to keep urine flow adequate and prevent renal shutdown.[40] Chronic fluid retention secondary to poor cardiac function, as well as fluid overload following bypass, also necessitate the use of diuretic agents in the postoperative period. Furosemide is utilized to induce diuresis in the presence of congestive heart failure, but increased fluid administration and osmotic diuresis with mannitol may be more effective if cardiac failure is absent.

Electrolytes and Glucose

Sodium is routinely administered in 5% dextrose in water at the rate of 2 meq/kg/24 hr, and potassium is added to the intravenous fluid after urine flow is established (1.5–2 meq/kg/24 hr). Calcium gluconate is administered intravenously in the rare event of hypocalcemia.

Hypoglycemia has been observed in small infants who are in congestive heart failure or under stress.[42,43] Blood glucose is measured at frequent intervals, and 10–20% dextrose in water is administered if a significantly low level is detected.

Antibiotic Therapy

Prophylactic antibiotics are routinely administered to infants undergoing cardiac surgery. Although specific evidence regarding the efficacy of antibiotics in this situation is lacking, the rationale for prophylaxis seems reasonable.[44,45] The introduction of intracardiac "foreign bodies" such as sutures and patches, may leave the patient prone to endocardial infection in the early postoperative period, and once infection ensues in such cases, the prognosis for survival is poor.[46] Furthermore, cardiopulmonary bypass may alter host resistance[47] and repeatedly exposes the patient's entire circulating blood volume to environmental contamination.[44]

At this institution, antibiotic therapy for infants is routinely instituted with penicillin and kanamycin one day prior to surgery and continued for 5 days postoperatively. Subsequent alteration in the duration or choice of antibiotic treatment is based on specific indication. Bacterial endocarditis has not occurred postoperatively in the infant group of postsurgical patients at this institution.

RECOVERY PHASE

On the first postoperative day the chest tubes are removed and chest physio-therapy is begun. Extubation is considered if (1) the blood gases are normal on assisted ventilation, (2) the infant is alert, and (3) the cardiovascular status is stable. These criteria are usually fulfilled by the second or third postoperative day. Oral feedings are instituted after the infant has been extubated and is breathing without difficulty. Adequate time for uninterrupted sleep is provided. The need for digitalis or diuretic therapy is constantly reassessed and these agents are administered as indicated. In general, it has been our experience that if surgical intervention has successfully corrected or palliated the hemodynamic abnormality, the later postoperative period is one of rapid improvement of cardiac function to well beyond the preoperative status, without undue difficulties in management.

SUMMARY

The essential prerequisite for a successful outcome following surgery for infants with congenital heart disease, is an operation that achieves anatomic correction or palliation of the basic hemodynamic abnormality. In addition, however, careful perioperative medical management is required to prepare the critically ill infant for surgery, and to allow him to benefit from its technical accomplishment.

The goals during the preoperative period are twofold: to attain optimal cardiorespiratory status and to obtain an accurate diagnosis. Following surgery, physiologic data is meticulously monitored, and intensive supportive care is instituted.

This paper has presented an overall approach to perioperative care of the infant from the time that a congenital heart defect is suspected until the late post-surgical recovery period. The important aspects of management are outlined, and therapeutic problems during all phases of the pre- and postoperative period are discussed.

REFERENCES

1. Lambert, E. C., Canent, R. V., and Hohn, A. R.: Congenital cardiac anomalies in the newborn. Pediatrics 37:343, 1966.

2. Cooley, D. A., and Hallman, G. L.: Cardiovascular surgery during the first year of life. Amer. J. Surg. 107:474, 1964.

3. Fyler, D. C.: Diagnosis and treatment: the salvage of critically ill newborn infants with congenital heart disease. Pediatrics 42:198, 1968.

4. Stark, J., Hucin, B., Aberdeen, E., and Waterston, D. J.: Cardiac surgery in the first years of life: experience with 1049 operations. Surgery 69:483, 1971.

5. Segal, S.: Transfer of a premature or other high risk newborn infant to a referral hospital. Pediat. Clin. N. Amer. 13:1195, 1966.

6. Baker, G. L.: Design and operation of a van for the transport of sick infants. Amer. J. Dis. Child. 118:743, 1969.

7. Gersony, W. M.: Cyanosis in infancy: a practical diagnostic approach. Heart Bull. 20:8, 1971.

8. Burchell, H. B., and Ongley, P. A.: Supplement on complications of cardiac catheterization. Circulation 37:675, 1968.

9. Vaeghese, P. J., Celermajer, J., Izukawa, T., Haller, J. A., and Rowe, R. D.: Cardiac catheterization in the newborn: experience with 100 cases. Pediatrics 44:24, 1969.

10. Stanley, V., Hunt, J., Willis, K. W., and Stephen, C. R.: Cardiovascular and respiratory function with Cl-581. Anesth. Analg. (Paris) 47:760, 1968.

11. Dawes, G. S.: Fetal and Neonatal Physiology. Chicago, Year Book, 1968, p. 191.

12. Downes, J. J.: Resuscitation and intensive care of the newborn infant. Int. Anesth. Clin. 6:911, 1968.

13. Clark, H.: An evaluation of antibiotic prophylaxis in cardiac catheterization. Amer. Heart J. 77:767, 1969.

14. Gilladoga, A. C., Levin, A. R., Deely, W. J., and Engle, M. A.: Cardiac catheterization and febrile episodes. J. Pediatr. 80:215, 1972.

15. Bordalen, B. E., Wang, H., and Holtermann, H.: Osmotic properties of some contrast media. Invest. Radiol. 5:559, 1970.

16. Grieskin, A. B., Oetliker, O. H., Wolfish, N. M., Gootman, N. L., Bernstein, J., and Edelmann, C. M.: Effects of angiography on renal function and histology in infants and piglets. J. Pediatr. 76:41, 1970.

17. Gootman, N., Rudolph, A. M., and Buckley, N. M.: Effects of angiographic contrast media on cardiac function. Amer. J. Cardiol. 25:59, 1970.

18. Malm, J. R., Bowman, F. O., Jr., Jesse, M. J., Hayes, C. J., Steeg, C. N., and Gersony, W. M.: Techniques in management of infants requiring cardiopulmonary bypass. *In* Birth Defects: Original Article Series. Congenital Cardiac Defects—Recent Advances. Baltimore, Williams & Wilkins, 1972, p. 51.

19. Pierce, W. S., Raphaely, R. S., Downes, J. J., Waldhausen, J. A.: Cardiopulmonary bypass in infants: indications, methods and results in 32 patients. Surgery 70:839, 1971.

20. Hikasa, Y., et al.: Open heart surgery in infants with an aid of hypothermic anesthesia. Arch. Jap. Chir. 36:495, 1967.

21. Barratt-Boyes, B. G., Simpson, M., Neutze, J. M.: Intracardiac surgery in neonates and infants using deep hypothermia with surface cooling and limited cardiopulmonary bypass. Circulation 43 and 44: (Suppl. 1): 25, 1971.

22. Mohri, H., Dillard, D. H., Crawford, E. W., Martin, W. E., and Merendino, K. A.: Method of surface-induced deep hypothermia for open heart surgery in infants. J. Thorac. Cardiovasc. Surg. 58:262, 1969.

23. Downes, J. J., Nicodemus, H. F., Pierce, W. S., and Waldhausen, J. A.: Acute respiratory failure in infants following cardiovascular surgery. J. Thorac. Cardiovasc. Surg. 59:21, 1970.

24. Cheney, F. W., and Martin, W. E.: Effects of continuous positive-pressure ventilation on gas exchange in acute pulmonary edema. J. Appl. Physiol. 30:378, 1971.

25. Mellins, R. B., Chernick, V., Doershuk, C. F., Downes, J. J., Sinclair, J. C., and Waring, W. W.: Respiratory care in infants and children. Amer. Rev. Resp. Dis. 105:2, 1972.

26. Epstein, R. A.: A method of fixation of nasotracheal tubes in infants. Anesthesiology 33:458, 1970.

27. Aberdeen, E., and Behrendt, D. M.: Cardiac surgery in infants. Hosp. Manage. Suppl. 33:315, 1970.

28. Epstein, R. A.: The sensitivities and response times of ventilatory assistors. Anesthesiology 34:321, 1970.

29. Epstein, R. A.: Humidification during positive pressure ventilation of infants. Anesthesiology 35:532, 1971.

30. Sloan, H., Sigmann, J., Kahn, D., Stern, A., and Lennox, S.: Open heart surgery in infants: problems of extracorporeal circulation. *In* Cassels, D. E. (Ed): The Heart and Circulation in the Newborn and Infant. New York, Grune & Stratton, 1966, p. 364.

31. Hernandez, A., Goldring, D., and Hartmann, A.: Measurement of blood pressure in infants and children by the Doppler ultrasonic technique. Pediatrics 48:788, 1971.

32. Gersony, W. M., Bowman, F. O., Jr., Steeg, C. N., Hayes, C. J., Jesse, M. J., and Malm, J. R.: Management of total anomalous pulmonary venous drainage in early infancy. Circulation 43 (Suppl. 1): 19, 1971.

33. Bell, H., Stubbs, D., and Pugh, D.: Reliability of central venous pressure as an indicator of left atrial pressure. Chest 59:169, 1971.

34. Waldo, A. L., Ross, S. M., and Kaiser, G. A.: The epicardial electrogram in the diagnosis of cardiac arrhythmias following cardiac surgery. Geriatrics 26:108, 1971.

35. Talner, N. S., Sanyal, S. K., Gardner, T. H., Rivard, G., and Holloran, K.: The biochemical alterations associated with congestive heart failure in infancy. *In* Cassels, D. E. (Ed.): The Heart and Circulation in the Newborn and Infant. New York, Grune & Stratton, 1966, p. 162.

36. Strauss. J.: Fluid and electrolyte composition of the fetus and the newborn. Pediat. Clin. N. Amer. 13:1077, 1966.

37. Rubin, M. I., Bruck, E., and Rapoport, M.: Maturation of renal function in childhood. J. Clin. Invest. 28:1144, 1949.

38. Beall, A. C., Jr., Cooley, D. A., Morris, G. C., Jr., and Moyer, J. H.: Effect of total cardiac by-pass on renal hemodynamics and water and electrolyte excretion in man. Ann. Surg. 146:190, 1957.

39. Dobrin, R. S., Larsen, C. D., Holliday, M. A.: The critically ill child: acute renal failure. Pediatrics 48:286, 1971.

40. Powers, S. R., and Norman, J. C.: Renal failure following cardiopulmonary bypass. *In*

Norman, J. C. (Ed.): Cardiac Surgery. New York, Appleton-Century-Crofts, 1967, p. 467.

41. Haller, J. A., Jr., Talbert, J. L., White, J. J.: Monitoring massive fluid therapy in infants. Southern Med. J. 62:1334, 1969.

42. Benzing, G., Schubert, W., Hug, G., and Kaplan, S.: Simultaneous hypoglycemia and acute congestive heart failure. Circulation 40:209, 1969.

43. Schaffer, A. J., and Avery, M. E.: Diseases of the Newborn. Philadelphia, Saunders, 1971, p. 470.

44. Nelson, R. M., Jenson, C. B., Peterson, C. A., and Sanders, B. C.: Effective use of prophylactic antiobiotics in open heart surgery. Arch. Surg. 90:731, 1965.

45. Holswade, G. R., Dineen, P., Redo, S. F., and Goldsmith, E. I.: Antibiotic therapy in open heart operations. Arch. Surg. (Chicago) 89:970, 1964.

46. Gersony, W. M., and White, N. R.: "Patch embolization" following repair of ventricular septal defect. Amer. J. Cardiol. 26:315, 1970.

47. Engle, M. A.: Post operative syndromes. *In* Moss, A. J., and Adams, F. H. (Eds.): Heart Disease in Infants, Children and Adolescents. Baltimore, Williams & Wilkins, 1968, p. 1087.

Complete Correction of Cardiovascular Malformations in the First Year of Life

Brian G. Barratt-Boyes, John M. Neutze, Eve R. Seelye, and Marie Simpson

I T HAS BEEN FRUSTRATING for both cardiologists and cardiac surgeons to be unable to offer safe corrective surgery to neonates and infants with congenital heart disease when techniques using extracorporeal circulation have become routine in older children and adults. A glimmer of hope was raised by isolated reports of successful closure of ventricular septal defects, using miniaturized but otherwise conventional perfusion equipment and techniques;[1,2,3] but cardiologists have been slow to accept these results as reproducible, and have virtually insisted that the cardiac malformations of their neonatal and infant patients be palliated rather than corrected by the surgeon.[4]

Fortunately, it would now appear that intracardiac repair can be performed safely in neonates and infants, provided the heart is totally relaxed and completely empty of blood to allow accurate repair, and provided the duration of extracorporeal circulation is strictly limited to avoid metabolic and pulmonary complications. We have accomplished these ends by surface cooling the infant to low temperatures, correcting the defects during a period of total circulatory arrest and then rapidly rewarming the infant by a short period of total body perfusion.[5,6]

TECHNIQUE

Premedication consists of 0.1 ml/kg body weight of a mixture of pethidine 25 mg, chlorpromazine 6.25 mg, and promethazine 6.25 mg/ml. The infant is placed on a circulating water blanket, and anesthesia is induced by mask, using equal parts of nitrous oxide and oxygen plus 0.5%–1% halothane. Intravenous d-tubocurarine (1 mg/kg) is given and followed by insertion of an orotracheal airway and nasopharyngeal and rectal temperature probes. Ventilation is continued with nitrous oxide and oxygen and 0.5% halothane. Carbon dioxide (2.5%) is added to anesthetic and oxygenator gases at temperatures below 30°C.

Pressure monitoring lines are sited in the abdominal aorta and inferior cava via the left groin vessels, and cooling, which has already begun using the water blanket, is now accelerated by stacking plastic bags of crushed ice around the body, avoiding contact with peripheral parts. The ice bags are removed at 24°–25°C and the chest then opened through a sternal splitting incision. No important arrhythmia has occurred during the cooling phase.

The child is heparinized (3 mg/kg), the cavae taped and a single venous cannula inserted into the right atrial appendage, followed by a 10–12F catheter into

From the Cardiothoracic Surgical Unit, Green Lane Hospital, Auckland, New Zealand.

Brian G. Barratt-Boyes, M.B., Ch.M., F.R.A.C.S., F.A.C.S., F.R.S. (N.Z.): *Surgeon-in-Charge, Cardiothoracic Surgical Unit, Green Lane Hospital; and Professor of Surgery, University of Auckland, Auckland, New Zealand.* John M. Neutze, M.D., F.R.A.C.P.: *Cardiologist, Green Lane Hospital, Auckland, New Zealand.* Eve R. Seelye, B.A., F.F.A., R.C.S., F.F.A., R.A.C.S.: *Anesthetist, Green Lane Hospital, Auckland, New Zealand.* Marie Simpson, F.F.A., R.C.S., F.F.A., R.A.C.S.: *Anesthetist, Green Lane Hospital, Auckland, New Zealand.*

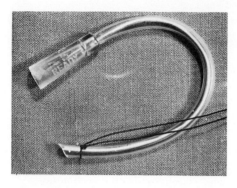

Fig. 1. A disposable plastic nasal suction catheter modified for use as the arterial perfusion cannula. A strong silk ligature is tied 5 mm from the obliquely cut tip and marks the depth to which the cannula is introduced into the aorta.

ascending aorta for arterial return (Figs. 1 and 2). These lines are connected to an infant perfusion circuit containing an efficient heat exchanger (Fig. 3) and primed with two units of fresh heparinized whole blood, to which 2 meq of potassium chloride and 5 meq of sodium bicarbonate are added. If the nasopharyngeal temperature has not by this stage fallen to a suitable level, total body perfusion is commenced at a flow rate of 100 ml/kg/min to complete the cooling, maintaining a temperature gradient of 6° C between the blood leaving the machine and the nasopharynx. In severely cyanosed infants, a short period of cooling perfusion is always used in order to oxygenate the tissues fully prior to circulatory arrest. At the appropriate temperature of 20°–24° C (depending on the expected circulatory arrest time) perfusion is stopped and blood drained from the infant into the machine to empty the heart and lungs. The caval snares are tightened and the aorta clamped above (distal to) the arterial cannula. The heart is now opened and the intracardiac repair carried out in a totally bloodless, completely relaxed heart.

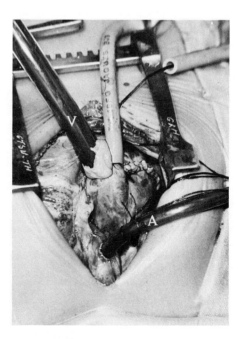

Fig. 2. Arterial (A) and single venous (V) perfusion cannulae in position in the ascending aorta and right atrial appendage, respectively.

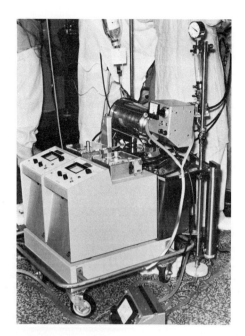

Fig. 3. **Extracorporeal circuit containing roller pumps, a disc oxygenator, and an efficient heat exchanger, which is mounted on the right of the machine.**

At the completion of the repair, air is flushed from the left heart by syringing isotonic saline solution through the left ventricle via a fine catheter introduced into the apex of this chamber, aspirating the solution through a connector on the arterial line and gently massaging the heart chambers. It should be noted that in patients with atrial baffle repair for transposition, the air is flushed from the right heart via the right atrial appendage and the venous return line moved to the left atrial appendage.

Rewarming bypass is now commenced and the infant rapidly rewarmed to 35° C. The temperature of the blood leaving the machine is rapidly raised to 30° C and within 3 min to 37° C and 2 meq potassium chloride plus 10 meq sodium bicarbonate are added to the circuit. The heart usually starts beating within moments of receiving warm blood, but if not, it is electrically defibrillated. Perfusion flows are kept at 100 ml/kg/min, and central venous pressure at 5–10 mm Hg to allow the contracting heart to contribute a normal arterial pulse (Fig. 4).

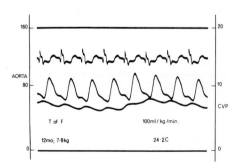

Fig. 4. **Aortic pulse contour recorded 4 min after commencing rewarming bypass at a flow rate of 100 ml/kg/min. The central venous pressure (CVP) at this time was 8 mm Hg.**

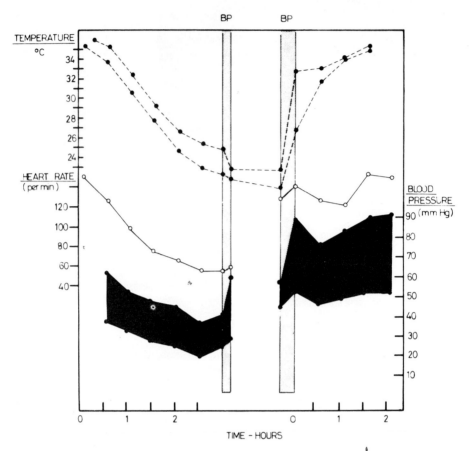

Fig. 5. Average changes in nasopharyngeal and rectal temperatures, heart rate and blood pressure in 40 infants up to 22 mo of age undergoing surface cooling followed by an average 5-min period of cooling bypass (BP), a 1-hr circulatory arrest period, and a 20-min period of rewarming bypass. Rectal temperature averaged 1.5°–2° C less than nasopharyngeal temperature. Changes in these variables have been plotted at 30-min intervals and at the beginning and end of the perfusion periods. During rewarming perfusion, blood pressure rose to normal levels within a few minutes (see Fig. 4).

At 35° C, perfusion is stopped and protamine sulphate given to neutralize the heparin. Central venous pressure is elevated to 10–15 mm Hg by giving blood through the arterial line into the aorta, and rewarming is continued with the water blanket during wound toilet and closure. To assist in rewarming the heart, the pericardial cavity is irrigated with warm Ringer's solution. The pericardium is drained with two tubes and left unsutured, and the pleural spaces are not drained unless they have been inadvertently opened. At the conclusion of operation the tubocurarine is reversed with an appropriate intravenous dose of a mixture of atropine 0.15 mg and neostigmine 0.3 mg.

This sequence is depicted in graphic form in Fig. 5, which shows average changes in nasopharyngeal and rectal temperatures, blood pressure, and pulse rate during cooling and rewarming for the first 40 infants under 2 yr of age.

POSTOPERATIVE CARE

The infant is moved from the operating room when the nasopharyngeal temperature returns to 35° C. Prior to this a chest x-ray is taken to ensure complete expansion of both lungs, and provided the respiratory and circulatory state are both stable, the orotracheal tube is removed. If assisted ventilation is considered necessary, a noncuffed plastic nasotracheal tube is inserted for this purpose.

In the intensive care area, infants under 6 mo of age are nursed in an incubator to maintain body temperature and supply a humidified atmosphere with an oxygen content of 30%–50%. In older infants, oxygen is given by a head cone or mask. A Bird respirator and a circuit with a reduced dead space (Q circuit) are utilized when assisted ventilation (IPPB) is required. During the first 12 hr, arterial blood samples are analyzed frequently for blood gases and potassium. Sodium bicarbonate is given if the base deficit exceeds 5 meq/liter and potassium chloride to maintain serum potassium levels between 4 and 5 meq/liter. Blood glucose is measured, but hypoglycemia has never been encountered.

Fluid requirements are met initially by intravenous administration of 2 ml/kg/hr of one-fifth normal saline in 4.2% dextrose until 1 meq/kg of sodium has been given and then changed to 5% dextrose solution. Lost blood is replaced with freeze-dried plasma and whole blood sufficient to keep central venous pressure between 5 and 10 mm Hg, since whole blood alone was found early in the series to produce too high an hematocrit, particularly in cyanotic infants.

Arterial and central venous pressures and also occasionally left atrial pressure are monitored continuously for 48 hr and, if necessary, longer. Indicator dilution cardiac outputs have not been measured during the postoperative period in these infants, for technical reasons. A urinary catheter is not used routinely but is inserted whenever there is doubt about urinary output or cardiac output. Isoprenaline infusion (0.5–1 microgram/min) is begun when a falling cardiac output is suspected and is used more frequently, therefore, than in older children and adults.

Oral feeding with water is begun on the evening of the first postoperative day, provided the infant is vigorous and not artificially ventilated and continued with increasing strengths of milk mixture. Digoxin and frusemide are given whenever there is evidence of a low cardiac output or fluid retention, but are not usually begun until the second day postoperatively, since during the first day or two isoprenaline, or sometimes adrenaline, are relied upon for circulatory support when this appears to be necessary.

METABOLIC ASPECTS

Physiological studies were made in 21 of the first 40 infants under 2 yr of age.[7] Arterial blood lactate, base deficit, pH and P_{CO_2} were measured at different stages of the procedure and whole-body oxygen consumption was calculated from the calibrated arterial pump flow and the arteriovenous oxygen-content difference. The blood lactate concentration was subtracted from the corresponding base deficit to yield the metabolic acid component not accounted for by lactate; this component is referred to as the residual base deficit.

Blood Lactate

During surface cooling, blood lactate was unchanged at a mean value of 1.45 meq/liter (SD 1.02 meq/liter). It rose slightly during the cooling bypass and more rapidly after the end of circulatory arrest and reached a maximum mean value of 5.68 meq/liter (SD 0.98 meq/liter) at the end of the rewarming bypass. Thereafter, except in one patient whose heart persistently fibrillated and who died, blood lactate began falling before the patient left the operating theater. At its height, therefore, the extracellular lactic acidosis was barely greater than the peak values reached in our adult patients during continuous total body perfusion with moderate hypothermia.[8]

Residual Base Deficit

As in our adult patients, big fluctuations were seen in the metabolic acid component not due to lactate. During the cooling bypass, residual base deficit fell by 11.0 meq/liter and during the rewarming bypass it rose by 11.3 meq/liter. In three infants who were surface cooled throughout, there was no significant change in residual base deficit during cooling, but a rise of 8.3 meq/liter occurred during the rewarming bypass. During final surface rewarming in all patients, there was no further significant change in mean residual base deficit. The observed changes do not appear to be artefactual and are thought probably to be due to hydrogen ion shifts between cellular and extracellular compartments.

Arterial pH varied during the operation between mean values of 7.29 and 7.43 (SD 0.08 and 0.05, respectively).

Whole-body Oxygen Uptake

The mean oxygen uptake during the cooling bypass was 1.26 ml/kg/min at a mean nasopharyngeal temperature of 22.9° C. Two minutes after the end of circulatory arrest, the mean oxygen uptake had risen to 3.73 ml/kg/min at 22.6° C. Oxygen uptake did not alter significantly from this higher value during rewarming bypass (mean duration 22 min) despite a temperature rise of 9.5° C. Internal evidence suggests that the oxygen uptake values obtained before circulatory arrest and at the end of the rewarming bypass were probably near to oxygen requirement. The uptake just after circulatory arrest, while the temperature was still low, indicates the repayment of oxygen debt incurred during the period of circulatory arrest.

The oxygen deficit incurred was calculated as the product of the mean oxygen consumption just before arrest and the mean duration of arrest in minutes (51 min). This value was compared with an estimate of lactate released up to 6 min after the end of circulatory arrest. The lactate "recovered" was only one-sixth of the expected amount; presumably the remaining lactate had yet to be washed out of ischemic tissues. It is surmised that this washout continued beyond the time when blood lactate began to fall at the end of the rewarming bypass; the higher body temperature and the establishment of natural circulation might be expected to increase the rate of lactate utilization considerably.

Table 1. Results of Corrective Surgery Using Profound Hypothermia From July 1969 to July 1971 *

Diagnosis	Age in mo			
	< 1	1–6	7–12	Total
VSD	0	8	3	11
Double outlet right ventricle	0	1	0	1
Partial atrio-ventricular canal	0	1	2	3
Total atrio-ventricular canal	0	2 (2)†	0	2 (2)
TAPVC	2	4 (1)	2	8 (1)
Truncus arteriosus	0	2 (1)	0	2 (1)
Tetralogy of Fallot	1	4 (1)	7	12 (1)
TGA	1	8 (1)	5	14 (1)
TGA + VSD	4 (3)	4 (1)	0	8 (4)
TGA + VSD + coarctation	2 (2)	1 (1)	0	3 (3)
Pulmonary atresia	2 (1)	0	0	2 (1)
Pulmonary atresia + VSD	0	1	0	1
Totals	12 (6)	36 (8)	19	67 (14)
Aortic stenosis	1 (1)	1 (1)	0	
Underdeveloped right ventricle	0	0	1 (1)	

* For abbreviations see text.

† Numbers in parentheses indicate hospital deaths.

RESULTS

All 67 infants operated upon during the first 2 yr of our experience with this technique, commencing in July 1969, are listed in Table 1. Three infants, two with aortic stenosis and endocardial fibroelastosis and one with an underdeveloped right ventricle had uncorrectable lesions. This was suspected preoperatively in each patient, and they are excluded from further analysis. Figure 6 graphs the ages and weights of the 27 acyanotic infants with a high pulmonary blood flow (including total anomalous pulmonary venous connection in this category) while in Fig. 7 similar data are shown for the 40 cyanotic infants. The causes of the 14 hospital deaths (within 3 mo of operation) are summarized in Table 2.

Fig. 6.   Weight and age and hospital mortality in infants with an increased pulmonary blood flow. Curved line represents third percentile weight averaged for boys and girls from the data supplied by the Children's Medical Center, Boston, Mass. Open circles, VSD; closed circles, DORV; open squares, partial AV canal; closed squares, total AV canal; open triangles, TAPVC; diamond, truncus arteriosus; and plus signs, hospital deaths.

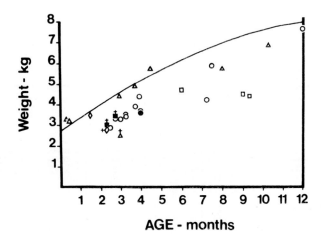

Table 2. Causes of Hospital Deaths in 14 Patients*

	Diagnosis	Age	Weight (kg)	Mechanism of Death	Time of Death
Surgical error	Total A-V canal	2 mo	3.0	Iatrogenic MI	2 days
	Truncus	2 mo	2.9	Iatrogenic PA stenosis and VSD	2 mo
	TGA + VSD	19 days	3.5	Iatrogenic TI	2 days
	TGA + VSD + PDA	4 wk	2.3	Ligation descending aorta	Operation
Pulmonary	Tetralogy of Fallot	6 wk	5.4	"Alveolar capillary block"	36 hr
	TAPVC	3 mo	2.5	Pneumothorax	36 hr
	TGA + VSD + PDA + hypoplastic arch	2 wk	3.3	Left lung collapse	24 hr
Tamponade	TGA + VSD	12 days	3.7	Clot lateral to right atrium	12 hr
Right heart failure	Pulmonary atresia	5 days	2.7	Unrelieved TS / Small RV?	7 hr
Uncertain	Total AV canal	2 mo	3.4	Low cardiac output	18 hr
	TGA	6 mo	6.2	Hypoxia	24 hr
	TGA + VSD	2 mo	3.4	Mucous plug?	6 days
	TGA + VSD + hypoplastic arch	11 days	3.0	Low cardiac output	15 hr
	TGA + VSD + PDA + coarctation	3 mo	4.2	?	Operation

* For abbreviations see text.

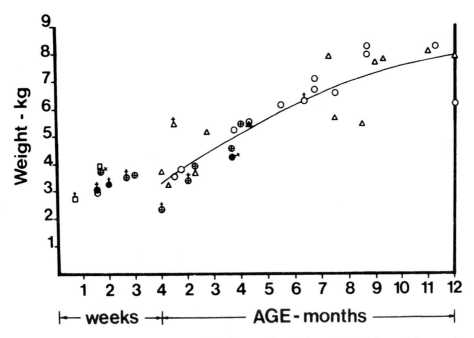

Fig. 7. Weight, age, third percentile weight line, and hospital mortality in infants with cyanosis. Open circles, TGV; partially closed circles, TGV and VSD; closed circles, TGV, VSD, and coarctation; open triangles, T of F; closed triangles, pulmonary atresia and VSD; open squares, pulmonary atresia; and plus signs, hospital deaths.

Table 3. Results of Repair of Ventricular Septal Defect Under Profound Hypothermia

Case No.	Age (mo)	Weight (kg)	Associated Defects	PA* (mm Hg)	Aorta† (mm Hg)	$Q_p^\ddagger/Q_s^\S$	PVR$^\|$	units (sq m)
1	2 1/2	2.9	ASD¶, PDA**	55	55	2.5		4.4‡‡
2	2 3/4	3.3		74	75	3		7
3	3	3.3	—	82	85	3		5‡‡
4	3 1/4	3.4	Coarctation	75	85	1.8		8
5	3 1/4	3.5	ASD dextrocardia	61	67	5		1.3
6	3 3/4	3.9	—	64	78	3.5		2.5
7	4	4.4	—	56	80††	2.5		3.0‡‡
8	4	3.7	PDA	75	75	4.5		2.5
9	7 1/4	4.2	—	52	88	3.5		2
10	7 1/2	5.8	PDA	60	100	4.5		1.5
11	12	7.6	—	82	84	2.3		4

* Pulmonary artery systolic pressure.

† Aortic systolic pressure.

‡ Pulmonary blood flow.

§ Systemic blood flow.

$\|$ Pulmonary vascular resistance.

¶ Atrial septal defect.

** Patent ductus arteriosus.

†† Femoral artery.

‡‡ Assumed oxygen consumption.

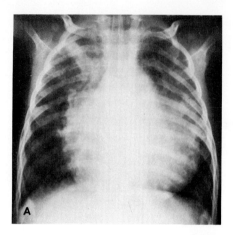

Fig. 8.   Chest x-rays of a 3-mo-old infant with
VSD (Case 6) 18 hr before operation, while on
IPPB, showing pulmonary edema (A), and 1 yr
postoperatively (B).

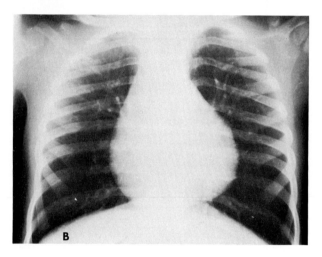

Ventricular Septal Defect (VSD)

These 11 infants are further detailed in Table 3. Closure of the defect was
undertaken in preference to pulmonary artery banding, and in all instances,
therefore, these children were in heart failure, which was not controlled by
digitalis and diuretics. All were under the third percentile for weight (Fig. 6).
At cardiac catheterization, pulmonary artery and aortic systolic pressures were
equal or within 10 mm Hg in seven (Table 3), and in five of these the pulmonary
vascular resistance was significantly raised (4–8 units-M^2). Cases 3 and 6 were in
frank pulmonary edema at the time of operation, and in Case 6 (Fig. 8) this was
treated by IPPB during the 24 hr prior to operation.

Other associated defects (Table 3) were closed at the time of operation, and
in Case 4 the coarctation had been repaired at 6 wk of age (Fig. 9). Case 11 was
the only example of multiple muscular defects, although the cineangiogram had
incorrectly suggested a double defect in one other (Case 9), and in both these
infants correction was postponed because of expected difficulties in repair and
in the hope that the shunt would lessen with growth. Repair in fact proved
straightforward.

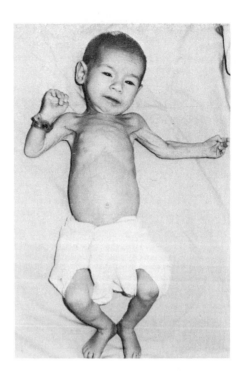

Fig. 9. A 3-mo-old infant with VSD and coarctation photographed before operation (Case 4, Table 3). This baby weighed 3.4 kg and was in severe heart failure that could not be controlled medically.

After VSD closure, which was performed through a ventriculotomy, right heart pressures fell to normal, or near normal, in all instances, and all infants survived operation and appear on clinical assessment to have satisfactory closure (Fig. 8). IPPB was required in two. One of these (Case 6) had been ventilated for 24 hr preoperatively and this was continued for a further 18 hrs postoperatively. In Case 5, IPPB was commenced following an unexpected cardiac arrest on the third day. While this child recovered and has normal cardiac findings, he is left with significant brain damage.

Atrio-Ventricular Canal

The three patients with partial A-V canal were in severe heart failure from a combination of a high pulmonary blood flow and severe mitral incompetence. They were markedly underweight for age (Fig. 6) and cachectic in appearance (Fig. 10), and as there was no palliative procedure available, their salvage by conventional repair (closure of the ostium primum atrial defect with pericardium and of the mitral leaflet cleft by direct suture) was as dramatic as any in the series. There were no postoperative complications. Clinical improvement was evidenced by reduction in heart size and pulmonary plethora (Fig. 11). Residual mitral incompetence is considered trivial in one and mild in two.

The two infants with total A-V canal were less fortunate, as both died postoperatively. Both had equalized right and left heart pressures due to a large ventricular communication and were in severe heart failure. The atrioventricular valve repair[9] was technically good in one infant, who was in extremis preoperatively, and died unexpectedly 18 hr postoperatively, but in the second the left atrial pressure tracing indicated important mitral incompetence, from which the baby succumbed after 48 hr.

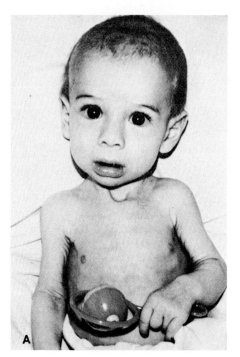
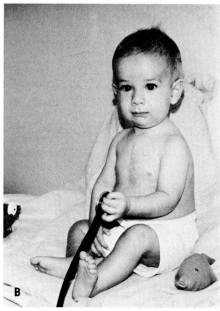

Fig. 10. Photographs of an infant with partial AV Canal. Preoperatively (A) this 6-mo-old weighed only 4.7 kg and was in severe heart failure with a pulmonary to systemic flow ratio of 3.3 and severe mitral incompetence. Three mo after operation (B) he weighed 6.9 kg.

Total Anomalous Pulmonary Venous Connection (TAPVC)

These eight infants ranged in age from 8 days–10 mo and in weight from 2.5–6.8 kg (Fig. 6). In two the anomalous connection was supracardiac, in four intracardiac and in two infradiaphragmatic. A 9-day-old baby had, in addition to TAPVC to the coronary sinus, an interrupted aortic arch with a large patent ductus arteriosus and a large VSD. All these defects were corrected successfully at one operation, using three periods of circulatory arrest.[10] One infant died

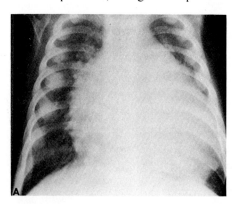
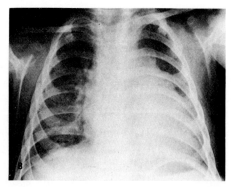

Fig. 11. Chest x-rays of a 9-mo-old infant with partial A-V canal and similar clinical findings to the child depicted in Fig. 10. (A) Before operation, (B) 14 mo after operation.

from the effects of a pneumothorax, which occurred during inexpert removal of the chest tube. Two required prolonged IPPB and tracheostomy, and one of these babies died later (4 mo postoperatively) from complications secondary to a tracheal stenosis. Autopsy in this child showed an excellent repair. The six surviving infants have had a good hemodynamic result.

Double Outlet Right Ventricle

This 4-mo-old infant was accurately assessed preoperatively, the cineangiogram showing a well-developed subaortic conus. She was in severe heart failure, and correction using a pericardial tunnel to direct flow from the left ventricle through the VSD and out to the aorta was carried out in preference to pulmonary artery banding. Recovery was uneventful.

Tetralogy of Fallot

The 12 infants with this anomaly ranged in age from 4 wk–12 mo and came foward for complete repair in preference to a palliative shunt because of cyanotic attacks. During the 2-yr period only one infant with tetralogy was shunted because, in this instance, it was inconvenient to stage an emergency profound hypothermic procedure. No patient was refused repair because of unfavorable anatomy. An outflow patch of pericardium was required in 7 of the 12 because of hypoplasia of the pulmonary ring and pulmonary trunk, and in one instance the patch was carried across the pulmonary artery bifurcation (Fig. 12). A woven teflon patch was used to close the VSD.

One 6-wk-old infant died 36 hr postoperatively from the effects of hypoxia. The lungs were difficult to ventilate during induction of the anesthetic and became progressively stiffer in the postoperative period in association with progressive cyanosis, despite IPPB with increasing concentrations of oxygen. Necropsy showed a good repair and did not elucidate the pathology in the lungs. It may be significant that in this infant in error, the gases in the ventilator were not humidified for the first 12 hr. One child remained in complete heart block for the first 8 days before reverting to sinus rhythm. IPPB was required for up to 36 hr in the four youngest patients, aged 4–9 wk, but not in the eight over this age.

All 11 survivors left the hospital in a satisfactory state and, with the exception of one who died later from unrelated epidemic diarrhea, have made good progress. None have a residual shunt on clinical assessment.

Transposition of the Great Arteries (TGA)

In Table 1 and Fig. 7, infants with TGA have been divided into three categories according to the complexity of the lesion.

Simple TGA: These 14 babies had an atrial baffle repair performed at varying intervals following balloon atrial septostomy. Two of the youngest, aged 11 and 55 days, had a large patent ductus arteriosus, and operation, which included ductus closure, was indicated because of persistent heart failure. The remainder had no other lesions and came forward for atrial baffle repair at this young age, either because of inadequate relief of cyanosis by septostomy (and as an alternative to repeat septostomy or septectomy) or, in most instances, electively.

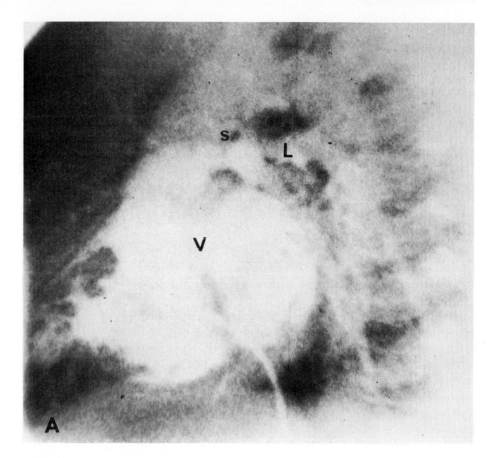

Fig. 12A. Left anterior oblique cineangiogram frame of an 8-mo-old infant with tetralogy of Fallot. This child had a severe infundibular stenosis (I) and a small pulmonary ring with distal tethering of the pulmonary valve leaflets producing supravalvular stenosis (S). The origins of the left (L) and right (R) pulmonary arteries were also hypoplastic. A pericardial patch was required to enlarge this region and extended from the distal right ventricle onto the origins of both pulmonary arteries. The large ventricular septal defect (V) is well seen.

There was one death 24 hr postoperatively, probably hypoxic in origin. This child was not artificially ventilated, arrested unexpectedly, and could not be resuscitated. One 55-day-old child remained in complete heart block for 8 hr postoperatively, and a 16-wk-old infant was first noted to have a left-sided weakness 2 mo postoperatively. This infant had a series of severe hypoxic spells preoperatively and it was suspected that he suffered a cerebral thrombosis at this time rather than cerebral damage at operation. There were no other significant complications and all have progressed well.

TGA and Large VSD: These eight infants, aged 12 days–4 mo, were in heart failure and in the six youngest, operation was an urgent matter (Fig. 13). Surgery consisted of closure of the VSD through a right ventriculotomy followed by placement of a pericardial atrial baffle through a right atriotomy. This complex repair was completed during a single circulatory arrest period, varying from 54–69 min at 20°C in six, but two separate periods of circulatory arrest separated by a 5-min period of perfusion were required in the other two.

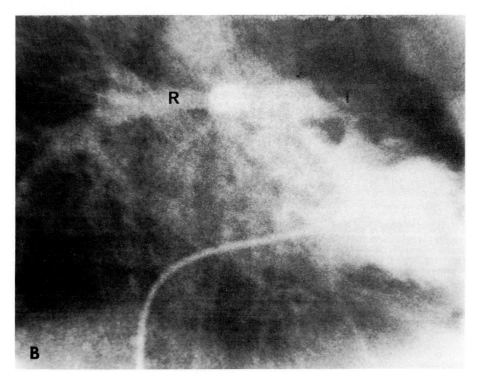

Fig. 12B. Right anterior oblique cineangiogram frame of same patient described in Fig. 12A. See legend of Fig. 12A for other details.

Four of the eight babies died and while three of these four deaths occurred in neonates, this factor may be fortuitous as each death was the result of an avoidable error in management (Table 2). Thus, the 12-day-old died from pulmonary venous obstruction from localized clot compressing the lateral right atrial wall;[11] the 19-day-old with an A-V canal type VSD, from surgically produced tricuspid incompetence; the 4-wk-old from massive pulmonary edema when cooling perfusion was commenced with a ligature around the descending aorta instead of the large patent ductus. The 2-mo-old infant arrested 3 days postoperatively, probably from a mucous plug in the main bronchus, and while he was being resuscitated, external cardiac massage was inadequately carried out, so that cerebral damage occurred, from which the child succumbed on the sixth day.

In two of these infants the VSD was very large, due to downward extension beneath the septal tricuspid leaflet (A-V canal type defect). As noted, one of these died from tricuspid incompetence because the teflon patch used in the repair proved too bulky and filled the crevice beneath the tiny septal leaflet. In the second such defect, therefore, pericardium was used for the VSD repair and this child has done well.

While complete heart block was common during the rewarming phase and periods of nodal rhythm not infrequent postoperatively, none of these babies presented rhythm problems. IPPB was used in four of the seven infants who left the operating room alive and two of the three who were not ventilated survived. One baby suffered a right phrenic palsy and subsequent right lower lobe pneu-

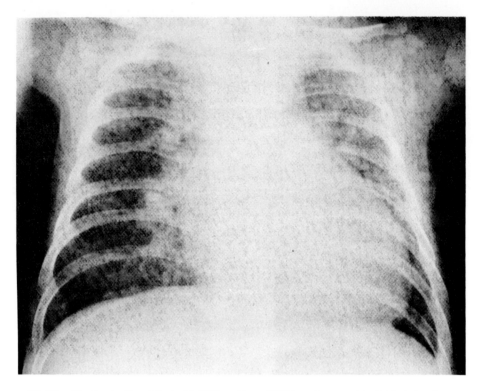

Fig. 13.   Chest x-ray of an infant with TGA and large VSD (age 4 mo, weight 5.4 kg) showing cardiomegaly and pulmonary plethora and representative of others in this category. Pressures were equal
in pulmonary artery and aorta, and there was severe heart failure. This child is now well.

monia, but there were no other respiratory problems. The four babies who left
the hospital have made good progress, although none has yet been restudied.

   TGA plus VSD plus Coarctation: These three babies presented an even more
formidable problem than those just detailed, but as our past results with coarctation repair and pulmonary artery banding in this group had been bad,[12] we
elected to attempt complete correction. All babies were in severe congestive
heart failure preoperatively and all died within 24 hr of operation (Table 2). In
two, the hypoplastic arch and coarctation were corrected 2 and 4 days prior to
the intracardiac repair (Fig. 14). In the third baby, the coarctation was repaired
first through a left thoracotomy with the child then being repositioned supine for
closure of the VSD and placement of the baffle through a sternal splitting incision, using two periods of circulatory arrest. This procedure was no more complex than that used successfully in the 8-day-old infant with interrupted aortic
arch and other anomalies referred to earlier,[10] and we therefore plan to continue with this approach.

Pulmonary Atresia

   The two infants with pulmonary atresia, an intact ventricular septum and an
apparently adequately developed right ventricle seen over this 2-yr period, both
came forward immediately for intracardiac correction. This consisted of closure

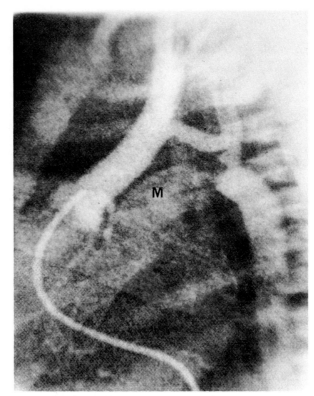

Fig. 14. Cineangiogram frame in lateral projection from an infant with TGA, large VSD and hypoplastic aortic arch (age 2 wk, weight 3.3 kg). The main pulmonary artery (M) is faintly outlined by flow through a patent ductus. The hypoplastic arch was corrected 4 days before the intracardiac repair by anastomosing the left subclavian artery to the side of the left common carotid artery. A dacron patch was also placed across the narrow aortic isthmus and coarctation.

of the patent ductus, wide opening of the atretic valve membrane through a pulmonary arteriotomy, excision of excessive muscular trabeculations in the right ventricular outflow and body through a limited transverse ventriculotomy, and closure of the atrial communication through an atriotomy. The tricuspid valve was examined, and if possible and appropriate, any leaflet fusion relieved.

The 5-day-old infant was left with a gradient across a small tricuspid valve (Fig. 15) but no gradient at pulmonary valve level. The effective right ventricular cavity was about two-thirds normal size and may have been too small (Fig. 16). This baby died 7 hr postoperatively in right heart failure, and, in retrospect, the atrial communication should have been left open.

The 11-day-old infant had a normal tricuspid valve and no gradient here or at the pulmonary valve level. The right ventricular cavity was virtually normal in size (Fig. 17). This infant remained in right heart failure for some weeks postoperatively, but 6 mo later is well and not requiring decongestive drugs.

Pulmonary Atresia with Large VSD and Truncus Arteriosus

Both these conditions require complete reconstruction of the right ventricular outflow and pulmonary trunk and are, therefore, considered together.

In a 4-mo-old infant with pulmonary atresia, the VSD was closed with teflon and the right ventricular outflow and pulmonary trunk reconstructed with a complete pericardial tube. This baby made an uneventful recovery and remains well, although the plain chest film suggests dilatation of the pericardial

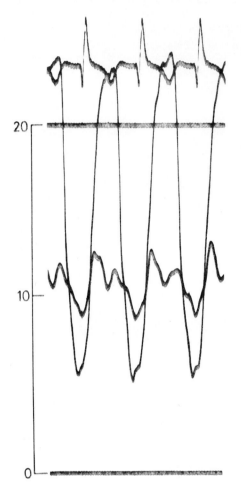

Fig. 15. Pressures recorded simultaneously from the right ventricle and right atrium at the end of operation in a 5-day-old infant with pulmonary atresia, who died postoperatively, showing an important gradient across the tricuspid valve.

tube. Encouraged by this experience, the next child to come forward, a Type II truncus arteriosus aged 9 wk, had a similar pericardial reconstruction. This baby redeveloped heart failure and required reoperation 2 mo later for stenosis at the distal pericardial anastomosis and a residual VSD. The pulmonary incompetence was not corrected at this second operation and this was at least partly if not chiefly responsible for the infant's death from right heart failure at the end of operation.

The next infant, aged 6 wk, with Type I truncus had a 16mm-diameter antibiotic sterilized aortic homograft valve and ascending aorta inserted to reconstruct the outflow. Recovery was uneventful. Since that time, two further infants (aged 1 yr and not included in the present series) have had a similar successful procedure. These grafts should be large enough to allow for considerable, if not complete, growth.

MORBIDITY

There has been no morbidity from postoperative bleeding or wound infection. A number of infants have developed tender matted areas beneath the skin of the

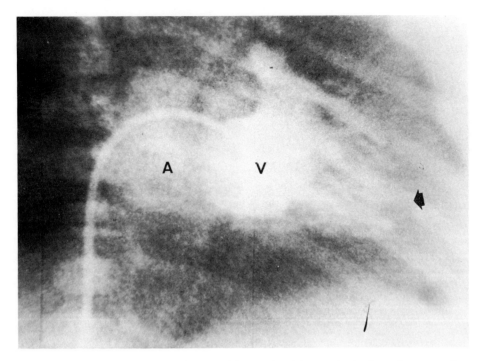

Fig. 16. Diastolic cineangiogram frame in right anterior oblique projection from the same patient as in Fig. 15. The effective right ventricular cavity (V) is smaller than normal as the portion adjacent to the apex (arrow) is heavily trabeculated. Coronary sinusoids were not demonstrated. There is some regurgitation of dye into the atrium (A).

front of the trunk in association with mild fever, and biopsy of one such area showed changes of fat necrosis. Spontaneous resolution has occurred in all instances.

Complete heart block has been common early in the rewarming phase, but in only two infants has it persisted for longer than a few hours. In one, with isolated VSD, it reverted to sinus rhythm on the first day, and in the other, with tetralogy of Fallot, on the eighth day.

Pulmonary Complications

A major advantage of this technique has been the virtual absence of major pulmonary problems, despite the fact that in many, recurrent respiratory infections were a preoperative problem and in some, infection had not been totally eradicated at the time of surgery. As noted in Table 2, only three hospital deaths were directly attributable to pulmonary complications, and pulmonary problems were unmanageable only in the infant with tetralogy of Fallot, who died of progressive cyanosis.

The aim has been to avoid IPPB whenever possible in the belief that intubation and ventilation carry a significant morbidity in the infant group. The number ventilated, either from the time of operation or subsequently (excluding those instances where IPPB was used only terminally) is shown in Table 4. IPPB was most often necessary in the neonatal group and was used in only 4 of the 40 infants over 2 mo of age. Two of these four required IPPB from the time of opera-

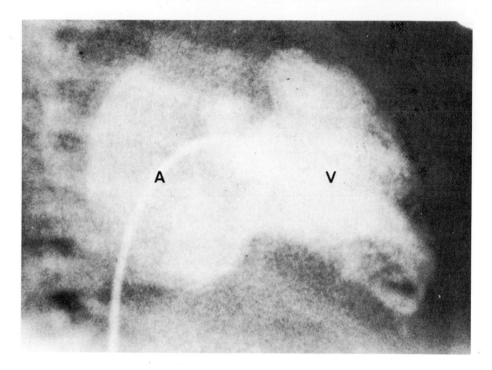

Fig. 17. Diastolic cineangiogram frame in right anterior oblique projection from an 11-day-old infant with pulmonary atresia who survived complete correction. The right ventricle (V) is virtually normal in size and in degree of trabeculation. The right atrium (A) is outlined by regurgitant flow from the ventricle.

tion, namely a 4-mo-old with TGA and VSD, who was slow in awakening, and a 3-mo-old with VSD, who had already been ventilated for 24 hr preoperatively. In the other two infants, ventilation was commenced on the first and third days for specific indications (development of pulmonary edema in a 4-mo-old with TAPVC and of cardiac arrest in a 3-mo-old with VSD).

There were 4 deaths among the 45 infants not ventilated, compared with 8 among the 20 who were. One of the former, attributable directly to total left lung collapse, which was present although unrecognized at the end of operation, could probably have been avoided if IPPB had been used. The practice of obtaining a chest radiograph in the operating room was commenced after this incident.

IPPB was required usually for less than 24 hr and in only two instances for more than a few days. Both these patients had TAPVC and were the only two requiring tracheostomy. In one, IPPB was required because of the onset of pul-

Table 4. Incidence of Assisted Ventilation (IPPB) in 65 Infants Leaving the Operating Room Alive

Age (mo)	IPPB	No IPPB	Totals
<1	9	2	11
1–2	7	7	14
3–6	4	17	21
7–12	0	19	19
Total	20	45	65

monary edema which gradually subsided in about 10 days, and was presumably due to compression or kinking of the pulmonary veins at the site of the posterior chamber anastomosis to the left atrium. In the second 8-day-old infant, with infradiaphragmatic anomalous drainage, IPPB was required from before the time of operation and it was never clear why he could not be extubated, although his postoperative course was complicated by severe diarrhea with failure to thrive. As already noted, this infant developed a tracheal stricture, from which he died at 4 mo of age.

Cerebral Complications

It was very difficult to assess the intelligence of many of these infants preoperatively, because they were severely ill, and intelligence testing has not yet been carried out postoperatively. However, the cerebral status has been questioned in only 3 of the 65 infants leaving the operating room alive. In two of these the cerebral state was not questioned until after resuscitation from cardiac arrest on the third day. One of these babies with TGA and VSD died on the sixth day, and the other with VSD alone shows severe mental retardation at 14 mo of age.

In only one instance was cerebral damage related either to the duration of circulatory arrest or to possible air embolization. In this infant preoperative development had been markedly retarded. She underwent repair of tetralogy of Fallot at 9 mo of age and required one 71-min period of circulatory arrest at 22°C. The development of uncoordinated movements and abnormal posture in the postoperative period indicated brain stem damage. These signs had disappeared by 5 wk, and at 16 mo of age developmental progress was encouraging, although physical milestones were still delayed. She could not crawl or pull herself erect, but could point to objects on request and was beginning to talk.

From our experience so far, it would appear that the maximal safe circulatory arrest time after surface cooling in infants lies between 60 and 65 min at 22°C and between 70 and 75 min at 20°C. When more than one arrest period is used, the safe interval is not known, but one infant has tolerated three periods of arrest of 25, 29, and 45 min duration at 22° C, separated by 5-7 min periods of perfusion at this same temperature.[10]

DISCUSSION

There have been two conditions only in which the result has been disappointing, namely total A-V canal and complex transposition. Nine of the total 14 deaths occurred in these two categories. If these two complex anomalies are excluded, there is a less marked difference in mortality with age than that depicted in Table 1, i.e. under 1 mo, six patients with one death (17%); 1–6 mo, 29 patients with four deaths (14%); and from 7–12 mo, 19 patients with no deaths. If patients in the second year of life are added to this last group and, although not included in this present series, in our view this is appropriate as they require surgical treatment with identical techniques, there were 36 patients aged 7–22 mo with three deaths (8%). While others reporting results of surgery in infancy have repeatedly emphasized a higher operative risk in smaller and younger babies,[13–15] our material does not really support an increasing risk factor with decreasing age and weight. Indeed, we suspect that once the detrimental effect of prolonged extracorporeal circulation is removed and ideal operating conditions are provided inside the heart, age becomes unimportant at least beyond the first month. Decreasing age assumes importance only in so far as it decreases the margin for error, both intraoperatively and postoperatively. Nearly all the deaths in this series were the result of avoidable error usually in the postoperative period and those that were not, bore little relation to the child's age or weight (Table 2). Moreover, only one death, in a 6-wk-old tetralogy of Fallot patient, appeared to be directly related to the perfusion.

There has been criticism of this technique on the grounds that surface cooling is too time consuming and inconvenient, and that the circulatory arrest period may result in cerebral damage. In our experience, the total anesthetic time in the under-1-yr-old patients seldom exceeds 4 hr and cerebral damage does not occur following surface cooling, provided the circulatory arrest time is closely related to nasopharyngeal temperature. The advantages of the technique lie in the operating conditions it provides for the surgeon, namely a totally bloodless, relaxed and still heart and in the short period of extracorporeal circulation required, regardless of the complexity of the heart defect. While it is clear from our experience and that of others, that infants can tolerate at least 1 hr of total body perfusion, it is probably true that the younger the child, the shorter the permissible perfusion time, and the shorter the perfusion the fewer the complications.

The alternatives to the method used by us are as follows: (1) Conventional bypass at normothermia or mild hypothermia without circulatory arrest. This does not fulfil any of the criteria just outlined, and despite miniaturization of equipment and attention to detail, has provided inferior results, particularly in complex conditions requiring longer perfusions.[13-15] Indeed, it is the cardiac surgeons' poor results with this technique that have convinced cardiologists that infants with tetralogy of Fallot and transposition must not undergo corrective surgery, and that pulmonary artery banding is preferable in isolated VSD.

(2) Profound hypothermia produced by bypass cooling (core cooling) rather than by surface means and followed by circulatory arrest and bypass rewarming. This technique has been used in older patients for many years,[16,17] and has recently been tried in infants with encouraging results.[18,19] Core cooling, however, approximately doubles the perfusion time to a total of 50–60 min and probably results in a greater metabolic acidosis than surface cooling. These could be important disadvantages in the neonatal group and the safe circulatory arrest time is not necessarily the same as that following surface cooling. The only advantage of this technique is a shortening of operating room and anesthetic time, which in small infants amounts to about 30 min. We are at present using this method in a group of infants to compare the metabolic changes with those found after surface cooling.[7]

(3) Surface cooling, circulatory arrest and surface rewarming. This method is advocated by Mohri et al.[20] but as used by them has the disadvantages of water-bath cooling and rewarming, explosive ether anesthesia, a prolonged anesthetic and total operating room time, and the need for manual cardiac massage during rewarming, which may damage the myocardium. The results obtained

may be superior to those using conventional perfusion, but the numbers operated upon are not sufficient to establish this point.[21] The metabolic data available with this technique[22] would indicate more severe metabolic acidosis than with surface cooling and bypass rewarming.

There is experimental support for the superiority of surface cooling combined with core rewarming over other methods of temperature manipulation.[23] Thus, with core cooling, core organs including the heart and liver are cooled rapidly, perfusion of the warm muscle mass is markedly reduced and the resultant temperature gradient persists to some extent throughout the period of arrest. A temperature gradient also occurs with surface cooling, but continued adequate cardiac output and liver function and more efficient cooling of the muscle mass limit the metabolic acidosis that occurs during the period of arrest. With bypass rewarming, cardiac output and liver function improve rapidly. Ballinger et al.[24] showed that a warm liver could correct the metabolic acidosis that results from cooling of the periphery. Our studies[7] showed rapid repayment of oxygen debt and early control of lactic acidosis during rewarming with the result that acidemia was minimized.

Based on the results reported here, some comments can be made on selection of patients for early correction.

In our view, one stage correction is clearly preferable to pulmonary artery banding in large VSD with uncontrollable heart failure, the one possible exception being an extensive "swiss cheese" anomaly with multiple perforations in the whole of the muscular septum. Despite the absence of surgical mortality in our VSD group, surgery is postponed if failure is controlled with decongestive therapy, in the hope that the defect will decrease in size with growth. In view of the risk of progressive pulmonary vascular disease and the continued morbidity in these patients, however, it is doubtful if this approach can be justified, and our future selection of candidates for operation in infancy may be less conservative Double outlet right ventricle can be regarded as a complex variety of VSD and, at least in its usual forms, can be handled in a similar fashion to uncomplicated VSD.

In TAPVC, palliative balloon atrial septostomy may not improve the clinical state, and even when it does appear to help, unexpected death can occur. For these reasons, early one-stage repair is carried out in all these infants regardless of their response to septostomy. The site of the amomalous connection has not affected the surgical mortality in this series, and it would seem that we can now look forward to a negligible mortality in this disease.

In tetralogy of Fallot, it is accepted practice in most clinics to delay intracardiac repair until 4 or even 5 yr of age and to use a shunt procedure in any infant who may demand relief of cyanosis.[25] This form of management stems from bad results with correction in infants using total body perfusion.[13] In contrast, our results would support a one-stage corrective approach, for the mortality has been considerably less than that which has followed palliation and a later second-stage repair. Indeed, review of the literature would indicate that the mortality of palliation in the neonate and infant with tetralogy is approximately 25%;[26] and this figure takes no account either of death during the subsequent waiting period or of morbidity from inadequate relief, strokes and cerebral abscess. Needless to say, corrective tetralogy surgery must first be learned in older patients, before it can be applied safely to the infant group.

In TGA the advisability of early corrective surgery is less controversial than in tetralogy of Fallot, for balloon atrial septostomy may not provide adequate palliation,[27] and there is an appreciable mortality and morbidity during the waiting period if repair is postponed until even 1 yr of age.[12] For these reasons we now carry out elective atrial baffle repair of simple TGA between 3 and 6 mo of age, and earlier than this if progress is unsatisfactory. In TGA with VSD, while the 50% salvage achieved is disappointingly low, early one-stage correction will probably prove preferable to septostomy and pulmonary artery banding, with later second-stage correction, at least in experienced hands. In TGA with a large VSD and pulmonary stenosis, early repair has not been attempted so far. However, followup of these infants indicates a disappointingly high mortality in the years following a palliative shunting operation[12] and corrective surgery might therefore be preferable at a younger age. Certainly the immediate results achieved following repair of truncus arteriosus and pulmonary atresia with large VSD using a homograft aorta and valve reported here, would indicate that a Rastelli procedure[28] would be feasible in the infant group.

SUMMARY

This article describes a surgical technique for correction of cardiac anomalies in infancy, which utilizes surface cooling to low temperatures, intracardiac repair during a 1-hr circulatory arrest period, and rapid rewarming by total body perfusion. The metabolic changes occurring with this technique and the postoperative management are detailed.

There were 14 hospital deaths among the 67 infants with correctable lesions operated upon in the first year of life (21%). For infants under 1 mo, the mortality was 50%, for those aged 1–6 mo it was 22%, and for those aged 7–12 mo it was 0%. Mortality was highest in two complex conditions, namely total A-V canal and transposition of the great vessels when combined with a a large ventricular septal defect (with or without coarctation of the aorta). If these two conditions were excluded, hospital mortality fell to 9%, and the apparent increase in risk with decrease in age became much less important.

Only one infant suffered cerebral damage from the circulatory arrest period, and this was minor. An important feature of the technique has been the virtual absence of major pulmonary problems.

In view of the results achieved, it is considered that one-stage correction is preferable to palliation, regardless of age, in almost all correctable conditions. In particular, this is so in large ventricular septal defect, total anomalous pulmonary venous connection, partial A-V canal, truncus arteriosus, and pulmonary atresia with large ventricular septal defect, tetralogy of Fallot, and transposition of the great vessels.

REFERENCES

1. Kirklin, J.: Ventricular septal defect with pulmonary vascular disease. New Zeal. Med. J. 64:34, 1965.

2. McGoon, D.C.: Treatment of septal defects in infancy and childhood. *In* Cassels, D. (Ed.): The Heart and Circulation in the Newborn and Infant. New York, Grune & Stratton, 1966, p. 332.

3. Sloan, H., et al.: Open heart surgery in infants: problems of extracorporeal circulation. *In* Cassels, D. (Ed.): The Heart and Circulation in the Newborn and Infant. New York, Grune & Stratton, 1966, p. 364.

4. Nadas, A. S.: Management of infants with ventricular septal defect, a controversy. Pediatrics 39:1, 1967.

5. Barratt-Boyes, B. G., Simpson, M., and Neutze, J. M.: Intracardiac surgery in neonates and infants using deep hypothermia with surface cooling and limited cardiopulmonary bypass. Circulation 43:25, 1971.

6. Okamoto, Y.: Clinical studies for open heart surgery in infants with profound hypothermia. Arch. Jap. Chir. 38:188, 1969.

7. Seelye, E. R., Harris, E. A., Squire, A. W., and Barratt-Boyes, B. G.: Metabolic effects of deep hypothermia and circulatory arrest in infants during cardiac surgery. Brit. J. Anaesth. 43:449, 1971.

8. Harris, E. A., Seelye, E. R., and Barratt-Boyes, B. G.: Respiratory and metabolic acid–base changes during cardiopulmonary bypass in man. Brit. J. Anaesth. 42:912, 1970.

9. Rastelli, G. C., Ongley, P. A., Kirklin, J. W., and McGoon, D. C.: Surgical repair of the complete form of persistent common atrioventricular canal. J. Thorac. Cardiovasc. Surg. 55:299, 1968.

10. Barratt-Boyes, B. G., Nicholls, T. T., Brandt, P. W. T., and Neutze, J. M.: Aortic arch interruption associated with patent ductus arteriosus, ventricular septal defect and total anomalous pulmonary venous connection. Total correction in an eight-day-old infant using profound hypothermia and limited cardiopulmonary bypass. J. Thorac. Cardiovasc. Surg. 63: 367, 1972.

11. Clarke, C. P., and Barratt-Boyes, B. G.: The cause and treatment of pulmonary oedema after the Mustard operation for correction of complete transposition of the great vessels. J. Thorac. Cardiovasc. Surg. 54:9, 1967.

12. Clarkson, P. M., Barratt-Boyes, B. G., Neutze, J. M., and Lowe, J. B.: Results over a ten-year period of palliation followed by corrective surgery for complete transposition of the great arteries. Circulation. 45:1251, 1972.

13. Ching, E., DuShane, J. W., McGoon, D. C., and Danielson, G. K.: Total correction of cardiac anomalies in infancy using extracorporeal circulation. J. Thorac. Cardiovasc. Surg. 62:117, 1971.

14. Cooley, D. A., and Hallman, G. L.: Surgery during the first year of life for cardiovascular anomalies: a review of 500 consecutive operations. J. Cardiovasc. Surg. (Torino) 5: 584, 1964.

15. Baffes, T. G.: Total body perfusion in infants and small children for open heart surgery. J. Pediat. Surg. 3:551, 1968.

16. Drew, C. E.: Profound hypothermia in cardiac surgery. Brit. Med. Bull. 17:37, 1961.

17. Belsey, R. H. R., Dowlatshahi, K., Keen, G., and Skinner, D. B.: Profound hypothermia in cardiac surgery. J. Thorac. Cardiovasc. Surg. 56:497, 1968.

18. Cartmill, T.: Personal communication, 1972.

19. Hamilton, D.: Personal communication, 1972.

20. Mohri, H., Dillard, D. H., Crawford, E. W., Martin, W. E., and Merendino, K. A.: Method of surface induced deep hypothermia for open heart surgery in infants. J. Thorac. Cardiovasc. Surg. 58:262, 1969.

21. Dillard, D. H., Mohri, H., and Merendino, K. A.: Correction of heart disease in infancy utilizing deep hypothermia and total circulatory arrest. J. Thorac. Cardiovasc. Surg. 61:64, 1971.

22. Baum, D., Dillard, D. H., Mohri, H., and Crawford, E. W.: Metabolic aspects of deep surgical hypothermia in infancy. Pediatrics 42:93, 1968.

23. Wolfson, S. K., Jr., Yalav, E. H., and Eisenstat, S.: An isothermic technique for profound hypothermia and its effect on metabolic acidosis. J. Thorac. Cardiovasc. Surg. 45:466, 1963.

24. Ballinger, W. F., II, Vollenvieder, H., Templeton, J. Y., III, and Pierucci, L., Jr.: Acidosis of hypothermia. Ann. Surg. 154:517, 1961.

25. Kirklin, J. W., and Karp, R. B.: The tetralogy of Fallot from a surgical viewpoint. Philadelphia, Saunders, 1970, p. 152.

26. Pickering, D., Trusler, G. A., Lipton, I., and Keith, J. D.: Waterston anastomosis. Comparison of results of operation before and after age six months. Thorax 26:457, 1971.

27. Tynan, M.: Survival of infants with transposition of the great arteries after balloon atrial septostomy. Lancet 1:621, 1971.

28. Rastelli, G. C., McGoon, D. C., and Wallace, R. B.: Anatomic correction of transposition of the great arteries with ventricular septal defect and subpulmonic stenosis. J. Thorac. Cardiovasc. Surg. 58:545, 1969.

Cardiomyopathies in Infants and Children

Leonard C. Harris and Quang X. Nghiem

IN THE PAST FEW YEARS increased attention has been devoted to the subject of myocardial disease in the pediatric age group. Pediatric cardiomyopathies are characterized by a high degree of morbidity and mortality.

There have been different approaches to the definition and nomenclature of the different myocardial diseases constituting the cardiomyopathies. A physiologic classification as proposed by Goodwin[1] does not commit one to a system that is dependent on an understanding of the etiology. It avoids the pitfall of using the term "chronic myocarditis" when referring to myocardial disease of obscure etiology. The authors have found it convenient to modify Goodwin's definition because of the different spectrum of myocardial disease in children when compared with adults.

In this communication the term "cardiomyopathy" is used to designate an intrinsic disease of the myocardium, which is not caused by shunts or valvular disease. Excluded from the cardiomyopathies are cases of known congenital morphologic anomalies.

The term "primary cardiomyopathy" is used to indicate disorders not known to be secondary to systemic disease, to disease in other organs or other systems. Usually the etiology is obscure.

The term "secondary cardiomyopathy" designates an intrinsic myocardial disease that is secondary to or associated with systemic disease, diseases of other organs or in other systems. Where myocardial disease coexists with skeletal muscle disease as in muscular dystrophies, the cardiomyopathy has been regarded as secondary, since the presenting and main clinical features usually are those of the skeletal myopathy. Also, the existing terminology of muscular dystrophy is well established. The course of the disease in the secondary cardiomyopathies usually is acute or subacute, rather than subacute or chronic as in the primary pediatric cardiomyopathies.

For the *classification of pediatric cardiomyopathies*, see Table 1.

PRIMARY CARDIOMYOPATHIES

Endocardial Fibroelastosis (EFE)

The disease is characterized by the presence of fibroelastic tissue over the endocardium. Usually the left ventricle, the left atrium, or both, are involved, and characteristically there is invasion of subendocardial tissue. The endocardial surface usually is covered homogeneously by a glistening white layer

From the Department of Pediatrics, Division of Pediatric Cardiology, The University of Texas Medical Branch, Galveston, Texas.

Supported by NIH Grant HE-49, 180 CR, and by Grants from the National Foundation Birth Defects Center and the Southeast Texas Health Foundation.

Leonard C. Harris, M.D.: *Professor of Pediatrics; Director, Division of Pediatric Cardiology, The University of Texas Medical Branch, Galveston, Texas.* Quang X. Nghiem, M.D.: *Associate Professor of Pediatrics; Assistant Director, Division of Pediatric Cardiology, The University of Texas Medical Branch, Galveston, Texas.*

Table 1. Classification of Pediatric Cardiomyopathies

Primary cardiomyopathies
  Nonobstructive
    Endocardial fibroelastosis of infancy
    Idiopathic non-obstructive cardiomyopathy
  Restrictive cardiomyopathy
    Hypertrophic type, with marked ventricular hypertrophy and small ventricular cavities
    Endomyocardial fibrosis (EMF of tropical type with endocardial destruction and dense fibrosis)
  Obstructive
    Idiopathic hypertrophic subaortic stenosis
Secondary cardiomyopathies
  Infective
    Virus
    Trypanosomal myocarditis
    Myocardial abscesses in bacterial endocarditis
    Diphtheritic myocarditis
  Of known metabolic etiology
    Glycogenosis type II (Pompe's disease)
  Associated with generalized neurologic or muscular disease
    Friedreich's ataxia
    Muscular dystrophy-Duchenne type.
  Collagen disorders
    Disseminated lupus erythematosis
    Dermatomyositis
  Neoplastic
    Leiomyofibroma
    Lymphoma
    Myxoma

that resembles an iced cake. The distribution, however, may be patchy. Endocardial fibroelastosis is often associated with congenital anomalies of the heart, particularly coarctation of the aorta, aortic stenosis, aortic atresia, or Pompe's disease. These types of EFE will be excluded from this review by definition. According to Blumberg and Lyon,[2] associated congenital anomalies are found in about $\frac{1}{4}$ to $\frac{1}{2}$ of cases. EFE of the left ventricle has been classified into two types: (1) the dilated variety with a large left ventricle; and (2) contracted type with a small or contracted left ventricle. In rare instances, there is fibroelastosis of the right ventricle. Endocardial fibroelastosis may involve the mitral, and, less commonly, the aortic valve.

Age Group: EFE is seen typically in the first year of life but cases have been reported at or beyond puberty. At this age, care must be taken to differentiate EFE from idiopathic nonobstructive cardiomyopathy or endomyocardial fibroelastosis.

Clinical Picture: Typically, infants with EFE develop symptoms between about 4 and 10 mo of age. The patient seems to be well until he develops signs of left heart failure, which may be preceded by a respiratory infection. No significant murmurs are heard initially, although mitral insufficiency and occasionally aortic insufficiency may subsequently develop. The chest roentgenogram shows cardiac enlargement, mainly of the left ventricle, and pulmonary venous congestion. The typical electrocardiographic picture is that of left ventricular hypertrophy with inverted T waves over the left precordial leads. Unusual electrocardiographic findings include signs suggesting myocardial infarction, first, second, or third degree heart block or various arrhythmias. [3]

Less commonly, the disease may present in the neonatal period. In these instances, EFE is more likely to be of the contracted type although the dilated type has been reported in the neonatal age group. In the contracted type of disease, the picture is often one of left-sided obstructive disease, particularly if the mitral valve is small. Left atrial pressure is elevated with pulmonary artery pressure near systemic arterial levels. The electrocardiogram[4] usually shows right ventricular hypertrophy with right axis deviation, but left heart overload may be seen.

The authors recently observed a baby who was born with massive ascites and pericardial effusion, as well as generalized edema. He had endocardial fibroelastosis of the left ventricle and died at approximately 36 hr of age. This was a case of cardiac failure in utero.

Diagnosis: The diagnosis is usually easily made due to the characteristic clinical findings, although atypical cases have been reported. The differential diagnosis includes anomalous left coronary artery, Pompe's disease, and acute myocarditis. Acute myocarditis is diagnosed mainly on the basis of clinical findings and associated electrocardiographic changes of tachycardia, small QRS voltage, and T and ST segment abnormalities. Most important, there are no signs of ventricular hypertrophy. The typical electrocardiogram and chest roentgenograms of Pompe's disease are seen in Figs. 1 and 2. In addition, the frog position and large tongue may point to this diagnosis (Figs. 3A and 3B). Anomalous left coronary artery is characterized by left heart failure. If infarction has occurred, shock or the signs of mitral insufficiency due to papillary muscle infarction may be present. The typical electrocardiogram of this condition is shown in Fig. 4.

Prognosis: Except for EFE presenting in neonates, when the prognosis is extremely poor,[5] the prognosis of EFE now appears to be more favorable than was thought a decade or more ago.

Some patients die within weeks or months of the onset. However, many survive the acute illness and live up to and through puberty. This course is more likely to occur when the disease presents in late infancy or in early childhood years. One of our patients with EFE first presented with cardiac failure at 2 yr of age, and initially responded to digitalis therapy. Mitral insufficiency appeared and its severity gradually increased until at 11 yr of age, mitral valve replacement was necessitated. Left atrial biopsy performed at surgery revealed endocardial fibroelastosis (Fig. 5). The patient has less cardiac enlargement than previously and pursues normal activities, short of strenuous exercise (Figs. 6A and 6B). This appears to have been a case of relatively mild endocardial fibroelastosis. Severe mitral insufficiency developed, presumably indicating that papillary muscle insertion in the left ventricle was situated high, resulting in a more transverse direction of traction on the chordae tendineae by the papillary muscles.[8]

Hemodynamic Features: The hemodynamic features have been studied by Lynfield et al.[9] and, more recently, by McLoughlin et al.,[10] who reported on 22 patients. In three of their cases, the diagnosis was verified by biopsy, the remainder being diagnosed on clinical grounds. Mean left atrial and mean pulmo-

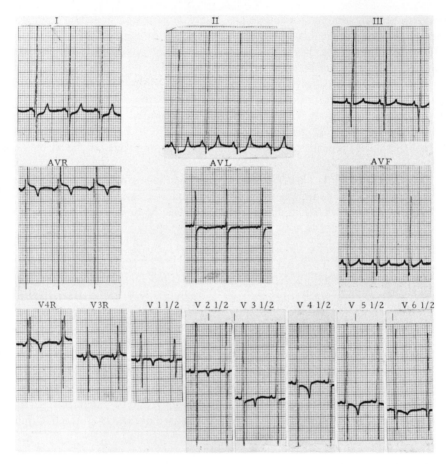

Fig. 1. Pompe's disease. Electrocardiogram of 5-mo-old girl. QRS voltage is markedly increased, indicating right and left ventricular hypertrophy.

nary artery pressures were moderately elevated. Both total pulmonary and pulmonary arteriolar resistances were increased in slightly more than half of the cases. Left ventricular stroke work was diminished in one third of the cases, and left ventricular dp/dt was diminished in all cases studied. Stroke volume at rest was low in only 9% of the cases. The ratio of left ventricular cavity to wall thickness was low in 75% of patients studied, indicating considerable hypertrophy in spite of dilated left ventricles.

Moller et al.[8] found that 14 of their 21 cases examined by left ventricular angiography had mitral insufficiency. Left ventricular volume appeared to change very little between systole and diastole in 14 cases. In more than 11 patients, systolic murmurs of mitral insufficiency were heard and in one half of these, apical diastolic filling murmurs, suggestive of mitral stenosis, were present. Mitral valvuloplasty in one case resulted in improvement.

Pathogenesis of EFE: Table 2 shows a summary of the most important theories regarding etiology of this condition.

Since some patients now are surviving the childhood years, the occurrence of

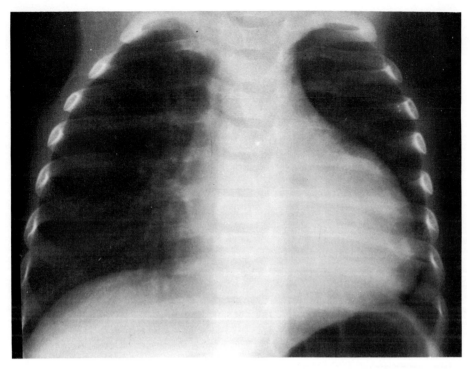

Fig. 2. Pompe's disease. Chest roentgenogram of same patient as in Fig. 1. Note the enlarged cardiac silhouette and the "left shoulder" contour of the left cardiac border, a sign of left ventricular hypertrophy.

mitral insufficiency is of great importance because it may limit patient survival in the adult years. The assumed mechanism is mentioned above. In addition, it is well known that when mitral insufficiency is marked, "mitral insufficiency begets mitral insufficiency," and its degree gradually becomes worse.

Recently Ainger[21] emphasized the occurrence of aortic insufficiency due to involvement of the aortic valve by the fibroelastosis. Prior to the development of mitral insufficiency the major hemodynamic abnormality appears to be impaired left ventricular contraction due to splinting by the fibroelastic layer. In addition, the subendocardium often is infiltrated by fibrosis, which tends to impair myocardial contractility. Left ventricular hypertrophy becomes marked[10] in spite of the degree of left ventricular dilatation present. While left ventricular hypertrophy helps to sustain cardiac output, hypertrophic muscle is less efficient than normal myocardium. Moreover, the benefit of hypertrophy occurs at the expense of elevated left ventricular end-diastolic pressure and volume, and the left ventricular myocardium operates progressively higher on the Starling curve. Eventually, when left ventricular wall tension is inadequate to sustain cardiac output, cardiac failure occurs.

Management: In caring for patients with EFE, digitalis should be continued several years after the disappearance of symptoms. This point is extremely important, since premature discontinuation of digitalis therapy in EFE can result in cardiac failure, which may not respond when digitalis is readministered. On the

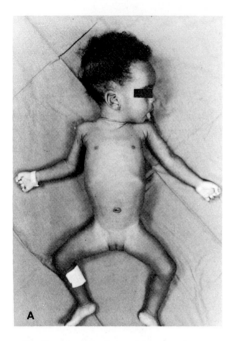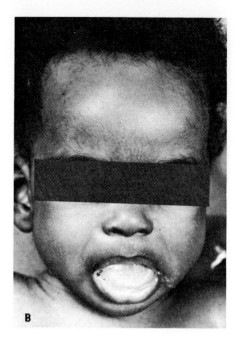

Fig. 3.   Pompe's disease. Same patient as in Figs. 1 and 2. Movement and tendon reflexes in both arms and legs were limited. Note the flaccid attitude and the large tongue. Cardiomegaly and hepatomegaly were present.

basis of past experience with rheumatic mitral insufficiency,[6,7] surgical replacement of the mitral valve may be indicated when estimated cardiac volume reaches at least twice the expected volume for age. Since subendocardial involvement is usually more extensive in EFE as compared to rheumatic mitral insufficiency, mitral valve replacement at an earlier stage may be indicated in EFE.

Idiopathic Nonobstructive Cardiomyopathy (INOC)

Stein et al.[22] first described this form of pediatric cardiomyopathy in 1964. At that time, the present authors had seen one patient with a cardiomyopathy similar to that described by Stein in South African Bantus. The clinical details and autopsy slides of this case were reviewed by Becker[23] who agreed that this disease was very similar to that seen predominantly in the Bantus in South Africa. INOC is very common in South Africa, accounting for 27% of all cases of heart disease among Zulus and 37.5% in urbanized Bantu in Johannesburg. We have studied nine cases in Texas. One patient was found at autopsy to have some atherosclerotic changes in the coronary arteries, and, although the disease had all the features of the congestive type of idiopathic nonobstructive cardiomyopathy her case was excluded from the series. This leaves eight cases that have been studied clinically, with cardiac catheterization, and in some cases, with angiographic procedures.[24,25]

Most patients presented with marked cardiac enlargement and failure, but no immediate clue as to cause could be seen. In some cases there had been a history of fever and pneumonia with several weeks or months of hospitalization for cardiac failure. A 5-yr-old patient presented with hemiplegia due to a cere-

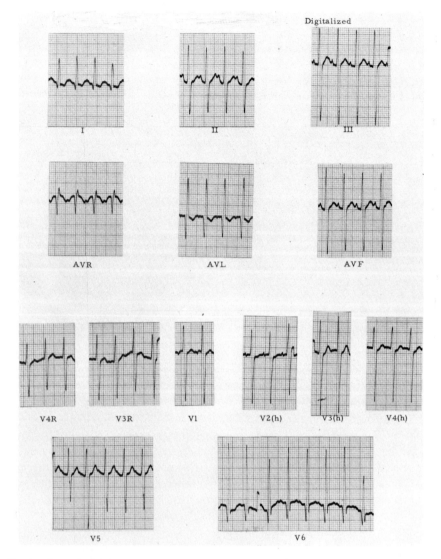

Fig. 4. Anomalous left coronary artery. Electrocardiogram of a 5-mo-old girl. Note wide, deep Q waves in AVL and V6. There was evidence of right atrial enlargement. Positive T waves over the right precordium were interpreted as reciprocal changes to T wave changes in V6.

bral embolus as the first sign of illness. Cerebral embolism occurred in two other cases in our series, being transient in one with disappearance of neurologic signs after 2 days.

Etiology of Idiopathic Cardiomyopathy: Theories as to the etiology of congestive idiopathic nonobstructive cardiomyopathy include:

(1) *Infective agent (Braimbridge et al.*[26]*).* Braimbridge et al. postulated an infective agent was responsible for this type of cardiomyopathy, after examining specimens of myocardium from seven patients with congestive cardiomyopathy. All specimens contained peculiar structures that were seen in only one of 120

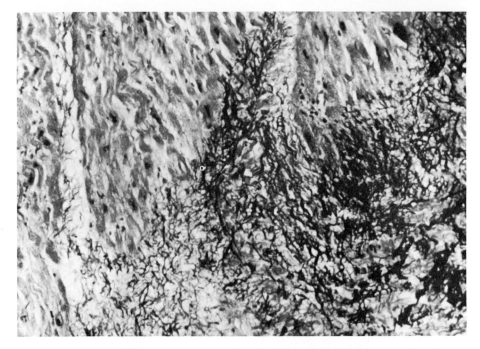

Fig. 5. Endocardial fibroelastosis: Left atrial biopsy of a black boy 10 yr and 9 mo old. Verhoeff-van Gieson stain. Note the irregular network of elastic fibers of different density, and interstitial fibrosis. This appearance is characteristic of endocardial fibroelastosis.

myocardial biopsies obtained from patients undergoing surgery for other reasons. The structures were recognized by their metachromatic staining and pleomorphism. The larger structures were called "mark bodies." The authors stated that the bodies grew in tissue culture, that injections of myopathic tissue into mice proved fatal and that chromatic particles could be observed in the mice. They claimed Koch's four postulates were fulfilled and thought the bodies might be an etiologic infective agent for cardiomyopathy. Rodin et al.[27,28] observed similar bodies in myocardial tissue from one child.

The theory of Braimbridge et al. has not been confirmed to date.

(2) *Deficiency of magnesium and potassium (Cadell[29])*. Cadell observed that endomyocardial fibrosis (EMF) occurred in members of low income groups who, because of malnutrition and chronic enteritis, were liable to have low magnesium and potassium. Selye[30] found potassium and magnesium administration to be effective in the prevention of myocardial necrosis in rats subjected to experimental stress. When deprived of potassium and magnesium and subjected to stress, the animals developed lesions like those commonly seen in EMF.

(3) *Genetic factors (Barritt and Al-Shamma'a[31])*. Barritt and Al-Shamma'a found a family history of heart disease in 4 of 11 cases of cardiomyopathy. One pair of siblings was seen in the present authors' cases.

(4) *Malnutrition (Gillanders[32])*. In South Africa Gillanders studied 30 cases of congestive cardiomyopathy in adult Bantus. Living on a deficient diet, the patients were malnourished. All recovered on a regime of digitalis, mercurial diuretics, yeast and normal diet. In 24 Bantu children with INOC, only one was

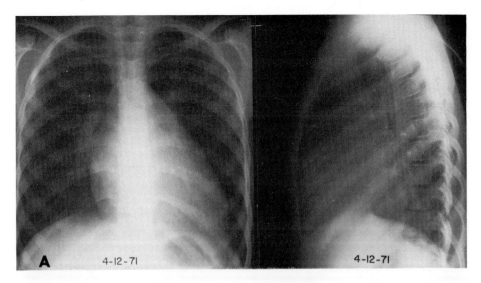

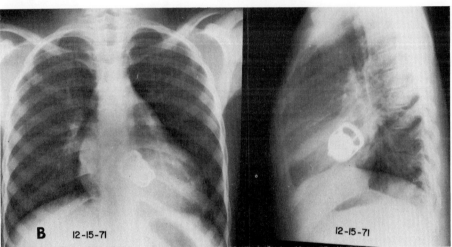

Fig. 6   Endocardial fibroelastosis. Same patient as in fig. 5. (A) The cardiac volume was 689 ml
or 98% above the upper limits of normal (95% confidence limits). Enlarged left ventricle, left atrium
and congestion in the right hilar area were evident. Patient required digitalis. (B) After mitral replacement, the cardiac volume decreased to 482 ml but was still 30% above the upper limits of normal. The largest reduction in size is seen on the lateral projection. The patient no longer needs
digitalis and his exercise tolerance has improved. Prognostic and hemodynamic significance of cardiac volume in the course of rheumatic mitral insufficiency has been studied.[6] In 6 children with
severe rheumatic insufficiency, who were not subjected to surgery, survival time was less than 2 yr
after the cardiac volume reached a figure of twice the normal value.[6,7]

found to be malnourished. This theory is unlikely to be the single cause of
INOC in children. Since INOC also occurs in well-nourished adults, malnutrition is unlikely to be a cause at any age.

(5) *Excessive plantain intake (Parry[33])*. Plantain is rich in 5-hydroxytryptamine,
and it was thought that INOC may be analagous to carcinoid heart disease.
Points against this theory are that 5-hydroxytryptamine does not reach the left

Table 2. Summary of the Current Theories of the Etiology of Endocardial Fibroelastosis (EFE)

Author	Date	Theory	Evidence For	Evidence Against
Kreysig [11]	1816	Fetal endocarditis		
Johnson [12]	1952	LV hypoxia	Foramen ovale frequently closed	May occur in absence of LV hypoxia
Keith, Rowe and Vlad [13]			Occurs with aortic atresia, but not with mitral atresia	Foramen ovale may be open and may be no obstruction to LV flow
Keith, Rowe and Vlad [13]	1968	Oxygen excess	Occurs more on left side, with patent mitral valve, and in non-cyanotic heart disease when associated with congenital cardiac anomalies	
Rosahn [14]	1955	Genetic factor—	High familial incidence	
Nielsen [15]	1965	autosomal recessive		
McKusick [16]		—	Described 6 siblings affected in one family in Amish tribe	
Fruhling [17]	1964	—	Occurrence in triplets; two identical members affected, one not affected. Occurrence in 1 pair of identical twins.	In 9 twin sets, only 1 affected in pair

Fruhling[17]	1964	Virus infection especially Coxsackie B 3 in utero or ex utero	High incidence of + myocardial cultures, mostly Coxsackie B in autopsied cases of EFE. 13 Positive cultures in 28 autopsied cases of EFE 113 Infants with suspected virus infections, 22 + cultures for Coxsackie. Passes placenta in animals. Histologic evidence of myocarditis in cases of EFE.	Some workers have found no histologic evidence of myocarditis in cases of EFE, e.g. Gross 1941, Himelfarb 1943.
Szanto[18]	1964	—		
Gerne[19]	1971	Mumps endocarditis	Chick eggs were inoculated with mumps virus. At 1 yr of age subendocardial fibroelastosis found in chicks. A woman known to have had mumps in 1st trimester had infant develop EFE at 22 mo of age.	
Black-Shaffer[20]	1957	EFE secondary to high wall stress which increases directly as the cube of the radius of the enlarged chamber		

side of the heart, where EMF may occur. In West Africa, plantain is not con-
sumed in large quantities, yet EMF occurs. Feeding plantain to patients does
not elevate 5-hydroxyindoleacetic acid excretion, and this theory has now
largely been discounted.

(6) *Deficiency of succinic dehydrogenase (Kobernick[34]).* Rodin, et al.[27,28] were
unable to demonstrate histochemically a deficiency of succinic dehydrogenase
in myocardial tissue obtained from a case of INOC. Normal dehydrogenase
activity was found in the myocardium of this patient. Other theories have been
listed previously.[25]

Pulsus Alternans[24]:   All of the cases studied by this group of investigators
had pulsus alternans at some time in the course of their disease. In one there was
a clinically undetectable 62mm difference between the peak pressure of large
and small beats resulting in the impression, when feeling the pulse, of marked
bradycardia. In addition, hypertension in the large beats was documented in
two patients (Figs. 7A and 7B). The degree of pulsus alternans as judged by the
difference between the peak pressures of large and small beats was variable in
the same patient. One patient improved simultaneously with disappearance of
pulsus alternans but died suddenly at home, and no autopsy could be obtained.
In two other patients, pulsus alternans disappeared with clinical recovery. This
physical sign is therefore not necessarily indicative of a grave prognosis. It is,
rather, an indication of myocardial dysfunction, which occurs most commonly
in progressive disease states. In one patient, pulsus alternans disappeared but
could be provoked by exercising the patient. The clinical recognition of pulsus
alternans may be extremely difficult, and frequently the diagnosis can only be
made with external carotid pulse recordings or cardiac catheterization. Pulsus
alternans appears to be an important and useful diagnostic sign of INOC of the
congestive type, but it is not pathognomonic for this cardiomyopathy, having also
been reported in one case of endocardial fibroelastosis.[21] By pacing the right
atrium and the right ventricle, it was shown that pulsus alternans could not be
abolished by changing the conduction path. However, its severity decreased during pacing, only to become worse when pacing was terminated. The end-diastolic volume was measured in three of the authors' patients and was found to be
extremely high. In other patients, evidence also indicated that end-diastolic
volume was much increased.

Hemodynamic Features: Our data have been reported previously.[24,25,27,28]
Pulsus alternans was concordant when both right and left heart pressures were
recorded. Cardiac output was normal or low at rest, increasing by an average of
40% in five patients to whom isoproterenol was administered intravenously,
largely, however, as the result of increased heart rate rather than increased
stroke volume. Pulmonary artery and right ventricular pressures were moderately elevated, the degree of elevation corresponding to the height of the left
atrial or pulmonary artery wedge pressure. Right atrial pressure was normal or
slightly elevated. Quantitative angiocardiography was performed in three children, and end-diastolic volume was markedly increased. Ejection fractions were
low.

Course and Prognosis of the Disease: Five of our eight cases pursued a fluc-
tuant but downhill course, eventually dying with chronic myocardial failure.

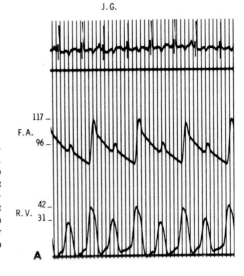

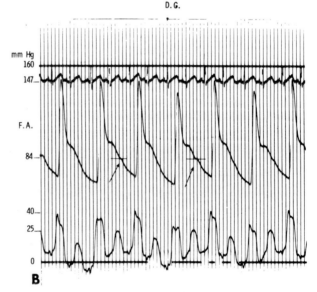

Fig. 7. Nonobstructive cardiomyopathy: Pulsus alternans occurring in two brothers. **(A)** J. G. aged 8 yr and **(B)** D. G. aged 5 yr. Note the concordance of pulsus alternans in right ventricular **(RV)** and femoral arterial **(FA)** tracings. At times the alternans was so severe that small beats were barely visible (arrows). When feeling the pulse this may be mistaken for bradycardia. (By permission of the American Heart Association, Inc.[24])

Two patients appeared to have recovered from the disease, are symptom-free, have no pulsus alternans and are able to carry out normal play activities. One of these had been estimated during cardiac failure to have a total cardiac volume[7] of twice the normal value estimated for his weight. In both of these patients the electrocardiogram returned to normal.

Prophylactic Use of Anticoagulants: In contrast to the cases of endomyocardial fibrosis occurring in Africa and other countries, the incidence of embolism in the congestive type of INOC is high. Correa et al.[35] found 14 cases with thromboembolism out of 28 autopsied cases with heart disease of undetermined etiology. Stein et al.[22] autopsied 12 of 14 fatal cases of INOC in children. Antemortem thrombi were found in the right ventricle in two and in the left ventricle in six cases. Higginson et al.[36] found intra-luminal thrombi in 48 of 80 patients of unspecified age, who were diagnosed as having the South African type of INOC. In the present series, three patients had cerebral emboli, and in two of these, emboli to other organs were also present.

Two of our patients were anticoagulated with sodium warfarin and maintained on anticoagulants in one case for 1 yr and in the other case for 3 mo. The sibling of one of these children had had a proven cerebral embolus, and the other patient had had a transient hemiplegia. Both children died of their disease, and neither showed any clinical signs of embolism during the periods of observation. Autopsy was obtained in only one of the two cases and revealed no antemortem thrombi in the heart. Therefore, it appears that further trials of anticoagulant prophylaxis are justified.

Histologic and Ultra-structural Changes: Histologic findings have been reported previously by Rodin et al.[25,27,28] and comments will be made only on our most recently performed study on a child with idiopathic nonobstructive cardiomyopathy. A biopsy of the right ventricle was obtained 1.5 yr before the child's death, and autopsy material was obtained 2 hr after death. Spindle shaped, metachromatic "mark" bodies[26,28] were present in myocardial tissue obtained from the left ventricle. Histochemical analysis revealed normal succinic dehydrogenase activity in the left ventricle.

Ultra-structural studies performed on right and left ventricular myocardium revealed some loss of cristae in the mitochondria. No comments can be made on these findings due to the possibility of postmortem autolysis. Thick, irregularly shaped Z bands were quite conspicuous. In addition, adjacent to an area of disruption and loss of myofibrils there was a small electron-dense mass resembling a portion of a degenerated Z band. Intercalated discs were irregularly arranged. Fibroblasts were seen in some areas containing collagen tissue.

Restrictive Cardiomyopathy

Biventricular Hypertrophy as a Restrictive Factor in Ventricular Filling: A 5-yr-old girl presented at the University of Texas Medical Branch with a history of recurring "asthma" followed by an attack of pneumonia. The jugular veins were distended and giant "a" waves were observed. In addition hepatomegaly was present. A grade III systolic murmur and a fourth heart sound were maximally heard at the apex. Electrocardiography (Fig. 8) showed evidence of marked biatrial enlargement, small anterior QRS forces, and left ventricular hypertrophy with depression of the ST segment over the left chest leads. First degree A-V block was present. In this patient cardiac catheterization showed tall "a" waves in both ventricles. No abnormal pressure gradients between the ventricles and their corresponding atria (Fig. 9) were present excluding mitral and tricuspid stenosis as possible causes of the tall "a" waves. Angiocardiography revealed a normal course of circulation with marked biatrial dilatation and decreased left and right ventricular cavitary volumes. This patient did not respond well to digitalis, and died at the age of 5 yr, 9 mo. Autopsy showed markedly dilated atria with small ventricular cavities and a thick interventricular septum. There was, in addition, a mild degree of interstitial fibrosis in both ventricles, which would be consistent with the presence of marked bilateral ventricular hypertrophy.

The possibility of this being a case of idiopathic hypertrophic subaortic stenosis

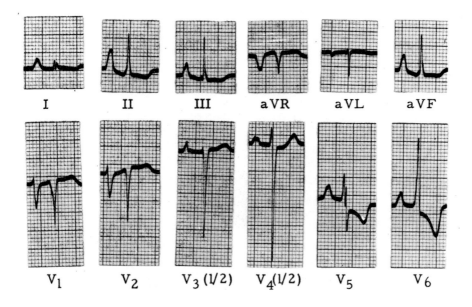

Fig. 8. Restrictive cardiomyopathy in a 5-yr-old white female. Electrocardiogram shows evidence of marked right and left atrial enlargement. QRS complexes suggest a left bundle branch conduction defect and/or left ventricular hypertrophy. (By permission.[25])

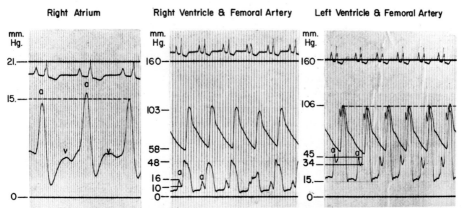

Fig. 9. Restrictive cardiomyopathy. Pressure tracing in a 5-yr-old, same patient as in Fig. 8. Note large "a" waves in the right and left ventricles, absence of pressure difference between "a" waves in the right atrium and right ventricle, and elevated ventricular diastolic pressure as in other forms of impedance to ventricular filling. (By permission.[101])

(IHSS) was considered. Isoproterenol was not administered to this child because of the severity of illness at the time the catheterization was performed. However there was no gradient in either ventricular cavity with the patient at rest and the degree of restriction to ventricular filling would have been unusual in IHSS, as would the very marked dilatation of both atria. This patient is regarded as a case of restrictive cardiomyopathy of unknown etiology. There was no family history of cardiomyopathy in this Caucasian family. No evidence of a similar case could be found in the available literature.[25]

Endomyocardial Fibrosis (EMF): Although Edington and Jackson[37] have questioned whether or not endomyocardial fibrosis and the congestive type of idiopathic nonobstructive cardiomyopathy are the same entity, there is now a great deal of evidence that these two conditions represent different disease states. Although the great majority of reported cases in Africa have been in native Africans, a number of cases have been reported in people of European descent, who have lived in the tropics, left that environment, and developed the first manifestations of the disease in a country in which this type of disease is not normally seen.[38] Brink and Weber[39] reported a case of EMF in a Caucasian who had previously lived in the Belgian Congo throughout his life and developed the manifestations of his disease while later living in South Africa. Brink found this to be a unique case in his extensive experience of cardiomyopathy in South Africa, concluding that these two diseases represented entirely different pathologic entities. In Africa, Parry[33] found the geographic distribution of EMF to be largely in the hot, humid areas. Cases occur in East, Central, and West Africa but not in North Africa or the more temperate areas of Southern Rhodesia and South Africa. Cases of EMF have been reported in Malaya,[40] Ceylon,[41] Colombia,[35] and Brazil.[42]

Incidence of EMF in children: The incidence of the disease in children is difficult to gauge because of scanty case reports. Parry[33] reported one case in a 6-yr-old, and Brockington[38] stated the disease usually affects children and young adults with death at an average age of 22 yrs. Males and females are equally affected. Cadell et al.[29] cited six children with EMF predominantly manifested in the right ventricle and associated with mitral insufficiency. The main features of the disease are dense fibrosis particularly in the apical and the inflow tract regions of one or both ventricles, with resultant restriction of ventricular filling, especially on the right side. In addition, the papillary muscles may be tethered by connective tissue invasion of the posterior leaflet of the mitral valve, thus causing mitral insufficiency. When the tricuspid valve is insufficient, ascites and pericardial effusion are common. When the right heart is involved right ventricular cavitary volume may be almost obliterated, with central venous tone being primarily responsible for the maintenance of circulation. On the left side, cavity volume is not reduced to a comparable extent, and mitral insufficiency may be severe. Since the endocardium is destroyed and replaced by fibrous tissue in endomyocardial fibrosis, there is a much smaller risk of thromboembolism than in INOC.

Although the etiology is obscure, some interesting observations have been made as to pathogenesis. Hearts with EMF show thickening of the walls of small coronary arteries, resulting in narrow lumina. These vascular changes are considered by Brink and Weber[39] (who cite Connors) to be the first morphologic alteration in hearts with EMF. Narrowing of the coronary arteries is thought to lead to gradual atrophy of the subendocardial fibers, which become replaced by fibrous tissue.

Idiopathic Hypertrophic Subaortic Stenosis (IHSS)

Idiopathic hypertrophic subaortic stenosis or obstructive cardiomyopathy was first described by Schmincke[43] in 1907. It is less commonly diagnosed in the pediatric age group but occurs in infants and even in neonates. It is characterized by hypertrophy of the ventricular septum and by thickening of the free wall of the left ventricle and sometimes the right ventricle, into which the interventricular septum may bulge. Endocardial thickening may be present on the hypertrophied left ventricular septum and on a part of the mitral valve lying opposite it. The hypertrophied muscle may result in outflow tract obstruction in one or both ventricles during systole. On the left side, obstruction may be aggravated by endocardial thickening. The anterior leaflet of the mitral valve may be relatively immobilized by endocardial thickening, resulting in mitral insufficiency.[44]

Structure of the Myocardium: Light microscopy[45] is reported as showing hypertrophied and disorganized muscle fibers with fibrosis of variable degree. Electron microscopy by Pearse[46] showed an increased number of degenerating mitochondria, and an excess of lysosomes. Muscle fibers were greatly hypertrophied and displayed shortening with atrophic changes. Electron microscopic examination of ten cases revealed an increase in the number of mitochondria and marked variability of sarcomere length.[47]

Etiology: The disease may be sporadic or familial, and evidence for a congenital etiology has been advanced. Neufeld et al.[48] described two cases, one in a stillborn baby and one in a 1-mo neonate. The authors have studied a case of IHSS first seen at the age of 2 wk. Daoud et al.[49] described a confirmed case in a 1-yr-old child with a 40 mm pressure difference between the left ventricle and the ascending aorta. Wood et al.[50] described three cases in siblings aged 3, 6, and 9 yr old. Diagnosis in the latter two was confirmed by cardiac catheterization. Braunwald et al.[51] reported nine cases with murmurs in the first years of life and three with murmurs in infancy. Several authors have reported typical murmurs at under 10 yr of age. It should be noted that occurrence early in life, and occurrence in siblings or families does not prove genetic origin.

Braunwald[51] reported a predominance of males in young patients. In the age group 6–10 yr, there were nine cases, all males, and in six patients aged 10–15 yr, one was a female. IHSS has been reported in Caucasians, Negroes and in one Chinese patient.

Symptoms: Congestive heart failure occurs only rarely with IHSS. Most commonly, the disease presents with a murmur in the second decade, but a similar mode of presentation in the first decade is not uncommon. Sudden death may occur in previously asymptomatic children. Early symptoms are exertional dyspnea, palpitations, chest pain, or syncope, usually in that order. Older patients are more likely to be symptomatic.

Physical signs are similar to those seen in adults. The pulses are usually characterized by a brisk upstroke and pulsus bisferiens, but they may be normal. In babies it is difficult or impossible to record exterior carotid tracings, but exterior brachial pulses of good quality can be recorded without difficulty in neonates.[52] Since the disease is most often diagnosed in children on the basis of abnormal auscultatory findings, it is appropriate to review these features. The heart sounds may be normal, but frequently the second sound exhibits wide or paradoxical splitting.[50] Midsystolic clicks have been described, and an apical systolic ejection murmur is typical. In patients with associated right ventricular obstruction, a systolic ejection murmur over the pulmonary area may be audible. In the presence of mitral insufficiency, the characteristic apical holosystolic murmur of this lesion is present. In addition, a double apical thrust is frequently palpated. Diastolic murmurs may occur but are distinctly uncommon.

Eelctrocardiographic Features: In children, the rhythm is typically sinus,

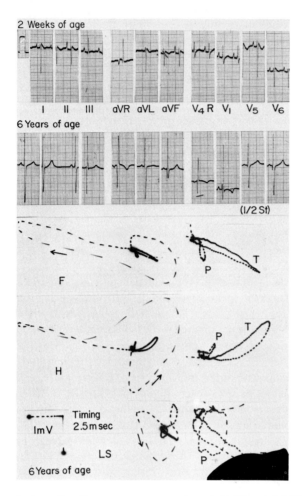

Fig. 10. Idiopathic hyperto- phic subaortic stenosis. Electro- and vectorcardiograms in in- fant aged 2 wk. In spite of se- vere left ventricular obstruction since infancy, patient had had signs of only right atrial en- largement and right ventricular hypertrophy from the age of 2 wk (upper panel) to 5 yr. At 6 yr, signs of left ventricular hy- pertrophy had become evident (lower panel). (By permis- sion.[102])

but as the disease progresses to adult life atrial fibrillation may occur. Electro- cardiographic signs of left ventricular hypertrophy with divergence of the QRS and T vectors are not uncommon. Deep Q waves in the lateral precordial leads frequently diminish with progression of the disease. Minimal criteria for the Wolff-Parkinson-White syndrome may be present. In infants electrocardio- graphic evidence of isolated right ventricular hypertrophy may be present despite severe left-sided obstruction (Fig. 10).[48]

Hemodynamics: The number of reported catheterized patients in the pedi- atric age group is small but four basic mechanical problems are characteristic: (1) Outflow tract obstruction in one or both ventricles; (2) impaired left ventricular filling due to either apposition of the anterior leaflet of the mitral valve with the interventricular septum in diastole or decreased left ventricular compliance re- sulting from left ventricular hypertrophy; (3) mitral insufficiency almost invari- ably present at some stage of the disease; and (4) decreased mechanical effi- ciency of the hypertrophied myocardium.

Pressure gradients as high as 85 mm Hg have been reported in children.[50] A notch may be seen on the ascending limb of the ventricular pressure curve, its height corresponding to peak pressure distal to the obstruction. Catheter entrapment may falsely elevate left ventricular pressures. This phenomenon demonstrates subendocardial pressures to be higher than intracavitary pressures and can be confirmed by selective angiocardiography (Fig. 11).

Pulsus alternans has been recorded in the body of the ventricle proximal to the obstruction.[51]

Course of the Disease: The course of the disease tends to be slowly progressive, but Nasser et al.[53] stress its variability. In general, children are less symptomatic than adults and often have a murmur for many years before symptoms occur. Occasionally there is spontaneous improvement.[45,53] Sudden death may occur in symptomatic or asymptomatic patients. An asymptomatic 11-yr-old patient of the authors had only a small pressure gradient in the right ventricle and none on the left side. He died suddenly during very strenuous activity and autopsy confirmed IHSS. Frank et al.[54] have also referred to sudden death in patients with small pressure gradients. It occurs equally in both the sporadic and familial type of disease according to Braunwald et al.,[51] but Goodwin[45] is of the opinion that sudden death is more common in familial IHSS. Bacterial endocarditis may affect the mitral valve.[45]

Management: The principles of medical management relate to the effect of interventions on ventricular volume and the contractile state of the myocardium.[45] Thus, if ventricular volume is decreased by blood loss, intraventricular gradients are increased but can be diminished by reinfusion. Increasing ventricular volume by hypervolemia or by systolic overload, as in peripheral vasoconstriction, increases ventricular volume and diminishes the tendency for intraventricular obstruction.

Increasing the power of contraction of the left ventricle exaggerates the pressure gradient. This may occur with exercise or by administration of digi-

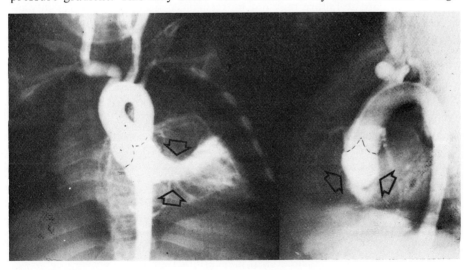

Fig. 11. Idiopathic hypertrophic subaortic stenosis: Same patient as Fig. 10 at age of 6 yr, now with recognizable phenotypic Turner's syndrome. Note the hypertrophic myocardium (arrows) forming an obstructive ring below the aortic valve (broken lines). Mild mitral insufficiency is responsible for slight regurgitation of contrast material into the left atrium. (By permission.[102])

talis or isoproterenol, which are contraindicated for the treatment of IHSS. β-Adrenergic stimulation provokes a gradient and β-adrenergic blockade reduces or abolishes the pressure gradient. Surgical therapy is indicated only if medical therapy with β-adrenergic blockade is unsuccessful. Recently, Shand et al.[55] reported the case of an infant treated with propranolol for 3 yr with improvement. They stressed the value of determining blood propranolol levels. Other than failure of propranolol treatment, indications for surgery are marked myocardial hypertrophy, ventricular gradients of greater than 50 mm Hg, or an "effective valve area" of 0.5–0.7 sq cm/sq m BSA or smaller.

SECONDARY CARDIOMYOPATHIES

Acute Myocarditis

Many infectious diseases may be accompanied by minor electrocardiographic changes in the absence of clinical manifestations of myocarditis. In this section, the authors will refer to myocarditis caused by known organisms in which signs and symptoms of myocarditis occur.

Viral Myocarditis

Myocarditis Caused by Coxsackie B virus: Although outbreaks of epidemic myocarditis in neonates have been recognized since before 1952,[56] Coxsackie B virus was first established as the typical cause in 1952, following a neonatal nursery epidemic in Southern Rhodesia.[57] Subsequently, Coxsackie B viral myocarditis was documented in reports from South Africa,[58] Holland,[59] and the United States.[60]

Although low grade diarrhea may be the first symptom, the onset is usually sudden, and is characterized by high temperature, tachycardia, collapse, cyanosis, and in some cases, cardiac failure. The disease is often fulminant, and in this situation cardiac failure may not be recognized because of the rapidity of the course of the disease. Gallop rhythm is not uncommon but murmurs are usually absent. The heart initially may be normal in size but dilates as the condition worsens. The electrocardiogram shows ST and T changes, low voltage QRS complexes, and tachycardia.

The diagnosis of myocarditis is made by the clinical and electrocardiographic findings. Often the case occurs in the context of an epidemic of myocarditis in a neonatal nursery. The virus may be cultured from feces, blood, or throat swabs. Neutralizing antibodies can be determined and the titer followed, this being of particular importance when more than one virus is cultured. The mother is the usual source of infection.

Neonatal Coxsackie myocarditis is associated with a high mortality. Javett et al.[58] described ten cases of whom four died, and Suckling and Vogelpoel[61] reported a 50% mortality in 8 neonates with Coxsackie myocarditis. Three of their survivors were reexamined at the age of 13 yr and were clinically, electrocardiographically, and radiologically normal. Sanyal et al.[62] reported the death of an adolescent due to Coxsackie virus myocarditis type 4.

Histology[58] shows a patchy or diffuse infiltration of pleomorphic cells. The inner third of the myocardium is most involved with a large number of mononuclear cells, a moderate number of histiocytes, a few lymphocytes, and other white cells. Granules resembling inclusion cells have been found in histiocytes. The myocardium shows areas where stain initially is not taken up. Longitudinal striations gradually disappear as transverse striations widen, but these too disappear, leaving homogeneous looking fibers, which then disappear, leaving empty sarcolemmal sheaths. Nuclear morphology demonstrates progressive pyknosis followed by complete dissolution. Changes may occur in both ventricles, atria, and the interventricular septum.

Burch et al.[63] examined the hearts of 50 children, obtained at routine autopsy. These patients ranged in age from stillborn to 4 yr, and histologic findings characteristic for myocarditis were found in 58%. Immunofluorescent antibody staining revealed evidence of Coxsackie B virus antigens in 24%. It is evident that Coxsackie B myocarditis is not uncommon although it is rarely recognized clinically.

Coxsackie viral myocarditis may result from infection of the myocardium in utero, which is not manifest until after birth. Burch[64] believes that a virus acquired in utero may lie dormant only to be activated later in life, causing clinical manifestations of myocarditis at that time. Whether myocarditis results directly from invasion of the myocyte or rather from a hypersensitivity reaction is not known. In utero viral myocarditis is a possible cause of still-birth.

Management: Digitalis and diuretics should be administered for cardiac failure, and therapy continued until the heart size is normal, since heart failure may recur when digitalis is discontinued.

Myocarditis Caused by Rubella Virus

Ainger et al.,[65] aware of persisting virus excretion after birth in infants with the rubella syndrome, sought evidence of active myocardial disease in affected neonates. Of 47 infants with the rubella syndrome, 10 had electrocardiographic evidence of "myocardial death, injury, and ischemia," the changes being observed within the first 10 days of life. Of seven infants with the picture of active myocardial disease in the neonatal period, four died. Three infants survived with evolutionary changes similar to those seen in myocardial infarcts in adults with subsequent healing. Three other neonates had electrocardiographic changes at birth indicating healed myocardial infarction, suggesting to the authors that healing had occurred in utero.

Rubella virus was isolated from many tissues but not from the heart. Van der Horst and Gotsman[66] described the case of a 17-mo-old male with hypoplastic pulmonary arteries with coarctations, as well as a patent ductus. In addition, there was an aneurysm at the apex of the left ventricle. Circumstantial evidence indicated rubella myocarditis as the cause of the aneurysm.

Histologic examination reveals extensive myocardial involvement with loss of cross-striation, swelling of fibers and nuclear pleomorphism. The myofibrils are granular and demonstrate vacuolization. The endocardium and epicardium appear normal.

Available facts suggest that: (1) Active rubella myocarditis occurs in utero; (2) it may heal in utero leaving a damaged myocardium; (3) the myocarditis may progress after birth, leaving varying degrees of myocardial damage; and (4) the myocardial damage may result in an electrocardiographic picture of

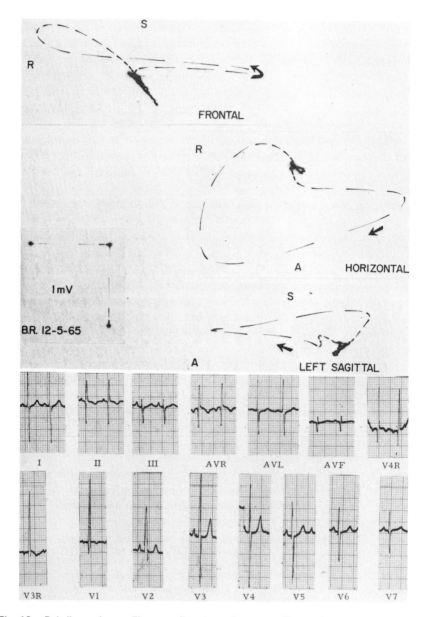

Fig. 12. Rubella syndrome. Electrocardiogram and vectorcardiogram in a neonate with patent ductus and cardiac failure. Note the initial counterclockwise loop and left axis deviation in the frontal plane in spite of evidence of right ventricular hypertrophy seen in the horizontal plane.

myocardial ischemia, injury or infarction, or conduction defect resulting in a counterclockwise loop with left axis deviation (Fig. 12).

The muscle may be weakened to such a degree that ventricular aneurysm results. In addition to myocardial damage, congenital cardiac anomalies often are present in the rubella syndrome.

Diagnosis: The diagnosis is suggested by the typical and reproducible clinical and electrocardiographic features. Serial studies of neutralizing antibodies usually confirm the diagnosis in young infants and the virus may be cultured from the nasopharynx, urine and blood.

Varicella Myocarditis

Varicella myocarditis is a rare condition which often has a rapid and fatal course. Moore et al.[67] described clinical myocarditis with heart failure in two children aged 16 mo and 2 yr. In these children, the signs of myocarditis were detected 3–4 days after the rash appeared. The clinical picture is characterized by severe vomiting, abdominal pain, tachycardia, gallop rhythm, and cardiac failure. Paroxysmal tachycardia may occur. Facial edema may be marked in young children with cardiac failure. Although the disease usually is acute, De Medeiros[68] described one case with a subacute course lasting 1 yr.

Focal perivascular round cell infiltration occurs, with occasional interstitial involvement and muscle fiber necrosis. Intranuclear inclusions in muscle fibers have been described. The diagnosis is made by observation of the typical chickenpox rash, isolation of the virus and by complement fixation tests.

Management: Diuretics are reported to be beneficial. Digitalis tends to cause toxicity[67] and indications for glycoside therapy are uncertain. If used, special precautions regarding toxicity are indicated. Moore et al.[67] recommend measuring central venous pressure as a guide to fluid therapy. The use of steroids is controversial, the objection being that fatal varicella dissemination has been reported with its use. Moore et al. used steroids in one patient who survived.

Myocarditis Caused by ECHO Virus

Bell and Grist[69] state that certain types of ECHO virus, notably 6 and 19, can cause myocarditis in humans. This is a less frequent cause of myocarditis than Coxsackie B virus. Maller et al.[70] recovered in high titer at autopsy, ECHO type 22 virus from the myocardium and pericardium of a 14-mo-old child. Pathologic studies revealed absence of plasma cells, and depleted immunoglobulins in the myocardial lymphocytic infiltration. This is a rare example of nonlymphopenic agammaglobulinemia with fatal ECHO viral infection and myocarditis. Cherry et al.[71] reported the case of a 7-wk-old infant with a diagnosis of paroxysmal tachycardia and electrocardiographic signs consistent with acute myocarditis, lasting for 15 mo. During the initial acute illness ECHO type 9 was isolated, and there was a rise in the serum antibody neutralizing titer.

Myocarditis Caused by Adenovirus

Henson and Mufson[72] described the case of an 11-mo-old child with an acute respiratory infection followed by cyanosis, collapse and cardiac arrest. The left ventricular myocardium was infiltrated with lymphocytes and plasma cells. Myocardial fibers were occasionally fragmented. Adenovirus 21 was isolated and neutralizing antibody titers supported the diagnosis of acute adenovirus myocarditis.

Trypanosomal Infections Causing Acute Myocarditis in Children

Myocarditis Caused by T. Cruzi: Chagas' Disease: Chagas' disease is caused by *Trypanosoma cruzi*, transmitted by *Triatoma infestans* or *Panstrong-*

ylus megistus, reduviid bugs that dwell in cracks in walls of primitively constructed houses in Latin America, where up to 7,000,000 people may be affected.[73,74] One case, with recovery of the organism has been described in the Corpus Christi area of Texas.[75] In other Southern states positive serologic evidence of infection has been found, and the reduviid bugs are present in Alabama, Georgia, Arizona and Florida.[75] For these reasons some of the Southern states are at risk.

The initial infection usually occurs in children. The infected bug bites the victim, usually on the face or mucous membranes, most commonly the eye or the mouth and this is followed by regional adenitis, usually preauricular, and unilateral bipalpebral edema. Symptoms are mild intermittent fever, sweating, muscular pains and at times diarrhea and vomiting. Weeks or months after the onset the heart may enlarge and cardiac failure may occur. Typically no murmurs are heard, but there may be a gallop rhythm and because of first degree block the first sound may be of diminished intensity.

The electrocardiogram shows tachycardia and premature atrial and ventricular contractions.

About 10% of cases are fatal in the acute stage, the cause of death being meningoencephalitis or cardiac failure. In patients surviving the acute stage, cardiomyopathy may occur after an interval of 10–30 yr. In Prata's[76] autopsy material, Chagas' disease was the cause of death in about 30% of all adults.

The diagnosis may be made in the acute stage by: (1) Typical clinical features; (2) Xenodiagnosis: "clean" bugs are fed on the patient and their feces examined for trypanosomes; and (3) Complement fixation tests may be positive within 6 wk of the onset.

Treatment: At least until recently there was no effective treatment. Mountain[77] reported the use in Brazil of an 8-aminoquinoline derivative known as 349 C 59. The results were regarded as promising.

Myocarditis Caused by Trypanosoma Rhodiense

The literature on African sleeping sickness makes little reference to myocarditis caused by *Trypanosoma rhodiense* in spite of its importance in determining the outcome of the disease.[78,79]

The clinical picture is manifested by evidence of "sleeping sickness" or encephalitis in Africa. A gallop rhythm and signs of cardiac failure may be noted and anemia may contribute to these findings. Electrocardiographically, T waves, ST changes, and a prolonged QT interval are noted.

The histologic picture[78,79] is characterized by myocardial hemorrhages, interstitial edema, mononuclear infiltration, and myocardial degeneration. The epicardium is thickened and shows cellular infiltrates which also occur in the coronary arteries and diffusely in the myocardium. Anitschkow cells and myocytolysis have been observed. In the end stages, mild fibrosis is present but not to the severe degree seen in Chagas' disease. Koten and de Raadt[79] note a general similarity between *Trypanosoma rhodiense* myocarditis and Chagas' myocarditis, which is of interest because both are *Trypanosomal* diseases. They mentioned specifically among their cases a child of 12 yr, and an infant 1-mo-old, who appeared to have had a transplacental infection.

Diagnosis is made by isolation of *Trypanosoma rhodiense* from the spinal fluid and by clinical and electrocardiographic findings of acute myocarditis.

Myocarditis Caused by Toxoplasma Gondii[5]

Toxoplasmosis may occur with or without an intact immunologic system and may be congenital or acquired. It may occur in families. The disease may be latent or overt.

Usually myocarditis is not recognizable clinically, being overshadowed by cerebral involvement, fever, and weakness. Disproportionate bradycardia, arrhythmias, cardiomegaly, or gallop rhythm may arouse suspicion of the diagnosis, which can be confirmed by electrocardiographic findings of T and ST changes, conduction defects or arrhythmias. In the neonate,[80] a dye test is a sensitive guide to toxoplasma infection. A dye test titer of 1:256 and a complement fixation titer of 1:32 are highly suggestive of a primary infection. At necropsy inoculation of tissue into animals may be performed. Pathologically, toxoplasma organisms are seen as minute ($5 \times 25\,\mu$ to $35 \times 100\,\mu$) basophilic masses within a pseudocyst in normal or damaged myocardial fibers. Cellular infiltration and interstitial fibrosis may occur.

A combination of pyrimethamine and triple sulfonamides has been advocated for treatment but effectiveness of this regimen has not yet been adequately evaluated.

Myocarditis Caused by Toxins

Diphtheritic Myocarditis: Diphtheria is still prevalent in the southwestern, western and northwestern portions of the United States. The incidence is greatest in nonwhites under 15 yr of age, usually unimmunized but sometimes partially or even fully immunized. In the latter the outcome is rarely fatal. In 1969 there were 254 reported cases of diphtheria in the United States with a mortality rate of 12.9%, and in 1970 there were 435 cases with a mortality rate of 6.2%.[81] In both 1969 and 1970, the greatest incidence was in the state of Texas. The great majority of fatal cases show electrocardiographic abnormalities which are a sensitive index of histologic changes.[82] Myocarditis is the most common cause of death[83] and since the diphtheria toxin has a special affinity for the conduction system, damage to it is the predominant feature of diphtheritic myocarditis.

Diphtheritic myocarditis is most reliably indicated by electrocardiographic changes. It occurred in 16.5%–84% of available recorded cases of diphtheria. Most observers, including the authors, find about one third of all cases of diphtheria have electrocardiographic abnormalities. The most common findings are ST and T changes occurring typically during the second week of the illness. In some cases ST and T changes are followed by right or left bundle branch block which in turn may precede total heart block (Fig. 13). Lesser degrees of heart block may occur. Arrhythmias, such as atrial or ventricular premature beats, supraventricular or ventricular tachycardia or atrial fibrillation are not uncommon. Occasionally the electrocardiographic pattern of myocardial infarction is present although these changes are completely reversible.[84] In about 50% of cases, electrocardiographic changes return to normal within 4 mo but

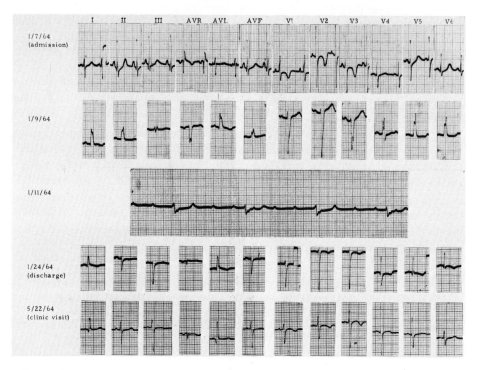

Fig. 13. Diptheritic myocarditis. A 5-yr-old boy. Within 48 hr after admission to the hospital, there was evidence of diminution of anterior forces, slurring of R-wave in V5-V6 with absent Q wave, slight ST depression and T inversion. Two days later (1/11/64) the patient had complete A-V block. He was successfully treated with intravenously infused isoproterenol to maintain an adequate heart rate. Three wk later, anterior forces were still diminished and inversion of T_{v_5}, v_6 was still present. Four mo later, the horizontal QRS axis had improved, T_{v_5}, v_6 being positive; the Q wave in v_5 was still absent.

in the remainder they may persist for up to 1 yr. Griffith and Herman[85] reported a case with persisting complete heart block.

Clinical signs, if present, are usually those of cardiac dilatation or a gallop rhythm. However, wide splitting of the first and second heart sounds occurs in right bundle branch block and signs of complete A-V block are easily detectable clinically.

Experimental studies have shown that diphtheria toxin alters protein and fatty acid metabolism in myocardial tissue. Burch et al.[86] studied the localization of toxin in the myocardium in a child who died of diphtheria on the 8th day. Widespread mitochondrial damage was seen by electron microscopy, although the probability of postmortem changes must be considered since the autopsy was performed about 2 hr after death. Large mononuclear and eosinophilic cells were seen in inflammatory areas. There was diminished activity of succinic and beta hydroxybutyric dehydrogenase activity, especially in conducting fibers. Diminished glycogen and increased lactic acid tended to occur with the prenecrotic phase of myofiber damage, in which there was a heavy accumulation of lipid droplets. These changes were not seen in normal or severely damaged fibers.

Immunofluorescent antibody staining showed diphtheria toxin to be mainly within large mononuclear cells in the necrotic areas; in myocardial fibers the distribution was patchy. Myofibrils were disrupted in scattered foci, leaving empty spaces.

In cases with ST and T changes the prognosis is usually good in the absence of involvement of the conducting system. In cases with right or left bundle branch block the mortality is about 50%. When total A-V block occurs, the mortality in four different series of reported cases averaged 84%, although in some series of cases all or almost all patients with complete heart block died. Examples are the reports by Stecher[87] wherein all of 19 cases died, and by Marvin and Buckley[88] with ten of eleven fatal cases. Therefore, this complication must be viewed with the utmost gravity.

Management: All patients with diphtheria should receive diphtheria anti-toxin and penicillin. Since the myocarditis is self-limiting, the approach to the patient with diphtheritic myocarditis should be one of intensive supportive care. If electrocardiographic abnormalities are already present, electrocardiograms should be performed daily until the patient is clinically stable. If no changes are present when the patient is first seen, electrocardiograms should be performed daily until the patient has passed the 3rd wk of the illness. If the electrocardiographic picture is changing, monitoring of the electrocardiogram should be continuous. Preparations should be made for the management of heart block if it should occur. This may involve intravenous infusion of isoproterenol by a pump at a rate of 0.03–0.08 μg/kg of body weight per min as necessary to maintain an adequate cardiac output. In one of our cases, isoproterenol was given for complete heart block with low cardiac output and was followed by conversion to sinus rhythm and later, recovery (Fig. 13). If isoproterenol is not effective in maintaining an adequate output, use of a pacemaker should be considered. Although the authors have no knowledge of pacemaker therapy in diphtheritic heart block, it has been used successfully in a patient with an assumed viral carditis with complete heart block.[89] In the authors' experience, overt cardiac failure without some degree of heart block or arrhythmias is not common. Congestive heart failure is preferably treated with diuretics rather than digitalis due to the increased sensitivity of the heart to cardiac glycosides during active diphtheritic myocarditis.

Intravenous lidocaine also should be available for treatment of ventricular tachycardia, which briefly preceded the death of another patient in the authors' series.

Muscular Dystrophy

Myocardial Involvement in Children: Progressive dystrophies consist of the Duchenne pseudo-hypertrophic type, the limb girdle dystrophy of Erb and facioscapulohumeral dystrophy (Landouzy-Dejerine). It may be impossible to differentiate the first two types.[90] The myocardium may be involved in the Duchenne dystrophy, but cardiac failure is rare during childhood.

Tachycardia is the earliest sign of cardiac involvement, arrhythmias may occur and murmurs are typically soft and heard best at the apex; but harsh murmurs may be heard at the pulmonary area. Perloff et al.[91] described the case of a 12-yr-old boy with Duchenne dystrophy, who had mitral insufficiency, attributed to papillary muscle dysfunction. Another child,[91] who had had Duchenne dystrophy since the age of 5 yr, died in cardiac failure at 18 yr.

The electrocardiogram may show tachycardia, a short PR interval, right, or commonly left ventricular hypertrophy. Abnormal Q waves may be seen in the left chest leads. Electrocardiographic abnormalities increase with age. Young patients may show minor changes or normal tracings. The Wolff-Parkinson-White syndrome may be present.[92]

Postmortem changes in children with Duchenne dystrophy rarely have been reported.[91] They consist of a flabby heart, slightly thickened and lengthened chordae tendineae and papillary muscles. Myocardial fibrosis and replacement of myocardial fibers by connective tissue may be seen but only on the left side. No specific treatment is available.

Generalized Glycogenosis (Type II) (Pompe's Disease)[93]

First reported[93] in 1932, and more recently reviewed by Nihill,[94] this rare disease is characterized by excessive deposition of glycogen in all tissues. Skeletal muscle weakness and involvement of anterior horn cells result in hypotonia, adoption of the frog position (Fig. 3A) and diminution or absence of tendon reflexes. The tongue is enlarged (Fig. 3B) due to glycogen deposition in about one-third of cases. Weakness of respiratory muscles results in recurrent respiratory infections, which may precipitate death. Involvement of the central nervous system may cause mental retardation.

Cardiac enlargement and failure may occur insidiously or be precipitated by a respiratory infection. Cardiac impulses usually are not forceful but the apex may be laterally and inferiorly displaced. Murmurs, present in about one-half of the cases, are systolic ejection in type and are possibly attributable to outflow tract obstruction. The electrocardiogram (Fig. 1) shows extremely tall, broad QRS complexes with a short PR interval (usually less than 0.09 sec). T wave changes may be present as well as left axis deviation in less than half of the cases. Chest roentgenograms show moderate to marked cardiac enlargement (Fig. 2). Endocardial fibroelastosis, and hypertrophy of the left ventricular free wall and septum with concomitant reduction in right ventricular cavitary dimensions are not uncommon.

The disease is known to result from a deficiency of acid maltase or 1–4 glucosidase, and the diagnosis is confirmed by documenting the enzymatic deficiency in lymphocytes, skeletal muscle or liver. The disease is transmitted as an autosomal recessive and is not sex-linked. Blood sugar is normal as are responses to epinephrine and glucagon. The heart usually is enlarged to a marked degree and cardiac failure is common. Light microscopy shows deposition of intracellular glycogen in the fibers, producing a lacework pattern. Electron microscopy shows the glycogen to be dispersed in the cytoplasm. Most patients with Pompe's disease die in the first year of life. Temporary improvement may result from the use of digitalis, but no effective definitive treatment has been found.

Friedreich's Ataxia With Myocardial and Coronary Artery Abnormalities[95]

Friedreich's ataxia is a hereditary, progressive degeneration of the posterior columns, spinocerebellar and pyramidal tracts of the spinal cord, brainstem and cerebellum. It may be associated with a cardiac condition apparently indistinguishable from IHSS, or there may be changes in the coronary arteries.

While the pathogenesis of the neurologic disease and the cardiac involvement is obscure, the characteristic central nervous system lesions are demyelinization and marked gliosis. Marked fibrosis is usually present in the myocardium with ventricular hypertrophy, vacuolization, or fatty degeneration of muscle fibers. Fibrosis of the conduction system and sinoatrial node may be noted. Medial hypertrophy and intimal proliferation of larger coronary arteries[96] and subintimal fibrosis in smaller vessels[97] has been reported. Recently, hypertrophic outflow tract obstruction has become known as a frequent association.[98-100]

Patients with Friedreich's ataxia and cardiac involvement may present with a systolic ejection murmur at the left sternal border, usually first detected near puberty. A third sound may be present and the heart noted to be enlarged. Chest pain due to coronary insufficiency has been reported but is not common.

Electrocardiographic findings include left or right ventricular hypertrophy, inverted or flattened T waves in AVF and the left precordial leads, and premature ventricular and atrial contractions. Atrial fibrillation and complete heart block have been reported.

Moore et al. described the case of a 9-yr-old child with Friedreich's ataxia and IHSS.[98] The pressure gradient in the left ventricle was exaggerated by administration of isoproterenol. Soulié et al.[99] catheterized the left ventricle in five children with Friedreich's ataxia. A pressure gradient within the left ventricular cavity was present in one at rest and in four after administration of isoproterenol. In two cases a pressure gradient within the right ventricular cavity was found. Similar findings have been reported in adults.[100]

In view of the possibility of IHSS or coronary artery abnormalities, cases of Friedreich's ataxia should be considered for cardiac catheterization, angiocardiography and coronary arteriograms. Medical or surgical treatment of IHSS may be mandatory.

CONCLUSION

The identification in 1952 of the Coxsackie virus as a cause of neonatal myocarditis, and subsequent demonstration that other viruses may similarly cause myocarditis represent discoveries which are presently beginning to broaden our knowledge of the pathogenesis of myocardial disease. This is especially apparent in rubella and Coxsackie viral myocarditis. The latter and the mumps virus appear to be able to cause EFE although additional causes are likely. It will be of great interest to follow cases of identified viral myocarditis to establish clearly whether or not they may cause "idiopathic" EFE, INOC and possibly EMF and other cardiomyopathies. Other etiologic factors, acting singly or in conjunction, have still to be investigated. The effects of stress on the myocardium and its control by magnesium and potassium require further study in population groups. Lack of knowledge as to etiology and pathogenesis must contribute to the high morbidity and mortality of the pediatric cardiomyopathies.

REFERENCES

1. Goodwin, J. F., Gordon, H., Hollman, A., and Bishop, M. B.: Clinical aspects of cardiomyopathy. Brit. Med. J. 1:69, 1961.

2. Blumberg, R. W., and Lyon, R. A.: Endocardial sclerosis. Amer. J. Dis. Child. 84:291, 1952.

3. Hastreiter, A. R., and Miller, R. A.: Management of primary endomyocardial disease. The myocarditis-endocardial fibroelastosis syndrome. Pediat. Clin. N. Amer. 11, 2:401, 1964.

4. Tingelstad, J. B., Shiel, F. O'M., and McCue, C. M.: The electrocardiogram in the contracted type of primary endocardial fibroelastosis. Amer. J. Cardiol. 27:304, 1971.

5. Rowe, R. D., and Mehrizi, A.: Myocardial disorders (cardiomyopathies). In The Neonate With Congenital Heart Disease. Philadelphia, W. B. Saunders, 1968, p. 265.

6. Harris, L. C., Nghiem, Q. X., and Schreiber, M. H.: Rheumatic mitral insufficiency in children: Course, prognosis, and effect of mitral valve replacement. Amer. J. Cardiol. 17:194, 1966.

7. Nghiem, Q. X., Schreiber, M. H., and Harris, L. C.: Cardiac volume in normal children and adolescents. Its application to patients with rheumatic mitral insufficiency. Circulation 35:509, 1967.

8. Moller, J. H., Lucas, R. V., Adams, P., Jr., Anderson, R. C., Jorgens, J., and Edwards, J. E.: Endocardial fibroelastosis. A clinical and anatomic study of 47 patients with emphasis on its relationship to mitral insufficiency. Circulation 30:759, 1964.

9. Lynfield, J., Gasul, B. M., Luan, L. L., and Dillon, R. F.: Right and left heart catheterization and angiocardiographic findings in idiopathic cardiac hypertrophy with endocardial fibroelastosis. Circulation 21:386, 1960.

10. McLoughlin, T. G., Schiebler, G. L., and Krovetz, L. J.: Hemodynamic findings in children with endocardial fibroelastosis. Analysis of 22 cases. Amer. Heart J. 75:162, 1968.

11. Kreysig, F. L.: 1816, quoted by Gross, P.: Concept of fetal endocarditis. Arch. Path. (Chicago) 31:163, 1941.

12. Johnson, F. R.: Anoxia as a cause of endocardial fibroelastosis in infancy. Arch. Path. (Chicago) 54:237, 1952.

13. Keith, J. D., Rowe, R. D., and Vlad, P.: Endocardial fibroelastosis. In Heart Disease in Infancy and Childhood (ed. 2). New York, McMillan, 1967, p. 858.

14. Rosahn, P. D.: Endocardial fibroelastosis: Old and new concepts. Bull. N.Y. Acad. Med. 31:453, 1955.

15. Nielsen, J. S.: Primary endocardial fibroelastosis in three siblings. Acta Med. Scand. 177:145, 1965.

16. McKusick, V. A.: A genetic view of cardiovascular disease. Circulation 30:326, 1964.

17. Fruhling, L., Korn, R., Lavillaureix, J., Surjus, A., and Foussereau, S.: Chronic fibroelastic myoendocarditis of the newborn and the infant (fibroelastosis). Ann. Anat. Path. (Paris) 7:227, 1962.

18. Szanto, P. B., Lacera, D., and Novak, G.: Fibroelastosis. An anatomic study. Quoted by Hastreiter, A. R., and Miller, R.A.: Pediat, Clin. N. Amer. 11:404, 1964.

19. St. Geme, J. W., Peralta, H., Farias, E., Davis, C. W. C., and Noren, G. R.: Experimental gestational mumps virus infection and endocardial fibroelastosis. Pediatrics 48:821, 1971.

20. Black-Shaffer, B.: Infantile endocardial fibroelastosis: A suggested etiology. Arch. Path. (Chicago) 63:281, 1957.

21. Ainger, L. E.: Mitral and aortic valve incompetence in endocardial fibroelastosis. Amer. J. Cardiol. 28:309, 1971.

22. Stein, H., Shnier, M. H., Wayburne, S., and Isaacson, C.: Cardiomyopathy in African children. Arch. Dis. Child. 39:610, 1964.

23. Becker, B. J. P.: Idiopathic mural endocardial disease in South Africa. Med. Proc. 9:124, 1963.

24. Harris, L. C., Nghiem, Q. X., Schreiber, M. H., and Wallace, J. M.: Severe pulsus alternans associated with primary myocardial disease in children. Circulation 34:948, 1966.

25. —, Rodin, A. E., and Nghiem, Q. X.: Idiopathic non-obstructive cardiomyopathy in children. Amer. J. Cardiol. 21:153, 1968.

26. Braimbridge, M. V., Darracott, S., Chayen, J., Bitensky, L., and Poulter, L. W.: Possibility of a new infective aetiological agent in congestive cardiomyopathy. Lancet 1:71, 1967.

27. Rodin, A. E., Harris, L. C., and Nghiem, Q. X.: Idiopathic, non-obstructive cardiomyopathy. Electron microscopic, histochemical and autopsy observations. Arch. Path. (Chicago) 91:62, 1971.

28. —, —, and —: Pediatric cardiomyopathies. J. Molec. Cell Cardiol. 3:63, 1971.

29. Cadell, J. L., Warley, A., Connor, D. H., D'Arbella, P.G., and Billinghurst, J.R.: Acquired heart disease in Ugandan children. Brit. Heart J. 28:759, 1966.

30. Selye, H.: Pathogens and conditioning factors. In The Chemical Prevention of Cardiac Necrosis. New York, The Ronald Press, 1958, p. 157.

31. Barritt, D. W., and Al-Shamma'a M.: Heart failure from unexplained cardiomyopathy. Brit. Heart J. 28:674, 1966.

32. Gillanders, A. D.: Nutritional heart disease. Brit. Heart J. 13:177, 1951.

33. Parry, E. H. O.: Endomyocardial fibrosis. In Ciba Foundation Symposium on Cardiomyopathies. Vol. I. Boston, Little, Brown, 1964, p. 322.

34. Kobernick, S. D., Mandell, G. H., Zirkin, R. M., and Hashimoto, Y.: Succinic dehydrogenase deficiency in idiopathic cardiomegaly. Amer. J. Path. 43:661, 1963.

35. Correa, P., Restrepo, C., and Quiroz, A. C.: Pathology of heart diseases of undetermined etiology which occur in Cali, Colombia. Amer. Heart J. 66:584, 1963.

36. Higginson, J., Isaacson, C., and Simson, I.: The pathology of cryptogenic heart disease. A study of the pathological pattern in 80 cases of obscure heart failure in South African Bantu Negro. Arch. Path. (Chicago) 70:497, 1960.

37. Edington, G. M., and Jackson, J. G.: The pathology of heart muscle disease and endomyocardial fibrosis in Nigeria. J. Path. Bact. 86:333, 1963.

38. Brockington, I. F., Olsen, E. G. J., and Goodwin, J. F.: Endomyocardial fibrosis in Europeans resident in tropical Africa. Lancet 1:583, 1967.

39. Brink, A. J., and Weber, H. W.: Endomyocardial fibrosis (EMF) of East, Central and West Africa compared with South African endomyocardiopathies. S. Afr. Med. J. 40:455, 1966.

40. LaBrooy, E. B.: Proc. Alumni Ass. Malaya 10:303, 1957. Quoted in Ciba Foundation Symposium on Cardiomyopathies. Boston, Little, Brown, 1964, p. 345.

41. Nagaratnam, N., and Dissanayake, R.V.P.: Endomyocardial fibrosis in the Ceylonese. Brit. Heart J. 21:167, 1959.

42. Andrade, Z. A., and Guimaraes, S. C.: Endomyocardial fibrosis in Bahia, Brazil. Brit. Heart J. 26:813, 1964.

43. Schmincke, A.: Üeber linksseitige muskulöse conusstenosen. Deutsch Med. Wschr. 33:2082, 1907.

44. Edwards, J. E.: Pathology of left ventricular outflow tract obstruction. Circulation 31:586, 1965.

45. Goodwin, J. F.: Obstructive cardiomyopathy. Cardiologia 52:69, 1968.

46. Pearse, A.G.E.: The histochemistry and electron microscopy of obstructive cardiomyopathy, In Ciba Foundation Symposium on Cardiomyopathies. Boston, Little, Brown 1964, p. 132.

47. Sonnenblick, E. H.: Correlation of myocardial ultrastructure and function. Circulation 38:29, 1968.

48. Neufeld, H. N., Ongley, P. A., and Edwards, J. E.: Combined congenital subaortic stenosis and infundibular pulmonary stenosis. Brit. Heart J. 22:686, 1960.

49. Daoud, G., Gallaher, M. E., and Kaplan, S.: Muscular subaortic stenosis. Amer. J. Cardiol. 7:860, 1961.

50. Wood, R. S., Taylor, W. J., Wheat, M. W., and Shiebler, G. L.: Muscular subaortic stenosis in childhood. Report of occurrence in three siblings. Pediatrics 30:749, 1962.

51. Braunwald, E., Lambrew, C. T., Rockoff, S. D., Ross, J., Jr., and Morrow, A. G.: Idiopathic hypertrophic subaortic stenosis. Circulation 30: (Suppl. IV) 3, 1964.

52. Harris, L. C., Weissler, A. M., Manske, A. O., Danford, B. H., White, G. D., and Hammill, W. A.: Duration of the phases of mechanical systole in infants and children. Amer. J. Cardiol. 14:448, 1964.

53. Nasser, W. K., et al.: Familial myocardial disease with and without obstruction to left ventricular outflow. Clinical, hemodynamic and angiographic findings. Circulation 35:638, 1967.

54. Frank, S., and Braunwald, E.: Idiopathic hypertrophic subaortic stenosis. Clinical analysis of 126 patients with emphasis on the natural history. Circulation 37:759, 1968.

55. Shand, D. G., Sell, C. G., and Oates, J. A.: Hypertrophic obstructive cardiomyopathy in an infant—propranolol therapy for three years. New Eng. J. Med. 285:843, 1971.

56. Stoeber, E.: Weitere untersuchungen über epidemische myocarditis (Schwielenherz) des Säuglings. Z. Kinderheilk. 71:319, 592, 1952.

57. Gear, J. H. S., and Measroch, V.: Annual report for 1952, South African Institute of Medical Research, p. 38.

58. Javett, S. N., et al.: Myocarditis in the newborn infant. A study of an outbreak associated with Coxsackie group B virus infection in a maternity home in Johannesburg. J. Pediat. 48:1, 1956.

59. van Creveld, S., and de Jager, H.: Myocarditis in newborns caused by Coxsackie virus. Clinical and pathological data. Ann. Paediat. 187:100, 1956.

60. Kibrick, S., and Benirschke, K.: Acute septic myocarditis and meningoencephalitis in newborn child infected with Coxsackie virus group B, type 3. New Eng. J. Med. 255:883, 1956.

61. Suckling, P. V., and Vogelpoel, L.: Coxsackie myocarditis of the newborn. Lancet 2: 421, 1970.

62. Sanyal, S. K., Mahdavy, M., Gabrielson, M. O., Vidone, R. A., and Browne, M. J.: Fatal myocarditis in an adolescent caused by Coxsackie virus, group B, type 4. Pediatrics 35: 36, 1965.

63. Burch, G. E., Sun, S., Chu, K., Sohal, R. S., and Colcolough, H. L.: Interstitial and Coxsackievirus B myocarditis in infants and children. JAMA 203:1, 1968.

64. —, and Giles, T. D.: The role of viruses in the production of heart disease. Amer. J. Cardiol. 29:231, 1972.

65. Ainger, L. E., Lawyer, N. G., and Fitch, C. W.: Neonatal rubella myocarditis. Brit. Heart J. 28:691, 1966.

66. Van der Horst, R. L., and Gotsman, M.S.: Left ventricular aneurysm in rubella heart disease. Amer. J. Dis. Child. 120:248, 1970.

67. Moore, C. M., Henry, J., Benzing, G., and Kaplan, S.: Varicella myocarditis. Amer. J. Dis. Child. 118:899, 1969.

68. De Medeiros Neto, G. A., de Almeida, D. B., and Facchini, F. P.: Myocarditis associated with chickenpox. Presentation of a case treated by corticosteroids. Rev. Hosp. Clin. Fac. Med. S. Paulo 16:427432, 1961.

69. Bell, E. J., and Grist, N. R.: ECHO viruses, carditis and acute pleurodynia. Lancet 1:326, 1970.

70. Maller, H. M., Powars, D. F., Horowitz, R. E., and Portnoy, B.: Fatal myocarditis associated with ECHO virus, type 22, infection in a child with apparent immunological deficiency. J. Pediat. 71:204, 1967.

71. Cherry, J. D., Jahn, C. L., and Meyer, T. C.: Paroxysmal atrial tachycardia associated with ECHO 9 virus infection. Amer. Heart J. 73:681, 1967.

72. Henson, D., and Mufson, M. A.: Myocarditis and pneumonitis with type 21 adenovirus infection. Association with fatal myocarditis and pneumonitis. Amer. J. Dis. Child. 121:334, 1971.

73. Editorial: Chagas' disease. Brit. Med. J. 1:1451, 1961.

74. WHO Technical Report Series, No. 102.

75. Older, J. J.: Clinical study of Chagas' disease. (*Trypanosomiasis cruzi*). Southern Med. J. 62:729, 1969.

76. Prata, A.: Chagas' heart disease. Cardiologia 52:79, 1968.

77. Mountain, J. C.: Chagas' disease. Proc. Roy. Soc. Med. 61:444, 1968.

78. de Raadt, P., and Koten, J. W.: Myocarditis in rhodesiense trypanosomiasis. E. Afr. Med. J. 45:128, 1968.

79. Koten, J. W., and de Raadt, P.: Myocarditis in *Trypanosoma rhodesiense* infections. Trans. Roy. Soc. Trop. Med. Hyg. 63:485, 1969.

80. Einchenwald, H. F.: The laboratory diagnosis of toxoplasmosis. Ann. N.Y. Acad. Sci. 64:207, 1956.

81. Center for Disease Control Surveillance Report, No. 11, 1971.

82. Ledbetter, M. K., Cannon, A. B., and Costa, A. F.: The electrocardiogram in diphtheritic myocarditis. Amer. Heart. J. 68:599, 1964.

83. Morgan, B. C.: Cardiac complications of diphtheria. Pediatrics 32:549, 1963.

84. Srivastava, S. C., Puri, D. S., and Lumba, S. P.: An electrocardiographic study of myocarditis in diphtheria. J. Ass. Physicians India. 14:365, 1966.

85. Griffith, G. C., and Herman, L. M.: Persistent complete heart block in diphtheritic myocarditis. JAMA 148:279, 1952.

86. Burch, G. E., Sun, S. C., Sohal, R. S., Chu, K., and Colcolough, H. L.: Diphtheritic myocarditis. A histochemical and electron microscopic study. Amer. J. Cardiol. 21:261, 1968.

87. Stecher, R. M.: Electrocardiographic changes in diphtheria: complete auriculoventricular dissociation. Amer. Heart J. 4:545, 1929.

88. Marvin, H. M., and Buckley, R. C.: Complete heart block in diphtheria. Heart 11: 309, 1924.

89. Johnson, J. L., and Lee, L. P.: Complete atrioventricular heart block secondary to acute myocarditis requiring intracardiac pacing. J. Pediat. 78:312, 1971.

90. Perloff, J. K., de Leon, A. C., and O'Doherty, D.: The cardiomyopathy of progressive muscular dystrophy. Circulation 33:625, 1966.

91. —, Roberts, W. C., de Leon, A. C., and O'Doherty, D.: The distinctive ECG of Duchenne's progressive muscular dystrophy. Amer. J. Med. 42:179, 1967.

92. —, de Leon, A. C., O'Doherty, D.: The cardiomyopathy of progressive muscular dystrophy. Circulation 33:625, 1966.

93. Pompe, J. C.: Over idiopatische hypertrophy van het hart. Nederl. Tijdschr. Geneesk. 76:304, 1932.

94. Nihill, M. R., Wilson, D. S., and Hugh-Jones, K.: Generalized glycogenosis type II (Pompe's disease). Arch. Dis. Child. 45:122, 1970.

95. Thorén, C.: Cardiomyopathy in Friedreich's ataxia. With studies of cardiovascular and respiratory function. Acta Paediat. 53:388, 1964.

96. Ivemark, B., and Thorén, C.: The pathology of the heart in Friedreich's ataxia. Acta Med. Scand. 175:227, 1964.

97. James, T. N., and Fisch, C.: Observations on the cardiovascular involvement in Friedreich's ataxia. Amer. Heart J. 66:164, 1963.

98. Moore, A. A. D., and Lambert, E. C.: Cardiomyopathy associated with muscular and neuro-muscular disease. In Watson H. (ed.): Paediatric Cardiology. St. Louis, C. V. Mosby Co., 1968, p. 766.

99. Soulié, P., et al.: Le coeur dans la maladie de Friedreich. Mal. Cardiovasc. 7:369, 1966.

100. Gach, J. V., Andriange, M., and Franck, G.: Hypertrophic obstructive cardiomyopathy and Friedreich's ataxia. Amer. J. Cardiol. 27:436, 1971.

101. Harris, L. C., et al.: Idiopathic nonobstructive cardiomyopathy in children. Amer. J. Cardiol. 21:162, 1968.

102. Nghiem, Q. X., Toledo, J. R., Schreiber, M. H., Harris, L. C., Lockhart, L. L., and Tyson, K. R. T.: Congenital idiopathic hypertrophic subaortic stenosis associated with phenotypic Turner's syndrome. Amer. J. Cardiol. In press.

Palliative Surgery in Infants With Congenital Heart Disease

Constantine J. Tatooles and Robert A. Miller

THE NEWBORN with congenital heart disease who is seriously ill should
be regarded as a medical and surgical emergency. Although the risks
of surgery are high in the sick newborn, when considered against the likelihood
of imminent death from the underlying malformation, there should be no
hesitation about proceeding with operation. Cardiac catheterization and angiocardiography may be indicated as early as the first hr of life.

There has been a continuing dialogue among pediatric cardiologists concerning the necessity for cardiac catheterization prior to cardiac surgery in the newborn and young infant. Those who feel that cardiac catheterization should not be
done feel that the diagnosis based on physical examination, x-ray of the chest,
and electrocardiogram is accurate enough to select infants for the surgical
procedures likely to be done in this age group. In addition, they point out that
the risk of cardiac catheterization in the newborn and sick infant is high and
that the infant's condition may deteriorate significantly during the cardiac
catheterization, making for a poorer risk patient at the time of surgery. However, because of rapid advances in surgical treatment of congenital heart disease
during the past few decades, correction or palliation of many cardiovascular
malformations previously considered incurable can now be effectively managed.
Accurate clinical diagnosis is more important today, since there is an array of
effective surgical procedures for the newborn child with congenital heart disease,
who, in the past, was doomed at infancy.

CARDIAC CATHETERIZATION

Infants are selected for cardiac catheterization, usually because cardiac
surgery may be imminent or because life threatening signs and symptoms of

From the Departments of Cardio-Thoracic Surgery and Pediatric Cardiology, Cook County Hospital, Chicago, Ill.

Supported by Chicago Heart Association Grant C72-34, NIH Research Grant HE08682, and by the Children's Heart Research Foundation, Hektoen Institute.

Constantine J. Tatooles, M. S., M.D.: *Chairman, Department of Cardio-Thoracic Surgery, Cook County Hospital, and Assistant Professor, Department of Surgery and Physiology, Loyola University Medical Center, Chicago, Ill.* Robert A. Miller, M.D.: *Chairman, Department of Pediatric Cardiology, Cook County Hospital, and Professor, Department of Pediatrics, Abraham Lincoln School of Medicine, University of Illinois, Chicago, Ill.*

heart failure are present. With accurate preoperative diagnosis, exploration at the time of thoracotomy is not necessary, thereby eliminating additional operative maneuvers that may be time consuming and detrimental to the patient. In addition, with the objective information obtained from the study, the severity of the cardiac malformation is understood, and the predictability of the operative result can be explained to the parents.

Cardiac catheterization and angiocardiography in the newborn and young infant can be done with little risk despite the presence of serious cardiovascular and metabolic symptoms. Of 163 infants catheterized in the past 2 yr in our laboratory, there were 3 deaths associated with the procedure (1.8%). Two infants died of progressive heart failure and the third from cardiac tamponade secondary to perforation of the heart.

The safety of the procedure is greatly increased by strict attention to details that are of special importance in the neonatal period. These include: (1) maintenance of body temperature—a continuously recording rectal temperature probe and a carefully regulated water mattress are required; (2) periodic determination of blood gases throughout the procedure; (3) correction of metabolic acidosis during the procedure; (4) accurate blood withdrawal measurements and hematocrit levels for replacement of whole blood when indicated; (5) test injection of contrast material to obtain critical placement of catheter for angiocardiogram, careful fixation of the catheter to the skin once the position has been established, and repeat test injections whenever the infant's position is changed; and (6) constant observation of the sick infant during the procedure by a nurse and the physician in charge of the procedure. Our experience has demonstrated that not only does cardiac catheterization rarely add to the subsequent risk of even an emergency operation, but may offer the opportunity to improve the condition of a baby who is in congestive heart failure, acidotic or anemic, when sent to the laboratory.

OPERATIVE THERAPY

Infants with congenital heart disease in failure who are unresponsive to medical management are candidates for operation regardless of age, weight, or severity of symptoms, if the anatomy present is suitable to restore or maintain physiologic and hemodynamic cardiopulmonary events. When septal defects are present between developed heart chambers or abnormal communications exist between the great arteries definitive operative procedures can correct these malformations. In addition, when abnormal exit of the great arteries from the heart or anomalous connection of the pulmonary veins to the heart are present, definitive operative therapy can correct these anomalies. However, in infants with lesions that produce obstruction to pulmonary blood flow with a proximal intracardiac shunt, the operative procedure is dependent upon the severity of the obstructing lesion. Depending upon the complexity of the lesion, a definitive or palliative procedure is utilized. Cardiac anomalies that remain uncorrected are primarily hypoplasia or atresia of one or the other atrioventricular valves, resulting in serious underdevelopment of the respective ventricle. Therefore, any condition that is characterized by absence, hypoplasia, or disease of the myocardium defies corrective operative therapy thus far, but,

**Table 1. Age Distribution of Infants Studied and Operated Upon
at Cook County Hospital (December, 1969-November, 1971)**

Age	Catheterized	Operated	Operative Deaths	Nonoperative Deaths	Total Deaths	Per cent Mortality Operative and Nonoperative
1–14 days	42	13	8	14	23	23/42, 55%
15–30 days	21	7	3	4	7	7/21, 33%
1– 3 mo	30	24	8	2	10	10/30, 33%
3– 6 mo	37	16	3	1	4	4/37, 11%
6–12 mo	33	13	2	1	3	3/33, 9%
Total	163	73	24	22	47	29%

depending upon the remaining anatomy, a palliative procedure may be attempted.

In general, the more complex cardiac lesions produce symptoms early in life, and the majority are inoperable. In our 2-yr review of 163 infants catheterized within the first yr of life, 42 were studied during the first 2 wk of life. Of the 42 infants, 15 patients had a hypoplastic left side syndrome. In the 29 infants not operated on, 14 died and 15 survived, while 8 of the 13 operated infants died. The total mortality for both the nonoperated and operated infants was 55% (Table 1).

Acceptable results in infant cardiac surgery are dependent primarily on events in the catheterization laboratory, operating rooms and in the pediatric intensive care unit. Painstaking care is essential in all areas pre- and post-operatively. A cardiac surgical resident, pediatric cardiology resident, and pediatric anesthesia resident or their equivalents should be available in these areas at all times to manage these patients in concert.

PATENT DUCTUS ARTERIOSUS

In 1907, Munro[1] first suggested surgical obliteration of the ductus arteriosus. In 1888, he demonstrated in an infant cadaver that the patent ductus arteriosus could be ligated. It was not until 1937 that Strieder[2] made the first attempt to close a patent ductus arteriosus. The closure was incomplete and the patient died. Gross,[3] in 1938, successfully closed the patent ductus in a 7-yr-old girl, thus opening the era for modern cardiac surgery. However, it wasn't until the early 1950s that a patent ductus was obliterated in an infant, nearly 60 yr after Munro's demonstration.

Infants with isolated patent ductus arteriosus are considered candidates for operation because of congestive heart failure or because cardiomegaly is present with a ductus that is patent beyond the first mo of life. However, in early infancy, there is a high incidence of additional cardiac anomalies, and closure of a patent ductus may be considered a palliative operative procedure until an associated cardiac anomaly can be corrected at a later age.

In a review by Panagopoulos et al.,[4] 55% of infants with a patent ductus the first 3 mo of life had associated cardiac anomalies, and 37% of those beyond 6 mo of age had additional cardiac anomalies. Of the 245 infants operated upon for patent ductus arteriosus within their 23-yr review, 109 had associated cardiac anomalies (43.5%). The total infant operative mortality was 19% (47/245). However, for 691 patients over the age of 1 yr, their operative mortality rate was less than 0.5%. In 12 infants operated upon for isolated patent ductus arteriosus within the past 2 yr at our institute, there was one death in a 2-mo-old with heart failure and pneumonia. With improved techniques for general anesthesia and meticulous postoperative management, the operative mortality rate in infants should approach that for children.

The surgical technique varies and some debate still exists as to whether the patent ductus arteriosus should be ligated or divided. However, for infants we prefer ligation of the ductus using two (1.2 mm diameter) ligatures. In those few cases where the ductus is wide (as wide as the aorta) and short, division and suture is utilized to avoid constricting the aorta.[5]

COARCTATION OF THE AORTA

Coarctation of the aorta has been successfully repaired in children and young adults since 1944, when Crafoord[6] resected a coarcted segment and rejoined the cut ends of the aorta. However, it wasn't until 1950 that Calodney and Carson[7] reported the seriousness of this lesion in infancy. Kirklin et al. in 1952 described a successful resection in a 10-wk-old infant.[8]

The anatomical features used for classification of coarctation are dependent upon the presence of a ductus arteriosus and the location of the coarctation above, at the level of, or below the ductus or ligamentum. The majority of infants with coarctation of the aorta have the preductal type. In a review of 333 patients with coarctation of the aorta by Tawes et al.,[9] 94 patients had preductal coarctation and 87 of these patients were under 1 yr of age. Of the 179 infants with coarctation of the aorta, 160 had associated anomalies (89%). At the time of operation, 37% of the total were age 3 mo or less. Patent ductus arteriosus is the most frequent lesion associated with coarctation of the aorta, followed by aortic valvular defects and ventricular septal defects. Multiple cardiac lesions and ventricular septal defects were more commonly associated with preductal coarctation and aortic arch atresia.

In infants, congestive heart failure that was worsening or not responding to therapy was a major indication for emergency operation. Medical treatment for congestive heart failure should be instituted early and continued. If the response to medical management is not satisfactory or if congestive heart failure increases after early favorable response, an emergency operation should be performed.

A left posterolateral thoracotomy through the third or fourth intercostal space allows for adequate exposure of the coarctation. In the majority of the patients, the coarctation can be resected and the aorta anastomosed end-to-end. However, in some patients a subclavian artery to descending aorta anastomosis or a variation of this procedure is necessary when a hypoplastic arch precludes an adequate primary anastomosis.[10] In those patients with preductal coarctation, ligation of the ductus arteriosus is the initial procedure. Following this, the coarcted segment can be excised, and the free ends of the aorta can be sutured end-to-end. Synthetic grafts are not used in infants.

Many of the associated multiple cardiac defects also require operative treatment. When a large left-to-right shunt with pulmonary hypertension from a ventricular septal defect is demonstrated, the pulmonary artery can be constricted during the operative procedure. In patients with transposition of the great arteries, atrial septostomy by the Rashkind[11] balloon procedure should be performed at the time of cardiac catheterization, and banding of the pulmonary artery in those patients with a ventricular septal defect can be decided upon prior to the time of operation.

The highest mortality in infants with coarctation of the aorta is in those with the preductal form. The mortality is greater early in life and decreases markedly after 6 mo of age.

If the infant survives the operation with preductal coarctation, the postoperative complications are few if meticulous care and awareness of airway obstruction is understood. Renal and spinal cord complications following cross clamping of the aorta rarely occur in infants. However, one of the common postoperative complications in infants is recoarctation. This can occur as early as 48 hr following operation, but is usually observed as a gradual development over mo to yr. The incidence of recoarctation in those infants operated varies from 8%–41%.[9,12]

Infancy alone is not a cause of high operative mortality. The mortality is usually dependent upon the lesion. Those infants with hypoplastic left side syndrome or with hypoplasia of the aortic arch have little chance for survival. Patients with an adequate aortic arch can survive despite the severity of the constriction of the coarcted segment.

The mortality rate in infants with coarctation who develop congestive heart failure is potentially high. Controversy has existed concerning medical treatment being more effective than surgical. The results of medical treatment alone have not been encouraging. In a comprehensive review, Mortenson et al.[13] reported a mortality rate of 64% among 134 infants in heart failure treated medically compared with a 37% operative mortality. Waldhausen et al.[14] reported a 71% mortality rate with medical management of infants with coarctation in congestive heart failure, but without an associated intercardiac lesion compared with a 15% operative morality rate. If an additional cardiac defect was present, none survived on medical therapy, while 45% were successfully treated by operation. In addition, Sinha et al.[15] reported a series of 75 patients in congestive heart failure with coarctation and associated cardiac defects with a mortality of 88% for those treated medically and 56% for those managed operatively. Therefore, operation is indicated if a satisfactory response to medical management is not obtained quickly (within 24–48 hr).

Infants with preductal coarctation present a special problem. The majority of these patients have multiple cardiac defects and resection of the coarctation alone does not insure survival. In the majority of patients with preductal coarctation and ductus only, the survival with operative therapy is approximately 50%. This is a considerable improvement since Glass[16] in 1960 and Cooley[17] in 1964 reported 90%–100% mortality rates in infants with congestive heart failure and preductal coarctation.

Recoarctation is a likely possibility, especially in infants under 6 mo of age, and those with a hypoplastic aortic arch. Because of the high incidence of associated cardiac anomalies and the development of recoarctation, the initial operation is considered a palliative form of therapy in infants.

INFANTS WITH INCREASED PULMONARY BLOOD FLOW

Muller and Dammann,[18] in 1951, introduced the procedure of constricting (banding) the pulmonary artery to decrease pulmonary blood flow in infants with excessive left-to-right shunts. Since then, the procedure has been increasingly utilized to treat intractable heart failure and to prevent the development of pulmonary vascular disease.[19-23]

The majority of infants with ventricular septal defects do not have symptoms. A small proportion develop heart failure and most of these infants can be treated satisfactorily by medical management. However, severe heart failure in the first mo of life may be present in patients with large left-to-right shunts or in patients with ventricular septal defects associated with other cardiac malformations.[24]

The indication for operation is failure of medical therapy judged mainly by continuous difficulties and inability of the baby to feed properly or to gain weight. The choice of whether to band the pulmonary artery or to perform definitive intracardiac surgery is in part dependent upon the experience of the operating team (pediatric anesthesiologist, cardiologist and surgeon) and the availability of pediatric-oriented intensive care personel. The surgical procedure best suited for an infant with congenital heart disease is that which will offer the most physiologic benefits with the least operative risk. If an institution performs an occasional operation upon an infant, then banding the pulmonary artery is a safer procedure. However, if an institution is geared toward infant cardiac surgery, then intracardiac repairs can be performed with satisfactory results, especially with ventricular septal defects.[25-27]

In patients with large left-to-right shunts and complicated malformations, such as single ventricle, truncus arteriosus, tricuspid atresia with increased pulmonary blood flow and common atrioventricular canal defects, pulmonary artery banding is indicated. Usually the palliative procedure will delay definitive cardiac reconstruction until a more favorable age and size.

The banding operation is performed from a left lateral thoracotomy through the third intercostal space. The ductus arteriosus or ligamentum is disected and ligated to insure closure of that structure. The pericardium is opened anterior to the phrenic nerve and the pulmonary artery disected and constricted with teflon or dacron bands. The effectiveness of pulmonary artery constriction is assessed by pressure measurements in the pulmonary artery beyond the constriction, in the right ventricle, and occasionally, in a peripheral artery. When pressure recordings are unavailable or imminent cardiac arrest demands prompt action, the pulmonary artery is constricted to one-third of its original diameter or to a diameter just short of that which produces bradycardia. Palpation of a thrill is also a helpful guide. When the pulmonary artery pressure is lowered sufficiently, (usually below 40 mm Hg), the band is secured. The pericardium is approximated almost completely and the chest closed with intercostal drainage.

The results obtained are clearly related to the cardiac lesion. In a review by

Table 2. Palliative Pulmonary Artery Banding at Cook County Hospital
(December, 1969–November, 1971)

No. Patients	Diagnosis	Age	Deaths
4	VSD*	1 mo–6 mo	—
2	Truncus	6 days–2 mo	1
9	A-V Canal† and PDA‡	1 mo–11 mo	2
2	VSD and PDA	1 mo–5 mo	1
2	VSD, PDA and ASD§	1 mo–2 mo	1
1	TGA‖, VSD and PDA	1 mo	1
1	VSD, PDA, ASD, Interrupted Aortic Arch Dextro-cardia, Situs Inversus	1 day	1
Total 21			7 (33%)

* Ventricular septal defect.
† Atrioventricular canal.
‡ Patent ductus arteriosus.
§ Atrial septal defect.
‖ Transposition of the great arteries.

Stark et al.,[24] patients with ventricular septal defects alone had a mortality rate of 2.2%. In patients with associated defects, the rate was much higher. In the past 2 yr, 21 patients have had banding of the pulmonary artery performed in our institution. There were no deaths in those infants with ventricular septal defect alone. In patients with additional anomalies the operative mortality was increased (Table 2). It should be emphasized that in selected patients in our series (5 patients), and those reported by others[25] with ventricular septal defects alone undergoing total intracardiac repair, none died, indicating the increased risk associated with more complex cardiac malformations in the infant. With continuing improvement in techniques of total operative repair with cardio-pulmonary bypass, more procedures will be performed in the very young.

INFANTS WITH DECREASED PULMONARY BLOOD FLOW

The subclavian pulmonary artery shunt, which was introduced by Blalock and Taussig[28] in 1945, began the era of palliative treatment for cyanotic congenital heart disease. Their shunt is still the procedure of choice in children with anomalies associated with obstructed pulmonary blood flow and a proximal right-to-left shunt. However, in infants whose anatomy does not allow this shunt to be made satisfactorily because of the limiting size of the vessels, a direct anastomosis between the aorta and pulmonary artery is required. It remained for Potts, Smith, and Gibson to devise an ingenious clamp and to develop the technique for this procedure.[29]

A Potts-Smith-Gibson anastomosis, which joins the decending aorta and left pulmonary artery, is effective but cannot be performed in patients with a right aortic arch and has proved a difficult palliative procedure to correct at the time of total cardiac repair. In addition, this shunt is fashioned in an area nearer a patent ductus arteriosus, which at times is the only vessel allowing blood to enter the pulmonary circulation. Therefore, for infants with small vessels, an anastomosis between the ascending aorta and right pulmonary artery was developed by Waterston in 1960 and reported in the foreign literature in 1962.[30]

Presently, there are two technically different approaches of ascending aorta right pulmonary artery anastomosis: the extrapericardial retrocaval approach (Waterston operation), and the intrapericardial technique published by Cooley and Hallman.[31]

Systemic pulmonary shunts are primarily palliative procedures for patients with anomalies that produce obstructed pulmonary blood flow with an intra-cardiac shunt proximal to the area of obstruction. However, for those patients whose anatomy does not allow for complete repair at a later date, it is a definitive procedure.

If an infant is severly cyanotic and is having cyanotic attacks or is unable to thrive clinically, then operation is indicated. In those infants who, after thorough study, are not amenable to an operation for restoring a normal circulation, then a palliative systemic pulmonary shunt is indicated. The choice of the shunt depends upon the size of the infant and the anatomy. Our preference is the Blalock-Taussig operation because the results are more predictable. However, for infants in whom the subclavian artery is too small for the establishment of a satisfactory anastomosis, the Waterston operation is at present the procedure of choice.

The Waterston operation is performed by entering the chest through the fourth right intercostal space through a widely opened incision that extends posteriorly. The main right pulmonary artery is dissected posterior to the superior vena cava, and the pericardium, which is anterior to the pulmonary artery, is incised exposing the posterior aspect of the aorta. The peripheral pulmonary artery branches are pulled laterally by heavy rubber ligatures. A partial occlusion clamp is placed with one jaw posterior to the right pulmonary artery and the other jaw anterior to the aorta. In order to prevent tenting of the pulmonary artery, the aorta is rotated laterally before the partial occlusion clamp is closed. The length of the aortic incision is measured in order to accurately determine the size of the anastomosis. In small infants, a 3-ml shunt is sufficient. In older infants, a 4-ml shunt should be established. Following the anastomosis with a fine continuous suture, the partial occlusion clamp is removed. The pulmonary artery appears full and a thrill is palpable in the right pulmonary artery. If the pulmonary artery is tense, then pulmonary artery pressure measurements are taken. When the pulmonary artery pressure is 60 mm Hg or more then two-thirds of the systemic pressure, the anastomosis is too large. A small difference in the diameter of the anastomosis can make a sizable difference in the shunt flow. Heart failure or unilateral pulmonary edema[32] are complications of too large an anastomosis in the early postoperative period. Immediate reoperation is necessary to decrease the size of the anastomosis.

In very small infants, the Waterston operation is technically easy and the incidence of shunt thrombosis is low. In addition, the potential of developing pericardial adhesions is minimal and the closure of the shunt following corrective procedures is technically easy. The prognosis for which palliative surgery is required is proportional to the underlying lesion. In tetralogy of Fallot, the results are excellent following total correction.

Pulmonary valvotomy or infundibular resection has achieved good palliation, especially in older patients with tetralogy of Fallot. Sellors[33] first performed closed pulmonary valvotomy in the tetralogy of Fallot, and his patient obtained satisfactory palliation. Brock first published an experience with this procedure, reporting his work in 1948.[34] Closed valvotomy and resection of infundibular musculature have been applied, primarily by Brock, to patients with tetralogy of Fallot.[35]However, for infants there seems to be more disadvantages than advantages to the Brock procedure and its immediate result is less predictable. It continues to be a useful palliative procedure in a few types of complex cyanotic congenital heart disease in which complete repair is not possible.

CONCLUSION

Palliative surgery continues to be an important part of infant cardiovascular care. Many such patients are now of sufficient size and age to have had corrective surgery that was not available or was far too risky when they needed help the most. Palliative procedures for transposition of the great arteries and for tetralogy of Fallot were being performed 10 yr before dependable correction of these anomalies could be done with acceptable risk. More recently, patients with truncus arteriosus, banded in the past, and those with pulmonary atresia and ventricular septal defect (pseudo truncus), shunted in the past, are now being corrected with aortic homografts.[36] Palliated patients with tricuspid atresia, Ebstein's anomaly and even more complex lesions may be corrected in the near future.

With the growing enthusiasum for total repair with hypothermia or cardiopulmonary bypass in infants, it would be wise to keep clearly in mind the purpose of all cardiac care—in infants—to keep them alive, healthy, and active either by repairing their defect, or by improving them with a low risk procedure, so that the infants will be alive when their lesion joins the group of those that can be completely repaired at low risk.

REFERENCES

1. Munro, J. C.: Ligation of the ductus arteriosus. Ann. Surg. 46:335, 1907.

2. Blalock, A., and Levy, S. E.: Discussion by John W. Strieder from Tuberculosis Pericarditis. J. Thorac. Surg. 7:151, 1937.

3. Gross, R. E., and Hubbard, J. P.: Surgical ligation of patent ductus arteriosus: A report of first successful case. JAMA 112:729, 1939.

4. Panagopoulos, G., Tatooles, C. J., Aberdeen, E., Waterston, D. J., and Benham Carter, R. E.: Patent ductus arteriosus in infants and children. Thorax 26 (2):137, 1971.

5. Gross, R. E.: Complete surgical division of the patent ductus arteriosus: Report of fourteen successful cases. Surg. Gynec. Obstet. 78:36, 1944.

6. Crafoard, C., and Nylin, G.: Congenital coarctation of the aorta and its surgical treatment. J. Thorac. Surg. 14:347, 1945.

7. Calodney, M. M., and Carson, M. J.: Coarctation of the aorta in early infancy. J. Pediat. 37:46, 1950.

8. Kirklin, J. W., Burchell, H. B., Pugh, D. G., Burke, E. C., and Mills, S. D.: Surgical treatment of coarctation of the aorta in a ten week old infant: Report of a case. Circulation 6:411, 1952.

9. Tawes, R. L., Aberdeen, E., Waterston, D. J., and Bonham Carter, R. E.: Coarctation of the aorta in infants and children: A review of 333 operative cases including 179 infants. Circulation 39 (Suppl. 1):173, 1969.

10. Blalock, A., and Park, E. A.: Surgical treatment of experimental coarctation (atresia) of the aorta. Ann. Surg. 119:445, 1944.

11. Rashkind, W. J., and Miller, W. W.: Creation of an atrial septal defect without thoracotomy: A palliative approach to complete transposition of the great arteries. JAMA 196:991, 1966.

12. Eshaghpour, E., and Olley, P. M.: Recoarctation of the aorta following coarctectomy in the first year of life: A follow-up study. J. Pediat. 80:809, 1972.

13. Mortenson, J. D., Cutler, P. R., Rumel, W. R., and Veassey, L. G.: Management of coarctation of the aorta in infancy. J. Thorac. Cardiovasc. Surg. 37:502, 1959.

14. Waldhausen, J. A., King, H., Nahrwald, D., Lurie, P. R., and Shumalsker, H. B., Jr.: Management of coarctation in infancy. JAMA 187:268, 1964.

15. Sinha, S. N., Muster, A. J., Cole, R. B., Kardatzke, M. L., and Paul, M. H.: Coarctation of the aorta with congestive heart failure in infancy: A pathophysiological review of seventy-five infants. Circulation 35, 36 (Suppl. II):239, 1967.

16. Glass, I. H., Mustard, W. T., and Keith, J. D.: Coarctation of the aorta in infants (a review of twelve years' experience). Pediatrics 26:109, 1960.

17. Cooley, D. A., and Hullman, G. L.: Cardiovascular surgery in the first year of life: Experience with 450 consecutive operations. Amer. J. Surg. 107:474, 1964.

18. Muller, W. H., Jr., and Dammann, J. F., Jr.: The treatment of certain congenital malformations of the heart by the creation of pulmonary stenosis to reduce pulmonary hypertension and excessive pulmonary flow. Surg. Gynec. Obstec. 95:213, 1952.

19. Albert, H. M., Fowler, R. M., Craighead, C. C., and Atik, M.: A treatment for infants with intractable cardiac failure due to interventricular septal defect. Circulation 23:16, 1961.

20. Goldblatt, A., Bernhard, W. F., Nadas, A. S., and Gross, R. E.: Pulmonary artery banding. Indications and results in infants and children. Circulation 32:172, 1965.

21. Hallman, G. L., Cooley, D. A., and Bloodwell, R. D.: Two-stage surgical treatment of ventricular septal defect: Results of pulmonary artery banding in infants and subsequent open-heart repair. J. Thorac. Cardiovasc. Surg. 52:476, 1966.

22. Morrow, A. G., and Braunwald, N. S.: The surgical treatment of ventricular septal defect in infancy: Technique and results of pulmonary artery constriction. Circulation 24:34, 1961.

23. Willmann, V. L., Cooper, T., Mudd, J. G., and Hanlon, C. R.: Treatment of ventricular septal defect by constriction of pulmonary artery. Arch. Surg. (Chicago) 85:745, 1962.

24. Stark, J., Aberdeen, E., Waterston, D. J., Bonham Carter, R. E., and Tynan, M.: Pulmonary artery constriction (banding): A report of 146 cases. Surgury 65:808, 1969.

25. Diacoff, G. R., and Miller, R. H.: Congestive heart failure in infancy treated by early repair of ventricular septal defect. Circulation 42 (Suppl. II): II–III, 1970.

26. Barratt-Boyes, B. G.: Cardiac surgery in neonates and infants. Circulation 44:924, 1971.

27. Malm, J. R., Bowman, F. O., Jr., Jesse, M. J., and Blumenthal, S.: Open heart surgery in the infant. Amer. J. Surg. 119:613, 1970.

28. Blalock, A., and Taussig, H. S.: The surgical treatment of malformations of the heart. JAMA 128:189, 1945.

29. Potts, W. J., Smith, S., and Gibson, S.: Anastomosis of the aorta to a pulmonary artery. JAMA 132:627, 1946.

30. Waterston, D. J.: Treatment of Fallot's tetralogy in children under 1 year of age. Rozhl. Chir., 41:181, 1962.

31. Cooley, D. A., and Hallman, G. L.: Intrapericardic Aortic-right Pulmonary Arterial Anastomosis. Surg. Gynec. Obstet. 122:1084, 1966.

32. Salem, M. R., Masund, K. Z., Tatooles, C. J., and Yanes, H. O.: Unilateral pulmonary qe dema following aorta to right pulmonary artery anastomosis (Waterston's Operation), Brit. J. Anaesth. 43:701, 1971.

33. Sellors, T. H.: Surgery of pulmonary stenosis: A case in which the pulmonary valve was sucessfully divided. Lancet 1:988, 1948.

34. Brock, R. C.: Pulmonary valvotomy for the relief of congential pulmonary stenosis: Report of three cases. Brit. Med. J. 1:1121, 1948.

35. — , and Campbell, M.: Infundibular resection or dilation for infundibular stenosis. Brit. Heart J. 12:403, 1950.

36. Wallace, R. B., Rastelli, G. C., Ongley, P. A., Titus, J. L., and McGoon, D. C.: Complete repair of truncus arteriosus defects. J. Thorac. Cardiovasc. Surg. 57:95, 1969.

Noninvasive Techniques in Pediatric Cardiovascular Disease

Richard A. Meyer and Samuel Kaplan

Richard A. Meyer and Samuel Kaplan

T HE ACCURATE DESCRIPTION of the anatomy and physiologic effects of congenital heart disease has traditionally depended on cardiac catheterization and selective angiocardiography. However, these procedures are not without hazard in small children and in neonates are associated with a significant risk.[1] Thus, noninvasive methods have a particular attraction in the diagnosis and management of cardiovascular disease in infants and children.

Noninvasive techniques are defined as those that can be applied without penetrating the skin or those that require simple venipuncture. In the broadest sense, noninvasive techniques include an accurate routine history and physical examination supplemented by phonocardiography, electrocardiography and chest roentgenography. These methods are sufficient to characterize several forms of congenital heart disease, including patent ductus arteriosus and ostium secundum atrial septal defect.

This discussion is limited primarily to the application of echocardiography to the diagnosis and management of heart disease in infants and children. A brief consideration of the venous pulse and systolic time intervals will also be included. Space will not permit discussion of the new and promising technique of radioisotope angiocardiography.[2-5] Other noninvasive methods that will not be presented in this review include recordings of the arterial pulse, precordial movements such as apexcardiography and kinetocardiography, impedance cardiography for measurement of cardiac output, radarkymography, ballistocardiography, magnetocardiography and plethysmography.

ECHOCARDIOGRAPHY

Echocardiography has been used successfully to record mitral and tricuspid valve motion,[6-9] to define the left ventricular outflow tract (LVOT) and aortic valve motion,[10] to detect pericardial effusions,[11] and to measure right and left ventricular dimension[12] as well as stroke volume.[12,13,31] However, most of the above work with diagnostic ultrasound has been confined to adults. Only recently have pediatric patients been studied using this technique.[14-18,20-24,27] The demonstration of the pulmonary valve by Gramiak et al.[25] should significantly aid the pediatric cardiologist. The purpose of this review is to present echocardiographic data obtained in infants and children with emphasis on its application in the neonate with congenital heart disease.

From the Department of Pediatrics, University of Cincinnati and The Children's Hospital, Cincinnati, Ohio.

Supported in part by USPHS Grant HL 05728, and by the American Heart Association, Southwestern Ohio Chapter.

Richard A. Meyer, M.D.: Assistant Professor of Pediatrics, University of Cincinnati, and The Children's Hospital, Cincinnati, Ohio. Samuel Kaplan, M.D.: Director, Division of Cardiology, Professor of Pediatrics, and Associate Professor of Medicine, University of Cincinnati, and The Children's Hospital, Cincinnati, Ohio.

Techniques and Findings in Normal Babies

The techniques used in obtaining echocardiograms were similar to that described previously [19,20] and will be outlined only briefly. Most commercial ultrasonoscopes embody similar design features; our studies were performed primarily with a Hoffrel instrument. The transducer used for children under the age of 5 yr had an outer diameter of $\frac{1}{2}$ inch and an active crystal diameter of $\frac{3}{8}$ inch, which was made of a PZT material. For neonates, a similar transducer was used; however, the crystal was fabricated from lead metaniobate.

The patients that we studied ranged in age from 5 hr to adolescence. For the most part, infants did not require sedation, and all patients were examined in a supine position. A composite that illustrates the transducer placement and anatomic structures encountered by the ultrasound beam is demonstrated in Fig. 1. The A mode is an amplitude–distance representation of the reflected echoes, while the motion mode is a time–distance representation of the same echoes. The calibration markers are 1 cm and 1 sec apart. Temporal events of the cardiac cycle and echoes produced by the septum, atrioventricular valves and left ventricular free wall are shown in Fig. 2. The echoes from the anterior leaflet of the mitral and tricuspid valves are identical in wave form.[8] A pincer effect is created when the septum and left ventricle come toward each other during systole.

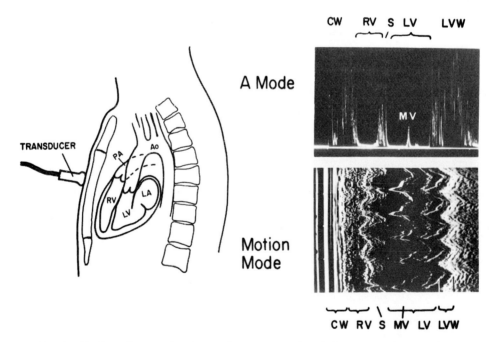

Fig. 1.   Idealized diagram showing cardiac structures in relation to transducer. Echograms illustrate the structures in A and motion modes. PA, pulmonary artery; Ao, aorta; LA, left atrium; CW, chest wall; RV, right ventricle; S, septum; MV, mitral valve; LV, left ventricular cavity; LVW, left ventricular wall.

Fig. 2. Idealized diagram showing normal characteristic wave forms of ultrasound cadiogram (echocardiogram) in relation to temporal events of the cardiac cycle. EKG, electrocardiogram; Phono, phonocardiogram; 1, first heart sound; 2, second heart sound; RS, right septal echo; LS, left septal echo; AV valve, atrioventricular valve echo; LV, left ventricle; endo, endocardial echo; epi, epicardial echo; peri, pericardial echo.

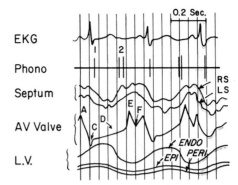

Normal values in babies (Table 1) were obtained from a study of 50 normal newborns.[20] This study served as a control for all other neonates with congenital heart disease. Echograms of normal neonates are shown in Figs. 3, 4, and 5. The ventricular cavities, septum, and anterior mitral leaflet (Fig. 3), the posterior mitral leaflet and the right and left septal echoes (Fig. 4), as well as the tricuspid valve with the ventricular septum and right atrial cavity posterior to the valve echo (Fig. 5), are all visualized. In every instance, an echo was obtained from the mitral and tricuspid valves.

Normally, the anterior mitral valve leaflet is attached to the mitral ring, which is contiguous with the posterior aortic ring. In its coapted position dur-

Table 1. Echocardiographic Findings in 50 Normal Neonates

	M* = 31	F+ = 19
	RANGE	MEAN
Age (in hours)	5 - 125	44
Wt. (in kg)	2.3 - 4.9	3.2
TV — Depth	2.4 - 3.2	2.8
TV — Velocity (mm/sec)	34 - 56	43
TV — Excursion	0.8 - 1.4	1.1
MV — Depth	3.1 - 4.7	3.8
MV — Velocity (mm/sec)	36 - 80	53
MV — Excursion	0.6 - 1.2	1.0
LA Diameter	0.6 - 1.3	0.9
LV Outflow tract	0.7 - 1.2	1.0
LV End diastolic	1.2 - 2.0	1.6
RV End diastolic	1.0 - 1.7	1.3

* Males.
+ Females.
    Abbreviations: TV, tricuspid valve; MV, mitral valve; LA, left atrium; LV, left ventricle; RV, right ventricle.

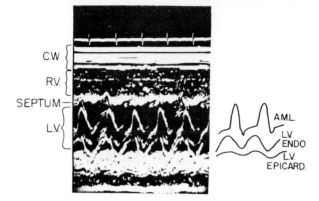

CW.
R.V.
SEPTUM
L.V.

A.M.L.
L.V. ENDO
L.V. EPICARD.

Fig. 3. Echocardiogram of newborn demonstrating the right and left ventricular cavities as well as the mitral valve echo. CW, chest wall; RV, right ventricle; LV, left ventricular chamber; AML, anterior mitral leaflet; LV endo, left ventricular endocardial echo; LV epicard, left ventricular epicardial echo.

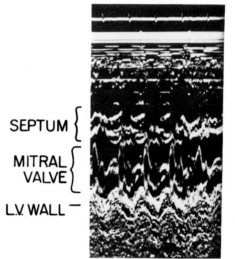

SEPTUM
MITRAL VALVE
L.V. WALL

A.L.
P.L.

Fig. 4. Echocardiogram of normal newborn showing the two septal echoes and the anterior and posterior mitral leaflets. LV wall, left ventricular wall; AL, anterior leaflet; PL, posterior leaflet.

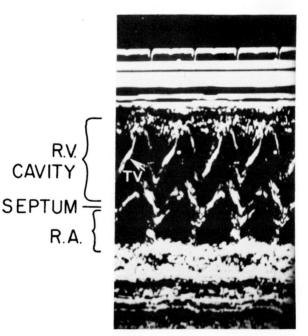

R.V. CAVITY
SEPTUM
R.A.

TV

Fig. 5. Echocardiogram of normal newborn showing the tricuspid valve. RV, right ventricular cavity; RA, right atrium; TV, tricuspid valve echo.

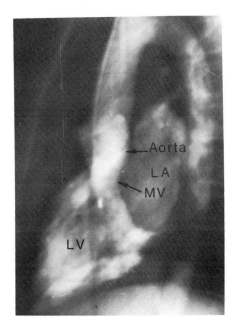

Fig. 6. Lateral left ventriculogram with mitral regurgitation demonstrating mitral-aortic continuity. LV, left ventricle; LA, left atrium; MV, mitral valve.

ing systole, the anterior mitral leaflet lies at the same depth from the anterior chest wall as the posterior margin of the aortic ring (Fig. 6). This anatomic relationship of mitral–semilunar valve continuity can be demonstrated by echocardiography (Fig. 7). From the mitral valve position, the transducer is slowly angulated medially and superiorly along the mitral valve leaflet towards its attachment to the mitral ring, which demarcates the posterior limits of the aortic root. The left ventricular outflow tract (LVOT) is formed by the anterior mitral leaflet and mitral annulus posteriorly, and the muscular and membranous ventricular septum anteriorly. Further superior angulation of the transducer records the anterior as well as the posterior margins of the aortic root (Fig. 8), while the posterior aortic cusp can be seen during diastole within the aortic root. Posterior to the aortic root lies the left atrium.[28] It was of interest that in our normal patients the aortic root and left atrium had similar dimensions, which persisted in all pediatric age groups.

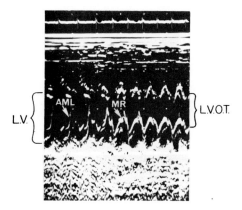

Fig. 7. Echocardiogram showing mitral-aortic continuity. Anterior movement of the mitral leaflet is diastolic, whereas anterior movement of the mitral ring is systolic. LV, left ventricular cavity; AML, anterior mitral leaflet; MR, mitral ring; LVOT, left ventricular outflow tract.

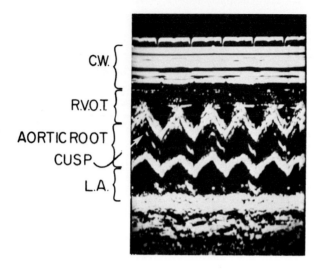

CW.

R.V.O.T.

AORTIC ROOT

CUSP

L.A.

Fig. 8. Echocardiogram of normal newborn showing the aortic root and left atrium posteriorly. The anterior movement of the aortic root is systolic. The posterior cusp is visualized in diastole. CW, chest wall; RVOT, right ventricular outflow tract; LA, left atrium.

Lundstrom[14] studied 45 children between the ages of 2 wk and 15 yr. He found the velocity of passive closure of the mitral and tricuspid valves was similar to that described in adults.[6-10,19] In our neonates, the mitral velocity was 53 mm/sec, while the tricuspid velocity was 43. The reason for the slowness is not readily apparent.

Congenital Heart Disease in the Critically Ill Neonate

Many neonates who are hypoxic, regardless of cause, may exhibit a shock-like picture that includes gray color, poor to absent peripheral pulses, hepatomegaly, and cardiomegaly. It is essential to differentiate cardiac and non-cardiac causes of this picture. Frequently neonates with *aortic atresia* and hypoplastic left ventricle cannot be distinguished clinically from those who have shock due to sepsis. However, neonates with aortic atresia have characteristically similar echocardiograms that are diagnostic of this syndrome.[20] The diagnostic criteria are: (1) absence of a normal mitral valve echo; (2) small to absent aortic root; and (3) a small posterior ventricle in the presence of a large anterior ventricle (Fig. 9). Usually the right ventricle is twice the normal dimension, while the left ventricle is one-third or less of the normal size. A distorted but recognizable mitral valve echo may be recorded within the posterior chamber, although frequently it is absent. Identification of the aortic root is accomplished by directing the transducer superiorly along the tricuspid valve until the margins of the aortic root are recognized (Fig. 9). It is important to recognize that the tricuspid valve is continuous with the anterior margin or the aortic root. Even though a LVOT is unidentifiable, an aortic root may be present and should be recordable. In our experience with 14 patients, the dimension of the aortic root has been one-half or less the normal size. The left atrium generally was of normal size. The tricuspid valve echo in a patient with aortic atresia is usually easily identifiable (Fig. 10). The above echocardiographic findings have enabled the diagnosis of aortic atresia to be made without resorting to cardiac catheterization or angiography. At our institution,

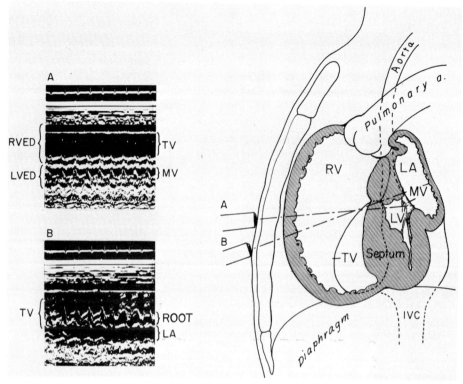

Fig. 9. Idealized diagram in sagittal view of patient with aortic valve atresia. Echogram A depicts the structures recorded from transducer position A. Echogram B depicts the structures recorded as the transducer is rotated from position A to position B. RVED, right ventricular end diastolic dimension; LVED, left ventricular end diastolic dimension; TV, tricuspid valve; MV, mitral valve; ROOT, aortic root; LA, left atrium; LV, left ventricle; IVC, inferior vena cava.

the last eight patients with this disease have been diagnosed by echocardiography alone, and this diagnosis was confirmed at autopsy in each instance.

Total anomalous pulmonary venous drainage is frequently considered in the differential diagnosis of a seriously ill baby with radiologic evidence of pul-

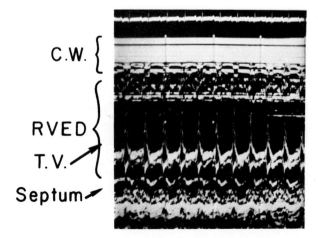

Fig. 10. Echocardiogram of patient with aortic atresia showing large right ventricle and easily identified tricuspid valve. CW, chest wall; RVED, right ventricular end diastolic dimension; TV, tricuspid valve.

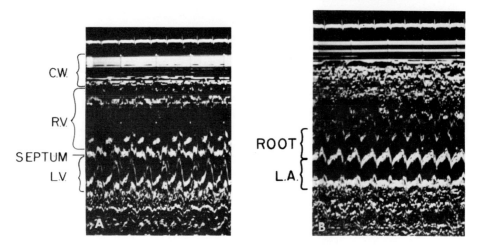

Fig. 11. Echocardiogram of patient with infradiaphragmatic total anomalous pulmonary venous drainage showing: (A) large right ventricle and small left ventricle, which contains a normal mitral valve echo; (B) normal left ventricular outflow tract and smaller than normal left atrium. CW, chest wall; RV, right ventricle; LV, left ventricle; ROOT, aortic root; LA, left atrium.

monary edema. This malformation has characteristic echocardiographic features (Fig. 11). Although this condition is frequently associated with a relatively small left ventricle, there are typical findings that distinguish this disease entity from others with a hypoplastic left ventricle. These consist of (1) a mitral valve echo that is normal in wave form and velocity although the amplitude may be diminished; (2) a left ventricle that, though small, generally exceeds the dimensions associated with aortic atresia; and (3) a LVOT and, hence, an aortic root echo that is easily obtainable and measures within the lower limits for normal neonates. It is of interest that, when these patients have a left ventricular dimension one-half or less of the normal mean dimension, they are poor surgical risks. In these patients the ventricular septal echo usually moves normally because there is right ventricular hypertension resulting from the pulmonary venous obstruction. In conditions with right ventricular volume overload, the septal motion is abnormal.[21,24] However, the septal motion remains normal if right ventricular hypertension exists.[21] The left atrial dimension is usually within the lower limits of normal.

Symptomatic patients with *single ventricle* may demonstrate minimal cyanosis and have clinical findings indistinguishable from patients with a large ventricular septal defect and pulmonary hypertension, atrioventricular canal, or transposition of the great vessels with a large ventricular septal defect. In our patients the application of ultrasound has been quite helpful in excluding or arriving at the diagnosis of single ventricle. Regardless of the anatomic classification,[29,30] functionally the heart behaves as a single ventricular chamber.

Van Praagh et al.[30] demonstrated that in most patients with single ventricle a morphologic septum can be identified, although it is markedly displaced. However, for practical purposes, it is nonexistent, and the single most important echocardiographic finding is the absence of a ventricular septal echo (Fig. 12). In these patients a septal echo is not identified even after careful search-

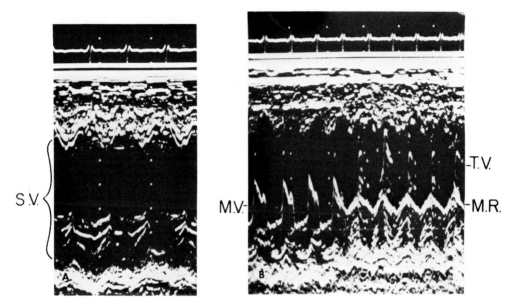

Fig. 12. Echocardiogram of patient with single ventricle and transposition of great arteries. (A) Septum was not identified; (B) shows two atrioventricular valves. SV, single ventricle; TV, tricuspid valve; MR, mitral ring.

ing, and the echogram is the same whether infundibular inversion is present or not.

Elliott et al.[29] described four possible combinations of the atrioventricular valves in single ventricle. The most common was a separate mitral valve and a tricuspid valve. Two separate valves may be demonstrated at different depths (Fig. 12). It is possible that the echo identified as the mitral ring may originate from a muscle bundle, which rarely arises between the basal leaflets of the tricuspid and mitral valves. The majority of our patients with single ventricle had two atrioventricular valves. However, if only a single atrioventricular valve is present, the echo produced by the valve has an excessive anterior excursion.

It has been suggested that single ventricle cannot be distinguished from malformations with hypoplastic left or right ventricles. In our experience this has not been a problem, since in the latter conditions there was echocardiographic continuity of one atrioventricular valve and the aortic root. In neonates with single ventricle, continuity with an atrioventricular valve and the pulmonary root echoes was not demonstrable. Furthermore, an aortic root or pulmonary root echo was not obtainable in any of our neonates. Therefore, these two echocardiographic findings as well as failure to demonstrate a septal echo assume diagnostic significance and strongly suggest the diagnosis of single ventricle.

In our experience the only entity that is difficult to distinguish from single ventricle is corrected or L transposition of the great vessels. The difficulty arises because the ventricles lie side by side, and the septum assumes a position perpendicular to the anterior chest wall. Thus, the transducer beam is parallel to the septum and fails to record it.

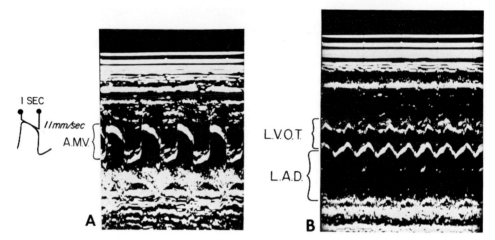

Fig. 13. Echogram of 18-mo-old patient with coarctation of the aorta. (A) Valve echo is thick, and velocity is quite slow. (B) Left atrium is large. This study confirmed suspected mitral stenosis. AMV, anterior mitral valve leaflet; LVOT, left ventricular outflow tract; LAD, left atrial dimension.

Congenital mitral stenosis, whether isolated or associated with other diseases, may readily be diagnosed by the slow mitral valve closure (Fig. 13). Orifice size and speed of closure of the mitral valve has not been correlated in children as it has in adults.[7] However, a velocity of 11 mm/sec is severely retarded compared to normal neonates.

Uncomplicated *tricuspid atresia* may readily be diagnosed by ultrasound in the neonate. The three characteristic echocardiographic findings are: (1) absent tricuspid valve; (2) a small anterior ventricular chamber; and (3) a LVOT and aortic root identified by mitral–semilunar valve continuity (Fig. 14). The small right ventricle contrasts with the large left ventricle and the mitral valve echo is easily demonstrable within the left chamber. Of great significance is the fact that, after careful searching, a tricuspid valve echo is unobtainable, although it is easily demonstrated in every normal newborn.[20]

Mitral–semilunar valve continuity and the aortic root are demonstrated in Fig. 14B. These findings assume diagnostic importance in differentiating tricuspid atresia from patients with aortic atresia and single ventricle. In aortic atresia the atrioventricular valve echo is continuous with the anterior margin of the aortic root (Fig. 9B), and in single ventricle an aortic root or outflow tract is not recorded.

There are great clinical similarities between *Fallot's tetralogy and double outlet right ventricle with pulmonic stenosis*. Echocardiographically, the differential diagnosis of these two diseases depends upon demonstration of mitral–semilunar valve relationship and an overriding aorta. The normal mitral–semilunar valve continuity has been described above (Figs. 6 and 7). In patients with double outlet right ventricle there is discontinuity between the mitral valve ring and the semilunar valve (Fig. 15). Ultrasonically, this is demonstrated (Fig. 16) by rotating the transducer medially and superiorly along the anterior mitral leaflet when an abrupt anterior displacement of the posterior margin of

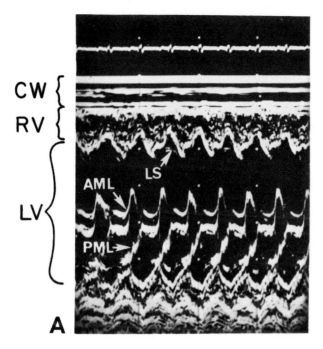

Fig. 14. Echocardiogram of a newborn with tricuspid valve atresia. (A) A minute right ventricular chamber is shown. Mitral valve echo is easily identified within the large left ventricular cavity. (B) Two adjoining polaroid pictures of same patient show mitral-aortic continuity. The aortic root is twice the normal size. CW, chest wall; RV, right ventricle; LV, left ventricle; AML, anterior mitral leaflet; PML, posterior mitral leaflet; LS, left septal echo; MV, mitral valve.

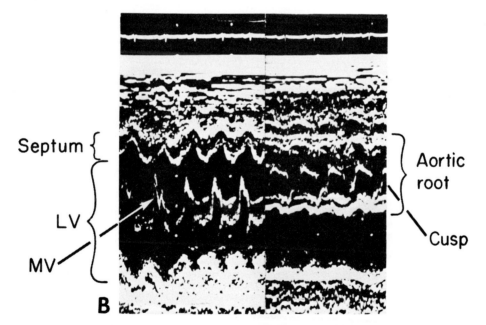

the aortic root is visualized. In patients with Fallot's tetralogy (Fig. 17) there is overriding of the aorta, but mitral–semilunar valve continuity is preserved. Overriding of the aorta can be demonstrated by discontinuity between the margin of the ventricular septum and the anterior wall of the aorta.

Other common forms of congenital heart disease in the symptomatic neonate

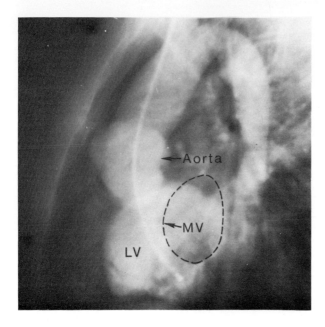

Fig. 15. Left ventriculogram demonstrating discontinuity of the mitral valve ring and the aortic root. MV, mitral valve ring; LV, left ventricle.

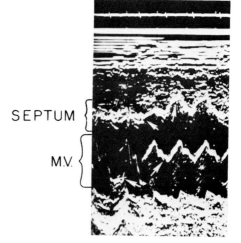

Fig. 16. This echogram shows discontinuity of mitral valve and aortic root. There is abrupt anterior displacement of aortic root from systolic position of mitral valve (lower arrows). Anterior displacement of the aorta is shown by the upper arrows. The septal and anterior aortic root echoes should be at the same depth. MV, mitral valve.

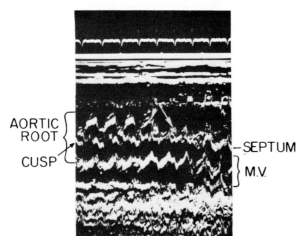

Fig. 17. Tetralogy of Fallot. There is continuity of mitral–aortic valves; however, aortic overriding of septum is shown (arrows). MV, mitral valve.

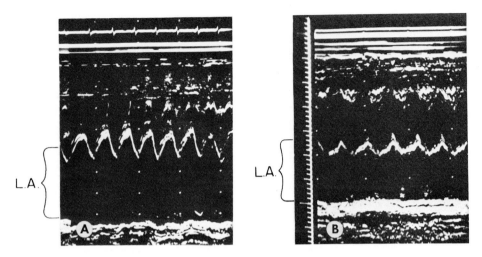

Fig. 18. Preoperative (A) and postoperative (B) echograms of 3½-yr-old boy with patent ductus arteriosus. The interval between (A) and (B) was 3 days. Depth markers are the same in both echograms. Size of left atrium in (A) decreased by one-half in (B).

do not have diagnostic echocardiograms. These include transposition of the great arteries, the coarctation syndrome, patent ductus arteriosus, and large ventricular septal defect. However, echocardiography is useful in the measurement of chamber size in these patients (Fig. 18) as well as evaluating associated atrioventricular and aortic valve disease.

Congenital Heart Disease in Older Children

Recently, conditions associated with right volume overload, which include *atrial septal defects, ostium primum defects, total anomalous pulmonary venous return, pulmonic insufficiency and tricuspid insufficiency*, have been studied by ultrasound. Diamond et al.[21] described two echocardiographic features associated with this condition in adults. Meyer et al.[24] confirmed these findings in 21 children prior to and following correction of their lesions. These features are abnormal septal motion and an increased right ventricular end-diastolic dimension. Preoperatively, all patients with right ventricle volume overload had an increased right ventricular end-diastolic dimension (RVED) (Fig. 19). The normal adult value[6] is 0.7 cm/sq m of body surface. After correction of the defects, the RVED generally diminishes by one-third within 6 mo of surgery.[24]

The normal ventricular septum (Fig. 20) moves posteriorly or towards the left ventricular wall during systole and anteriorly or away from the posterior wall during diastole. Practically all patients with right volume overload exhibit abnormal septal motion. More commonly, the septal motion is reversed and moves anteriorly in systole (Fig. 19A). Occasionally, an intermediate septal motion is recorded with little movement of septum so that the echo remains straight (Fig. 20) during systole. Following correction of the defects, the septal motion reverted to normal (Fig. 19B) when the RVED decreased by approximately one-third of the preoperative value.

The abnormal septal motion depends upon right volume overload in the presence of normal pulmonary vascular resistance and right ventricular pres-

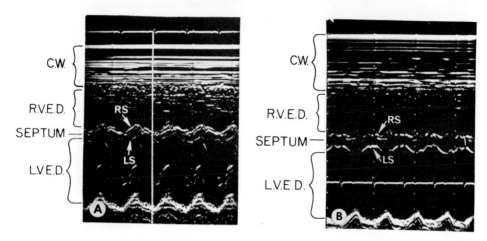

Fig. 19. Preoperative (A) and postoperative (B) echograms of a patient with secundum atrial septal defect (ASD). Preoperative echogram shows reversal of septal motion and enlarged right ventricle (3.2 cm/sq m). White line corresponds to Q wave of electrocardiogram. Postoperative echogram showing return of septal motion to normal and diminished right ventricular size (2.5 cm/sq m). CW, chest wall; RVED, right ventricular end diastolic dimension; RS, right septum; LS, left septum; LVED, left ventricular end-diastolic dimension.

sure.[24] If the pulmonary resistance or right ventricular pressure increases, the RVED may be increased, but the septal motion will be normal.[21] This technique has been useful in patients as young as 4 mo of age.

Another disease that lends itself to echocardiographic diagnosis is *hypertrophic subaortic stenosis.*[32-38] Moreyra et al.[33] described apposition of the anterior mitral leaflet to the ventricular septum during systole. Shah et al.[32] observed abnormal mitral valve motion in the form of abrupt anterior movement of the anterior leaflet in mid systole with resultant narrowing of the left ventricular outflow space (Fig. 21). Patients with persistently abnormal systolic mitral valve movement had an average peak systolic pressure gradient of 78 mm Hg. Those with inconstant abnormality had an average peak gradient of 24 mm Hg, and those with no resting abnormality had no gradients at rest.[35]

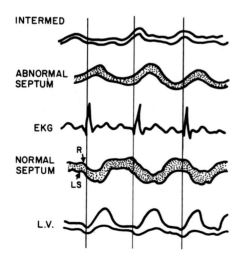

Fig. 20. Idealized diagram of the wave form and direction of the normal and abnormal types of septal motion in right ventricular volume overload. INTERMED, intermediate; EKG, electrocardiogram; R, right septal surface; LS, left septal surface; LV, left ventricular echo.

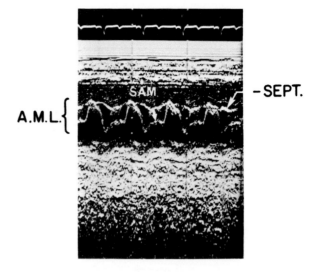

Fig. 21. Mitral valve echogram from 7-yr-old girl with idiopathic hypertrophic subaortic stenosis showing abrupt anterior bulge of the anterior mitral leaflet during mid and late systole, which narrows the left ventricular outflow. The anterior leaflet is in apposition with the septum during early diastole. AML, anterior mitral leaflet; SAM, systolic anterior movement; SEPT, septum.

In addition, Shah et al.[36] studied the long-term effects of ventriculotomy and oral propranolol therapy by echocardiography. The study showed no significant differences at rest between patients on propranolol and untreated patients, whereas most who underwent ventriculotomy did show improvement.

In children, *valvular aortic stenosis* is usually congenital in origin. Investigation of the aortic valve and root by ultrasound[10,39,40] in adults has provided useful information. Gramiak[10] measured various parameters of the aortic valve and root from echocardiograms of patients with and without aortic valve disease in an attempt to predict the severity of the stenosis. Unfortunately, valve area could not be determined ultrasonically. However, the presence of calcification could be detected. Calcification of the aortic valve has been recognized as an indicator of the severity of stenosis.[43] Gramiak found that when three or more echoes from the valve cusps were recorded during diastole, or the intensity of the cusp echoes equalled or exceeded the intensity of the wall echoes, then calcification was present, and the patient had significant valve

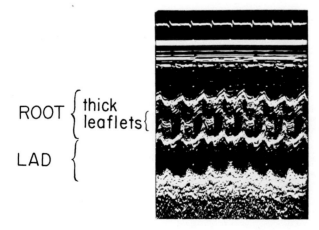

Fig. 22. Echogram of aortic root in 14-yr-old boy with severe aortic stenosis. There are multiple diastolic echoes, whereas in normals no more than three should be recorded. At surgery, this valve required replacement. ROOT, aortic root; LAD, left atrial dimension.

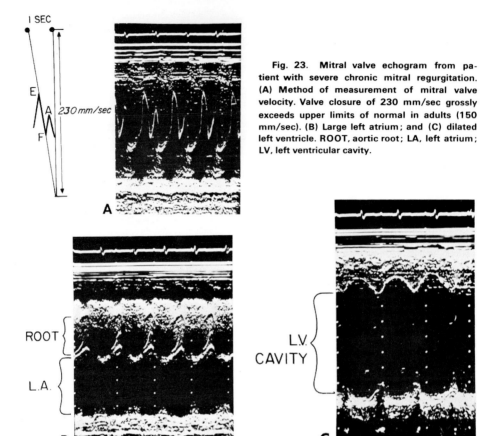

Fig. 23. Mitral valve echogram from patient with severe chronic mitral regurgitation. (A) Method of measurement of mitral valve velocity. Valve closure of 230 mm/sec grossly exceeds upper limits of normal in adults (150 mm/sec). (B) Large left atrium; and (C) dilated left ventricle. ROOT, aortic root; LA, left atrium; LV, left ventricular cavity.

stenosis. The multiplicity of diastolic echoes and the near equal intensity of the cusp and wall echoes can be demonstrated in pediatric patients (Fig. 23).

In addition to the above echocardiographic findings, measurement of the diameter of the aortic root provided useful information. It is possible to predict, within 1–2 mm, the size of the aortic valve ring. This may help the surgeon in planning the selection of the prosthesis and its size prior to operation. Knowledge of the size of the aortic valve ring has also been helpful in determining preoperatively whether transection of the ring will be necessary to relieve the obstruction.

Acquired Heart Disease

Mitral Valve Disease: To date there are no reports of echocardiography in pediatric patients with acquired mitral valve disease, although adults with mitral incompetence have been investigated.[29,44,45,56] The ultrasound finding most commonly examined in *mitral insufficiency* is the rapid closure of the anterior leaflet during passive ventricular filling. Measurement of the velocity of closure is shown in Fig. 23. Generally, adults with mitral valve closing velocities greater than 150 mm/sec have mitral insufficiency.[9] In our patients (5–15 yr) with documented mitral valve insufficiency, this value was not as

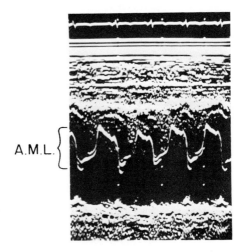

A.M.L.

Fig. 24. Mitral valve echogram from a 16-yr-old patient with mild mitral stenosis. The leaflet is slightly thickened and the velocity of diastolic closure is 28 mm/sec. AML, anterior mitral leaflet.

helpful, since one-half had velocities less than 150 mm/sec, and in many instances the values were less than 125 mm/sec. When normal valve velocities become available for various pediatric age groups, these values will be more meaningful. The other expected echocardiographic findings of mitral insufficiency include a large left atrium (Fig. 23B) and a large left ventricular end-diastolic dimension (Fig. 23C). The normal adult left atrial[14] and ventricular[6] dimensions are 2 cm/sq m and 4.5 cm, respectively.

A preliminary study[27] has suggested that the mitral valve closing velocity is increased in high output states and left to right shunts. These observations will be meaningful in the pediatric patient only when normal control values are available for various age groups beyond the neonate.

Although acquired *mitral valve stenosis* occurs infrequently in the pediatric patient, the echocardiographic findings would be expected to be similar to those for congenital mitral stenosis. These include a slow valve velocity (Fig. 24) and an enlarged left atrium. In adults, the rate of valve closure has been correlated with the valve areas and severity of stenosis.[7] Accordingly, the diastolic slope of 28 mm/sec shown in Fig. 24 would suggest that the patient had mild asymptomatic disease. Such correlations in children are as yet unavailable.

Echocardiography has been used to diagnose congenital or acquired *late systolic prolapse of the posterior mitral valve leaflet.* Dillon et al.[22] and Schwartz et al.[52] correlated clinical echocardiographic and hemodynamic data that show posterior displacement of the posterior mitral leaflet in mid and late systole. The valve leaflets behave normally during diastole (Fig. 25). It is not possible to record the abnormal posterior movement in every patient with prolapse of the posterior mitral valve leaflet. However, when this finding is recorded it is unique and therefore diagnostic.

Aortic Valve Incompetence: Echocardiography has been employed successfully to detect aortic insufficiency.[46–48,50] The ultrasonic features are mitral valve flutter (Fig. 26) and premature closure of the mitral valve (Fig. 27). Mitral flutter or diastolic oscillation of the anterior leaflet of the mitral valve is the vibration of the anterior leaflet resulting from the regurgitant jet striking the

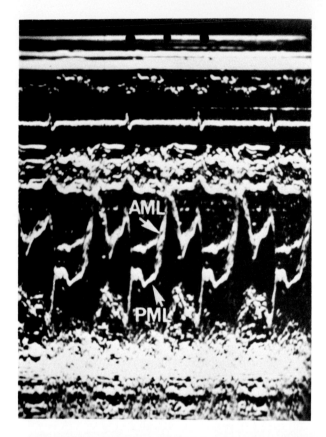

Fig. 25. Mitral valve echogram from patient with prolapse of posterior mitral leaflet. There is an abrupt posterior movement of posterior leaflet during mid and late systole. AML, anterior mitral leaflet; PML, posterior mitral leaflet.

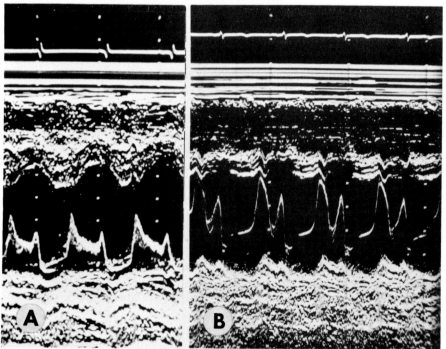

Fig. 26. Mitral valve echograms from patient with aortic incompetence (A) showing flutter of the anterior leaflet and from patient without aortic incompetence (B).

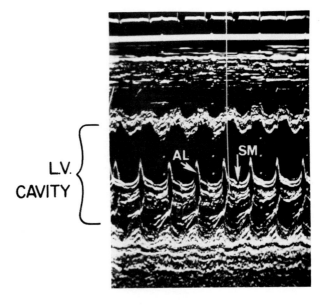

Fig. 27. Mitral valve echogram from a 12-yr-old boy with severe acute aortic insufficiency. The mitral valve closes before onset of the P wave, as indicated by white vertical line, and remains in closed position. Delay of opening movement of the mitral valve is also shown. AL, anterior leaflet; SM, onset of systolic movement.

anterior mitral leaflet.[47] The oscillations may begin during any part of the diastole but terminate with the onset of ventricular systole.

Winsberg et al.[47] estimated the frequency of classic fluttering to be 30–40 Hz. Atrial fibrillation also produces diastolic fluttering but of slower frequency. None of the 500 echocardiograms in their control patients exhibited classic fluttering. In several of our patients with acute rheumatic fever, classic fluttering was observed prior to the early diastolic murmur of aortic regurgitation. These patients subsequently developed the typical auscultatory findings of aortic valve disease associated with acute rheumatic fever.

In severe aortic regurgitation of acute onset the mitral valve closure is extremely premature and may precede the P wave (Fig. 27). Also, the mitral valve opening is delayed owing to superimposed failure of the left ventricle. Pridie et al.[50] explain the premature mitral valve closure on the rapid equilibration of the aortic and left ventricular pressures in acute aortic insufficiency. The steep rise in left ventricular pressure quickly exceeds the left atrial pressure and thus shuts the mitral valve prematurely. Prolongation of the systolic ejection time in severe aortic regurgitation delays the mitral valve opening. In patients with chronic regurgitation, obvious premature mitral valve closure is not seen, even in the presence of left ventricular failure.

Pericardial Fluid: One of the early applications of echocardiography that provided great impetus for developing the technique was the detection of pericardial fluid.[53-55] The technique has been proven to be highly accurate, safe and without risk. Therefore, the use of invasive methods are unnecessary for the diagnosis of pericardial effusion. Ordinarily, the pericardial echo fuses with the epicardial echo of the left ventricle. In the presence of pericardial fluid (Fig. 28), an echo-free space separates the nonmoving straight pericardial echo from the epicardial echo. Once the fluid has resorbed or been removed, this echo-free space is no longer visible (Fig. 28).

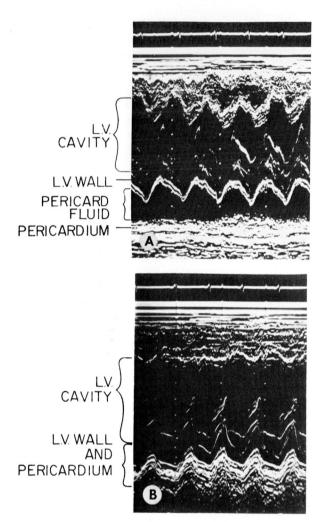

L.V. CAVITY

L.V. WALL

PERICARD FLUID

PERICARDIUM

A

L.V. CAVITY

L.V. WALL AND PERICARDIUM

B

Fig. 28. Echocardiogram of patient with pericardial effusion. (A) Large pericardial effusion showing fluid present. (B) Absence of pericardial fluid space after resorption of fluid. LV, left ventricular; PERICARD, pericardial.

THE VENOUS PULSE (EXTERNAL PHLEBOGRAM)

Inspection of the jugular venous pulse allows an analysis of the wave form and measurement of venous pressure. These physical signs yield considerable diagnostic information. Unfortunately, this simple bedside test may be neglected in children, especially in small, noncooperative patients who may have short necks. However, the extra time taken to analyze the jugular venous pulse is well worth the effort. Since excitement, crying, coughing, and the Valsalva maneuver increase the jugular venous pressure, it is essential that the child is relaxed during examination. The patient is propped in bed at an angle that reveals the maximum venous pulsation. This angle is frequently about 45°, but it may vary from 30–90°. Distention of the external jugular veins by constriction of their passage through the deep cervical fascia occurs in many normal children. Distention and pulsation of the jugular venous system above the sternal angle is abnormal and in many instances an increased venous pressure in the internal jugular vein appears as a venous pulsation without distention.

These pulsations accurately reflect the change in right atrial pressure at all stages of the cardiac cycle. The height of the central venous pressure is measured as the vertical distance between the top of the oscillating venous pulse and the sternal angle (i.e., the junction of the manubrium and body of the sternum). The normal jugular venous pressure oscillates at almost zero, and its peak seldom exceeds 3 cm of blood with reference to the sternal angle.

Venous pulsations in the neck may be readily distinguished from arterial pulsations.[65] Venous pulsations are diffuse, undulate, yield readily to pressure, and vary with the position of the patient, whereas carotid arterial pulsations are single, abrupt, only compressible with moderate pressure, and do not vary with the patient's position. The height of the venous pulse follows the intrathoracic pressure so that it drops during inspiration and rises in expiration. Abdominal pressure increases the height of the venous pulse and has little effect on arterial pulsations. Mild compression of the external jugular vein in the supraclavicular fossa abolishes venous pulsations and distends the veins, but will not affect carotid pulsations.

In each cardiac cycle the normal jugular phlebogram consists of two major positive crests, termed "a" and "v" (Fig. 29). Each of these waves is followed by negative troughs termed "x" and "y." The "c" wave, another crest, may interrupt the "x" descent. The "a" wave is produced by atrial systole, corresponds to right ventricular end-diastolic pressure, coincides with the P-R interval, and immediately precedes the upstroke of the carotid pulse. The first part of the "a" wave is due to passive filling of the atrium, and the latter is produced by atrial contraction. The "x" descent is caused by atrial relaxation. The "c" wave has been attributed to tricuspid valve closure or an artefact on the jugular phlebogram produced by the carotid pulse. It has been suggested that well-defined "c" waves due to tricuspid valve closure may be seen in atrial septal defects.[65] The "v" wave is produced by the inflow and accumulation of blood from the venous system into the right atrium. It is written during late ventricular systole and early diastole so that it corresponds to the interval between the onset of the T and P waves. The "y" descent is due to opening of the tricuspid valve with the escape of blood into the relaxed right ventricle.

Giant "a" Waves: In children giant "a" waves are seen most frequently in significant isolated valvular pulmonic stenosis (Fig. 29). Their presystolic timing is confirmed by the fact that these abrupt waves precede the upstroke of the carotid pulse and the first heart sound. These waves are produced by a powerful right atrial contraction necessitated by an increased resistance to right ventricular filling. The latter is due to either an increase in right ventricular end-diastolic pressure or decreased diastolic distensibility due to right ventricular hypertrophy and fibrosis. The diagnosis of tetralogy of Fallot is unlikely if giant "a" waves are present. Cyanotic children with large "a" waves usually have pulmonic stenosis, intact ventricular septum, and right-to-left atrial shunting. Giant "a" waves are also unusual in children with marked elevation of pulmonary vascular resistance secondary to ventricular septal defects or aortic–pulmonary communications. However, they may be seen in patients with severe pulmonary hypertension secondary to elevated pulmonary venous pressure in the absence of tricuspid incompetence. Large "a" waves are sometimes seen in

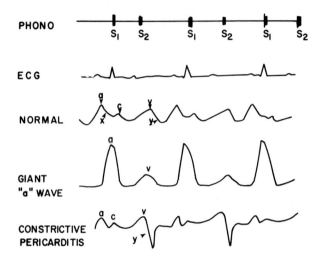

Fig. 29. Idealized diagram of the normal jugular phlebogram, giant "a" waves (e.g. due to severe pulmonic stenosis) and constrictive pericarditis (with deep "Y" deosis) and constrictive pericarditis (with deep "Y" descent). PHONO, phonocardiogram; S1, first heart sound; S2, second heart sound; ECG, electrocardiogram.

tricuspid stenosis or atresia, especially when the right to left shunt is restricted by a small opening in the atrial septum.

Right Ventricular Failure: The elevated systemic venous pressure is easily identified by observation of the jugular venous pulse in untreated right ventricular failure. The major venous pulse is either "v" or "y." Patients with incipient right ventricular failure and normal jugular venous pulse at rest have an elevation of jugular venous pressure with slight exertion that returns slowly to resting levels.

Tricuspid incompetence is associated with the large "v" waves, which are frequently transmitted to the liver, especially in the presence of atrial fibrillation. These are produced by transmission of right ventricular pressure to the right atrium through the incompetent tricuspid valve. If sinus rhythm is maintained, the large "v" waves may be preceded by recognizable "a" waves and "x" descents.

Complete heart block and other varieties of atrioventricular dissociation result in large pulsations (cannon waves), which are seen intermittently and irregularly in the jugular veins. They occur when the right atrium contracts against a closed tricuspid valve and correspond to P waves that fall within the Q–T interval of the electrocardiogram. Although independent "a" waves are seen in the jugular phlebogram which correspond to P waves, they are usually inconspicuous to inspection of the cervical veins.

Cardiac compression due to pericardial effusion or chronic constrictive pericarditis results in an elevated venous pressure throughout the cardiac cycle. The characteristic feature of the jugular phlebogram in patients with constrictive pericarditis is the deep "y" descent (Fig. 29). This is associated with diastolic collapse of the venous pulse, which follows the opening of the tricuspid valve as blood flows from the right atrium into the relaxing right ventricle. Following the "y" descent, the venous pressure rises sharply and rapidly, since right atrial and ventricular pressures equalize and further cardiac filling is limited by the pericardial compression.

Fever, anemia, or advanced liver disease in children may result in mild elevation of venous pressure, which has been attributed to the hyperkinetic circulation in these conditions. Significant elevations of the jugular venous pressure attributed to an increased blood volume occurs in many patients with *acute nephritis*. Superior vena caval obstruction raises venous pressure, but pulsations are maintained if the obstruction is incomplete. This is seen in patients who have had a partially functioning superior vena caval–right pulmonary anastomosis (*Glenn operation*) for the palliation of cyanotic congenital heart disease. After many years, right pulmonary artery perfusion can be impeded by narrowing of the distal branches of the pulmonary artery or by thrombosis of the anastomosis.

SYSTOLIC TIME INTERVALS

In adults, useful information concerning left ventricular function has been derived from measurement of systolic time intervals. These intervals are generally obtained from simultaneous fast speed recordings of the electrocardiogram, the indirect carotid or subclavian pulse and the phonocardiogram or apex-cardiogram (Fig. 30). Total electro-mechanical systole ($Q–S_2$) is the interval between the onset of ventricular depolarization (Q wave) to the initial high frequency vibration of the second heart sound (S_2). Left ventricular ejection time (LVET) is measured from the beginning of the upstroke to the dicrotic notch of the carotid pulse tracing. The preejection period (PEP) refers to the interval between the onset of ventricular depolarization and the beginning of left ventricular ejection and is obtained by subtracting LVET from $Q–S_2$. The measurement of systolic time intervals by these noninvasive methods compare favorably with corresponding intervals measured simultaneously during left ventricular and central aortic catheterization.[67]

There is much background physiologic information that supports the premise that systolic time intervals may be used to evaluate left ventricular function. $Q–S_2$ and LVET are abbreviated by tachycardia.[68,74] PEP is shortened by the increased heart rate of adrenergic cardiac stimulation but is unchanged with tachycardia induced by vagal blockade or atrial pacing.[68,69] LVET is prolonged,

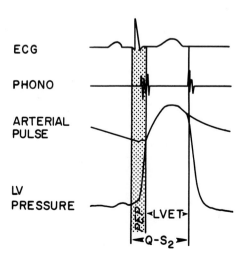

Fig. 30. Temporal events of cardiac cycle to illustrate method of measurement of systolic time intervals. PEP, preejection period; LVET, left ventricular ejection time; Q-S2, total electromechanical systole; ECG, electrocardiogram; PHONO, phonocardiogram; LV, left ventricular.

ECG

PHONO

ARTERIAL PULSE

LV PRESSURE

PEP shortened and $Q-S_2$ is generally unchanged when stroke volume is increased by enhanced ventricular filling.[70] PEP, LVET and Q–S are shortened by pharmacologic agents that induce positive inotropic effects.[69,71] PEP is inversely correlated with cardiac output and stroke volume.

Abnormal systolic time intervals have also been measured in patients with heart disease. In heart failure PEP is prolonged, LVET abbreviated, and $Q-S_2$ remains unchanged.[72] PEP is also prolonged in left bundle branch block.[73] LVET is increased in aortic stenosis. LVET is decreased by a lowered stroke volume and is increased when stroke volume is enhanced.

The ratio of PEP to LVET has been found to be especially useful, since it remains relatively constant in normal adults and is minimally affected by heart rate.[74] This ratio is inversely correlated with cardiac output and stroke volume. When myocardial disease is associated with diminished left ventricular function, PEP shortens while LVET lengthens so that PEP/LVET increases.

There are few reports of systolic time interval measurements in normal infants and children and those with cardiac disease. Harris et al. studied 146 children free of cardiovascular disease of which 47 were prematures, 50 were mature neonates, and 49 were older children.[75] They found that the duration of total electro–mechanical systole and left ventricular ejection time diminished linearly and in parallel with increasing heart rates up to 150/min. When the heart rate was above this level, these phases of systole diminished more gradually. However, the duration of PEP remained more or less constant and was unaffected by heart rates reaching almost 200/min. There was a wide distribution of the duration of systolic time intervals in premature babies. Left ventricular ejection time tended to be more prolonged at any level of heart rate in these babies. This was especially noticeable if the hemoglobin was less than 12 g/100 ml, which is a frequent occurrence in otherwise normal prematures.

Park, Dimich, and Steinfeld[76] measured systolic time intervals in 150 normal infants and 15 babies with clinical signs of left heart failure. They confirmed the inverse relationship between LVET and heart rate in normal infants. However, systolic time intervals in infants with left heart failure were different from those reported in adults. Babies in left heart failure due to large ventricular septal defects, or the coarctation syndrome, had prolonged ejection times with respect to heart rate, and PEP was normal.

This important preliminary report needs confirmation by the examination of a larger group of babies. Since major alterations in the duration of systolic time intervals accompany changes in stroke volume and heart rate, it is hoped that measurement of these intervals will be useful in evaluating changes in left ventricular function during the followup of infants and children with congenital heart disease.

SUMMARY

For the last 25 yr, the definitive diagnosis of congenital heart disease has depended upon cardiac catheterization and selective angiocardiography. Since these procedures are risky, especially in the severely ill neonate, noninvasive methods must be developed and widely applied.

Echocardiography in pediatrics is gaining popularity and as experience broadens, the degree of confidence in the method increases. A logical extension of the diagnostic application of the technique is to develop the method as a means of assessing cardiac function. Certainly, in adults, evaluation of left ventricular function has been initiated.[12,13,31,57-62] Similar information concerning very young children is not available at this time. The innovative application of cardiac scanning by Tanaka et al.[63] in Japan and King[64] in New York adds yet a further dimension to diagnostic ultrasound. Scanning produces a two-dimensional cross-sectional image of the intracardiac structures that provides a picture, as it were, of the heart. Development of this technique should markedly enhance the use of echocardiography as a noninvasive method for accurate anatomic diagnosis of congenital heart disease.

REFERENCES

1. Braunwald, E. and Swan, H. J. C. (Eds.): Cooperative study on cardiac catheterization. American Heart Association. Circulation 37 (Suppl. III), 1968.

2. Mason, D. T., Ashburn, W. L., Harbert, J. C., Cohen, L. S., and Braunwald, E.: Rapid sequential visualization of the heart and great vessels in man using the wide-field Anger scintillation camera. Circulation 39:19, 1968.

3. Graham, T. P., Jr., Goodrich, J. K., Robinson, A. E., and Harris, C. C.: Scintiangiocardiography in children. Rapid sequence visualization of the heart and great vessels after intravenous injection of radionuclide. Am. J. Cardiol. 25:387, 1970.

4. Kriss, J. P., Enright, L. P., Hayden, W. G., Wexler, L., and Shumway, N. E.: Radioisotopic angiocardiography. Wide scope of applicability in diagnosis and evaluation of therapy in diseases of the heart and great vessels. Circulation 43:792, 1971.

5. Hagan, A. D., Friedman, W. F., Ashburn, W. L., and Alazraki, N.: Further application of scintillation scanning technics to the diagnosis and management of infants and children with congenital heart disease. Circulation 45:858, 1972.

6. Popp. R. L., Wolfe, S. B., Hirata, S., and Feigenbaum, H.: Estimation of right and left ventricular size by ultrasound. Am. J. Cardiol. 24:523, 1969.

7. Edler, I.: Ultrasound cardiography in mitral valve stenosis. Am. J. Cardiol. 10:18, 1967.

8. Joyner, C. R., Hey, E. B., Johnson, J., and Reid, J. M.: Reflected ultrasound in the diagnosis of tricuspid stenosis. Am. J. Cardiol. 19:66, 1967.

9. Segal, B. L., Likoff, W., and Kingsley, B.: Echocardiography: Clinical application in mitral regurgitation. Am. J. Cardiol. 19:50, 1967.

10. Gramiak, R., and Shah, P. M.: Echocardiography of the normal and diseased aortic valve. Radiology 96:1, 1970.

11. Feigenbaum, H., Zaky, A., and Waldhausen, J. A.: Use of reflected ultrasound in detecting pericardial effusion. Am. J. Cardiol. 19:84, 1967.

12. Popp, R. L., and Harrison, D. C.: Ultrasonic cardiac echography for determining stroke volume and valvular regurgitation. Circulation 41:493, 1970.

13. Pombo, J. F., Troy, B. L., and Russell, R. O., Jr.: Left ventricular volumes and ejection fraction by echocardiography. Circulation 43:480, 1971.

14. Lundstrom, N. R., and Edler, I.: Ultrasound-cardiography in infants and children. Acta Paediatr. Scand. 60:117, 1971.

15. Chesler, E., Joffe, H. S., Vecht, R., Beck, W., and Schrire, V.: Ultrasound cardiography in single ventricle and the hypoplastic left and right heart syndromes. Circulation 42:123, 1970.

16. —, —, Beck, W., and Schrire, V.: Echocardiographic recognition of mitral–semilunar valve discontinuity: An aid to the diagnosis of origin of both great vessels from the right ventricle. Circulation 43:725, 1971.

17. Lundstrom, N.-R.: Ultrasound cardiographic studies of the mitral valve region in young infants with mitral atresia, mitral stenosis, hypoplasia of the left ventricle and cor triatriatum. Circulation 45:324, 1972.

18. Chesler, E., Joffe, H. S., Beck, W., and Schrire, V.: Echocardiography in the diagnosis of congenital heart disease. Pediatr. Clin. N. Am. 18:1163, 1971.

19. Feigenbaum, H.: Clinical applications of echocardiography. Prog. Cardiovasc. Dis. 14:531, 1972.

20. Meyer, R. A., and Kaplan, S.: Echocardiography in diagnosis of hypoplasia of

260 MEYER AND KAPLAN

left or right ventricle in neonatal congenital heart disease. Circulation 46:55, 1972.

21. Diamond, M. A., Dillon, J. C., Haine, C. L., Chang, S., and Feigenbaum, H.: Echocardiographic features of atrial septal defect. Circulation 43:129, 1971.

22. Dillon, J. C., Haine, C. L., Chang, S., and Feigenbaum, H.: Use of echocardiography in patients with prolapsed mitral valve. Circulation 43:503, 1971.

23. Lundstrom, N.-R: Ultrasoundcardiography in diagnosis of Ebstein's anomaly of tricuspid valve. Preliminary observations Proc. Ass. Europ. Pediatr. Cardiol. 3:44, 1971.

24. Meyer, R. A., Schwartz, D. C., Benzing, G., III, and Kaplan, S.: The ventricular septum in right ventricular volume overload. Am. J. Cardiol. 30:349, 1972.

25. Gramiak, R., Nanda, N. C., and Shah, P. M.: Echo detection of the pulmonary valve. Radiology 102:153, 1972.

26. Tajik, A. J., Gau, G. T., and Schattenberg, T. T.: Echocardiogram in total anomalous pulmonary venous drainage—report of a case. Mayo Clin. Proc. 47:247, 1972.

27. Ulta, L. B., Segal, B. L., and Likoff, W.: Echocardiography in congenital heart disease (Preliminary observations). Am. J. Cardiol. 19:74, 1967.

28. Hirata, T., Wolfe, S. B., Popp, R. L., Helman, C., and Feigenbaum, H.: Estimation of left atrial size using ultrasound. Am. Heart J. 78:43, 1969.

29. Elliott, L. P., Anderson, R. C., and Edwards, J. E.: The common cardiac ventricle with transposition of the great vessels. Br. Heart J. 26:289, 1964.

30. Van Praagh, V., Ongley, R. A., and Swan, H. J. C.: Anatomic types of single or common ventricle in man. Morphologic and geometric aspects of 60 necropsied cases. Am. J. Cardiol. 13:367, 1964.

31. Fortuin, N. J., Hood, W. P., Jr., Sherman, M. E., and Craige, E.: Determinations of left ventricular volumes by ultrasound. Circulation 44:575, 1971.

32. Shah, P. M., Gramiak, R., and Kramer, D. H.: Ultrasound localization of left ventricular (LV) outflow obstruction in hypertrophic obstructive cardiomyopathy (HOCM). Circulation 38 (Suppl. 6):6, 1968.

33. Moreyra, E., Klein, J. J., Schemada, H., and Segal, B. L.: Idiopathic hypertrophic subaortic stenosis diagnosed by reflected ultrasound. Am. J. Cardiol. 23:32, 1969.

34. Shah, P. M., Gramiak, R., and Kramer, D. H.: Ultrasound localization of left ven-

tricular outflow obstruction in hypertrophic obstructive cardiomyopathy. Circulation 40:3, 1969.

35. —, —, Adelman, A. G., and Wigle, E. D.: Role of echocardiography in diagnostic and hemodynamic assessment of hypertrophic subaortic stenosis. Circulation 44:891, 1971.

36. —, —, and Adelman, A. G.: Echocardiographic assessment of the effects of surgery and propranolol on the dynamics of outflow obstruction and hypertrophic subaortic stenosis. Circulation 45:516, 1972.

37. Popp, R. L., and Harrison, D. C.: Ultrasound in the diagnosis and evaluation of therapy of idiopathic hypertrophic subaortic stenosis. Circulation 40:905, 1969.

38. Pridie, R. B., and Oakley, C. M.: Mechanism of mitral regurgitation in hypertrophic obstructive cardiomyopathy. Br. Heart J. 32:203, 1970.

39. Hernberg, J., Weiss, B., and Keegan, A.: The ultrasonic recording of aortic valve motion. Radiology 94:361, 1970.

40. Gramiak, R., and Shah, P. M.: Echocardiography of the aortic root. Invest. Radiol. 3:356, 1968.

41. —, Shah, P. M., and Kramer, D. H.: Ultrasound cardiography: contrast studies in anatomy and function. Radiology 92:939, 1969.

42. Feigenbaum, H., Stone, J. M., Lee, D. A., Nassar, W. K., and Chang, S.: Identification of ultrasound echoes from the left ventricle by use of intracardiac injections of indocyanine green. Circulation 41:615, 1970.

43. Glancy, D. L., Freed, T. A., O'Brian, K. P., and Epstein, S. E.: Calcium in the aortic valve. Roentgenologic and hemodynamic correlations in 148 patients. Ann. Intern. Med. 71:245, 1969.

44. Joyner, C. R., Jr., Reed, B. E. E., and Band, J. P.: Reflected ultrasound in the assessment of mitral valve disease. Circulation 23:503, 1963.

45. Segal, B. L., Likoff, W., and Kingsley, B.: Echocardiography in combined mitral stenosis and regurgitation. Am. J. Cardiol. 19:42, 1967.

46. Pocock, W. A., and Barlow, J. B.: Etiology and electrocardiographic features of the billowing posterior mitral leaflet syndrome. Am. J. Med. 51:731, 1971.

47. Winsberg, F., Gabor, G. E., Hernberg, J. G., and Weiss, B.: Fluttering of the mitral valve in aortic insufficiency. Circulation 41:225, 1970.

48. Hernberg, J., Weiss, B., and Kugan, A.:

The ultrasonic recording of aortic valve motion. Radiology 94:361, 1970.

49. Fortuin, N. J., and Craige, E.: On the mechanism of the Austin Flint murmur. Circulation 45:558, 1972.

50. Pridie, R. B., Benham, R., and Oakley, C. M.: Echocardiography of the mitral valve in aortic valve disease. Br. Heart J. 33:296, 1971.

51. Zaky, A., Grabhorn, L., and Feigenbaum, H.: Movement of the mitral ring: A study in ultrasound cardiography. Cardiovasc. Res. 1:121, 1967.

52. Schwartz, D. C., Kaplan, S., and Meyer, R. A.: Late systolic mitral regurgitation in children. Am. J. Cardiol. 29:290, 1972.

53. Feigenbaum, H., Waldhausen, J. A., and Hyde, L. P.: Ultrasound diagnosis of pericardial effusion. JAMA 191:711, 1965.

54. —, Zaky, A., and Grabhorn, L. L.: Cardiac motion in patients with pericardial effusion. Circulation 34:611, 1966.

55. , —, and Waldhausen, J. A.: Use of reflected ultrasound in detecting pericardial effusion. Am. J. Cardiol. 19:84, 1967.

56. Joyner, C. R., and Reid, J. P.: Ultrasound cardiogram in the selection of patients for mitral valve surgery. Ann. N.Y. Acad. Sci. 118:512, 1965.

57. Murray, J. A., Johnston, W., and Reid, J. M.: Echocardiographic determination of left ventricular performance. Ann. Intern. Med. 72:777, 1970.

58. Pombo, J. F., Troy, B. L., and Russell, R. O., Jr.: Left ventricular volumes and ejection fraction by echocardiography. Circulation 43:480, 1971.

59. Krauntz, R. F., and Ryan, T. J.: Ultrasound measurements of ventricular wall motion following administration of vasoactive drugs. Am. J. Cardiol. 27:464, 1971.

60. Fischer, J. C., Chang, S., Konecke, L. L., and Feigenbaum, H.: Echocardiographic determination of mitral valve flow. Am. J. Cardiol. 29:262, 1972.

61. Smithen, C., Wharton, C., and Sowton, E.: Changes in left ventricular wall movement following exercise, atrial pacing and acute myocardial infarction measured by reflected ultrasound. Am. J. Cardiol. 29:293, 1972.

62. Cooper, R., Karliner, J. S., O'Rourke, R. A., Peterson, K. L., and Leopold, G.: Ultrasound determination of mean fiber-shortening rate in man. Am. J. Cardiol. 29:257, 1972.

63. Tanaka, M., et al.: Ultrasonic evaluation of anatomical abnormalities of heart in congenital and acquired heart diseases. Br. Heart J. 33:686, 1971.

64. King, D. L.: Cardiac ultrasonography. A stop-action technique for imaging intracardiac anatomy. Radiology 103:387, 1972.

65. Wood, P.: Diseases of the Heart and Circulation (ed. 3). Philadelphia, J. Lippincott, 1968.

66. Shabetai, R., Fowler, N. O., and Guntheroth, W. G.: The hemodynamics of cardiac tamponade and constrictive pericarditis. Am. J. Cardiol. 26:480, 1970.

67. Metzger C. C., Chough, C. B., Kroetz, F. W., and Leonard, J. J.: True isovolumic contraction time: Its correlation with two external indexes of ventricular performance. Am. J. Cardiol. 25:434, 1970.

68. Leighton, R. F., Zaron, S. J., Robinson, J. L., and Weissler, A. M.: Effects of atrial pacing on left ventricular performance in patients with heart disease. Circulation 40:615, 1969.

69. Harris, W. S., Schoenfeld, C. D., and Weissler, A. M.: Effects of adrenergic receptor activation and blockade on the systolic preejection period, heart rate, and arterial pressure in man. J. Clin. Invest. 46:1704, 1967.

70. Harley, A., Stermer, C. F., and Greenfield, J. C., Jr.: Pressure-flow studies in man: Evaluation of the duration of the phases of systole. J. Clin. Invest. 48:895, 1969.

71. Weissler, A. M., Gamel, W. G., Grode, H. E., Cohen, S., and Schoenfeld, C. D.: Effect of digitalis on ventricular ejection in normal human subjects. Circulation 29:721, 1964.

72. —, Harris, W. S., and Schoenfeld, C. D.: Systolic time intervals in heart failure in man. Circulation 37:149, 1968.

73. Adolph, R. J., Fowler, N. O., and Tanaka, K.: Prolongation of isovolumic contraction time in left bundle branch block. Am. Heart J. 78:585, 1969.

74. Weissler, A. M., Harris, W. S., and Schoenfeld, C. D.: Bedside technics for the evaluation of ventricular function in man. Am. J. Cardiol. 23:577, 1969.

75. Harris, L. C., Weissler, A. M., Manske, A. O., Danford, B. H., White, G. D., and Hammill, W. A.: Duration of the phases of mechanical systole in infants and children. Am. J. Cardiol. 14:448, 1964.

76. Park, S., Dimich, I., and Steinfeld, L.: Systolic time intervals in infants with heart failure. Circulation 42 (Suppl. 3):31, 1970.

Erythrocyte Oxygen Transport in Normal Infants and in Infants With Cardiovascular Disease

William W. Miller

THE MOVEMENT of oxygen from the external environment to the body cell involves several sequential and interrelated mechanical–chemical functions: pulmonary ventilation, blood loading in the lung, cardiac propulsion, arterial distribution to tissues, capillary blood unloading, and diffusion to and into the body cell. One or more of these transport components can be altered by a variety of physiologic changes, such as increased physical activity or abnormal environmental temperatures, and also can be affected by pathologic conditions, such as hypoxemia or congestive heart failure. Additional adaptations in oxygen transport occur in the normal human newborn as a result of the transition at birth from placental oxygen supply to air breathing.

This review will analyze certain aspects of the oxygen transport system which involve the erythrocyte of the human infant. The components of the system to be discussed are erythrocyte production, pulmonary oxygen loading, and tissue oxygen unloading. These components will be examined with reference to the fetus, the healthy newborn, and newborns with hypoxemia or with heart failure from congenital cardiac diseases.

Erythrocyte Structure and Function

The function of the erythrocyte is to transport oxygen, carbon dioxide, protons, and certain salts from one location to another within the vasculature. Most of its structure and metabolism provides for the maintenance of the hemoglobin molecule and for interactions between hemoglobin and other externally produced metabolic effectors. Hemoglobin makes up almost 95% of the protein of human erythrocytes, and most of the remaining 5% can be accounted for by enzymes that modulate its interaction with oxygen, carbon dioxide, protons, and salts. The three-dimensional structure of the hemoglobin tetramer is made up of four polypeptide chains bound by electro-chemical forces to four heme groups.

Oxygen Loading Capacity

Under normal circumstances of infancy, and even with most pathologic conditions, the oxygen loading capacity of blood is determined by the concentration of hemoglobin in each unit of blood flowing through the pulmonary capillaries. Although gross inequities of pulmonary ventilation and perfusion can modify pulmonary oxygen loading, extremely severe degrees of hypoventilation

From the Department of Pediatrics, University of Texas Southwestern Medical School, and the Division of Cardiology, Children's Medical Center, Dallas, Tex.

Supported by an Institutional Grant from the University of Texas Southwestern Medical School and by grants from the Dallas Heart Association and the American Heart Association, Texas Affiliate, Inc.

William W. Miller, M.D.: *Associate Professor of Pediatrics, Department of Pediatrics, The University of Texas Southwestern Medical School, Dallas, Tex. 75235.*

or heart failure are required, and even then hemoglobin concentration plays a significant role in oxygen transport.

The concentration of hemoglobin in blood is determined by the production of erythropoietin, secreted largely in the kidney, and by the availability of substrates for the synthesis of erythrocytes and hemoglobin in bone marrow. When both of these determinants operate, there are increases in both the number of erythrocytes and the concentration of hemoglobin. The stimulus for the production of erythropoietin is hypoxia. This response has been demonstrated as early as the eighth mo of fetal development, and, at birth, the marrow shows marked erythropoiesis, and erythropoietin can be measured in plasma. [1,2]

Recent refined measurements indicate that the molecular weight of adult hemoglobin (HB A) is approximately 64,460 g. [3] Each molecule of hemoglobin can combine with four molecules of oxygen (4 × 22.4 liter). Therefore, in quantitative terms the loading capacity of hemoglobin is 1.39 ml O_2/g. This same capacity applies to newborns, older children, and adults, since the molecular weights of fetal and adult hemoglobin molecules are only slightly different. [4,5]

Oxygen-Hemoglobin Equilibrium

The equilibrium between molecules of oxygen and hemoglobin is conveniently illustrated by a curve (Fig. 1), which identifies the relative amounts of hemoglobin combined with oxygen (oxyhemoglobin saturation) at various gas pressures of oxygen (oxygen tension). When oxygen loading is analyzed in relationship to hemoglobin mass, the term, oxyhemoglobin saturation, is useful. However, in most clinical circumstances, the actual oxygen content (ml O_2) of a specific volume of whole blood (100 ml) is a more meaningful measure of total oxygen load. The right–left position of each equilibrium curve is identified by the value for P50, the oxygen tension of the blood sample at which 50% of the hemoglobin mass is combined with oxygen. In healthy children and adults, the normal P50 is 26–27 mm Hg. [6]

Abnormalities of oxygen-hemoglobin affinity occur in a variety of diseases characterized by imbalances in oxygen supply and demand. They are recognized conveniently by shifts in the position of the oxygen-hemoglobin equilibrium curve to the right or left of the normal position (Fig. 2). Rightward shifts in the curve indicate decreased oxygen-hemoglobin affinity. They are identified by

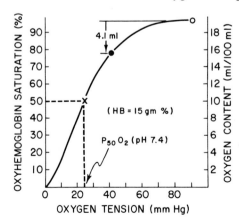

Fig. 1. The oxygen-hemoglobin equilibrium curve of normal adult blood. Position of the curve as defined by P50, the oxygen tension at 50% oxyhemoglobin saturation, is normally 26 mm Hg and the arterial-venous (open and closed circle, respectively) difference in oxygen content is 4.1 ml/100 ml blood flow with hemoglobin 15 g/100 ml.

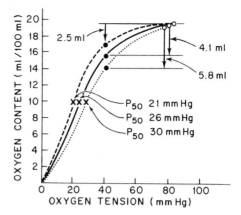

Fig. 2. Normal oxygen-hemoglobin equilibrium (P50 26 mm Hg) and oxygen unloading
capacity (4.1 ml/100 ml) is compared with a
rightward-shifted curve (P50 30 mm Hg) with
increased unloading capacity (5.8 ml/100 ml)
and a leftward-shifted curve (P50 21 mm Hg)
with decreased unloading capacity (2.5 ml/
100 ml).

higher values of P50. Leftward shifts in the curve indicate increased affinity of
hemoglobin for oxygen. They are represented by lower P50 values. The sigmoid
shape of the oxygen-hemoglobin equilibrium curve for human blood indicates
that, in the normal range of alveolar oxygen pressure (80–100 mm Hg), wide
shifts to the right or left of normal have little effect in changing the oxygen content of blood leaving the lung. In contrast, at the lower oxygen pressure of the
tissues (40 mm Hg), small changes in oxygen tension are associated with large
differences in oxygen content. Therefore, if the arteriovenous difference of oxygen content remains constant, a rightward shift is associated with an increase
in mixed venous oxygen tension and a leftward shift is accompanied by a decreased mixed venous oxygen tension. Alternatively, if mixed venous blood
oxygen tension remains constant, the arteriovenous difference in oxygen content increases with a rightward shift in the equilibrium curve and decreases
with a leftward shift. Since the rate of oxygen movement from capillary bed to
cell mitochondria is a function of the difference in oxygen pressure, it can be
assumed that the rightward shift of decreased oxygen affinity facilitates systemic oxygen transport and the leftward shift diminishes it. In this review,
measurements of oxygen content, oxygen saturation, and oxygen tension were
made at 37°C, and all P50 values have been corrected by calculations to a
standard pH of 7.4.[7]

The sequential and cooperative association and dissociation of four oxygen
molecules with one molecule of hemoglobin can be symbolized chemically by
an equation system of four consecutive and reversible reactions:

$$HB_4 + O_2 \underset{k_1}{\overset{k_1'}{\rightleftharpoons}} HB_4O_2 \tag{1}$$

$$HB_4O_2 + O_2 \underset{k_2}{\overset{k_2'}{\rightleftharpoons}} HB_4O_2 \tag{2}$$

$$HB_4O_4 + O_2 \underset{k_3}{\overset{k_3'}{\rightleftharpoons}} HB_4O_6 \tag{3}$$

$$HB_4O_6 + O_2 \underset{k_4}{\overset{k_4'}{\rightleftharpoons}} HB_4O_8 . \tag{4}$$

The distribution of the velocity constants for each of these eight reactions accounts for the sigmoid shape of the curve that is characteristic of human blood.[8] Shifts in the position of the equilibrium curve are the result of changes in the velocity constants for oxygen-hemoglobin dissociation (k) or association (k′).

The equilibrium between oxygen and hemoglobin is influenced by several interrelated physical and chemical factors, including temperature, carbon dioxide tension, hydrogen ion concentration, and DPG.[6,9-17] The effects of protons and of temperature have been known for some time. A decrease in oxygen-hemoglobin affinity with a rightward shift in the equilibrium curve occurs with acidemia and with hyperthermia. An increase in affinity with a leftward shift is associated with alkalemia and hypothermia. Increases in erythrocyte temperature result in rapid hemoglobin deoxygenation by increasing the hemoglobin binding of DPG in place of oxygen. The quantitative effect of temperature is represented by the equation, $\Delta \log P50/\Delta T = 0.024$. Increased hydrogen ion concentration has both an immediate, direct effect upon oxygen equilibrium and a slower, indirect effect through metabolic alterations of DPG concentration. The direct effect of acidemia is a rightward shift in the equilibrium curve (Bohr effect) due to changes in the dissociation constants. At a constant P_{co2} a change in pH of 0.10 is associated with a P50 difference of approximately 2.5 mm Hg. Carbon dioxide alters oxygen affinity directly by an instantaneous change in erythrocyte pH and indirectly by a less rapid, binding to hemoglobin as carbamate.

2,3-Diphosphoglycerate

A few years ago, it was discovered that two intermediates of erythrocyte glycolysis, 2,3-diphosphoglycerate (DPG) and adenosine triphosphate, profoundly change the affinity of hemoglobin for oxygen and carbon dioxide.[15-17] In human erythrocytes, DPG has the predominate chemical effect on affinity because its concentration (18 μ mole/g HB) is significantly greater than that of adenosine triphosphate (4 μ mole/g HB).[18-19] When DPG is excluded from reactions between hemoglobin and oxygen, there is a marked increase in the affinity between these two molecules, as demonstrated by a leftward shift in the equilibrium curve. If DPG is added to the hemoglobin-oxygen reaction, and in the concentration found in normal human erythrocytes, the affinity between hemoglobin and oxygen becomes identical to that found in normal intact erythrocytes. Several studies have shown that DPG is the primary chemical regulator of hemoglobin affinity for oxygen.[20,21] Indeed, throughout the physiologic range of DPG within human erythrocytes, there is a precise, direct, and statistically correlative relationship between DPG concentration and the position of the oxygen-hemoglobin equilibrium curve (Fig. 3).[22]

In intact erythrocytes DPG influences oxygen affinity both by a direct, instantaneous change in pH and by an indirect effect of specific interaction with the hemoglobin molecule.[23] At physiologic pH, DPG is a highly charged anion, and, according to the Gibbs-Donnan theory, it influences the distribu-

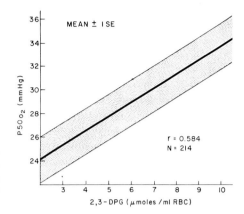

Fig. 3. Precise, statistically significant relationship between erythrocyte DPG concentration and the position of the oxygen-hemoglobin A equilibrium curve at 37°C and pH 7.4. (Modified after Lenfant.[22])

tion of protons on each side of the erythrocyte membrane. High levels of DPG are associated with lower erythrocyte pH and increased oxygen-hemoglobin dissociation. DPG also increases the rate of oxygen dissociation from hemoglobin as a result of a direct effect on the dissociation constants.[24] Measurements of the dissociation constants of erythrocytes with high DPG (61 μ mole/ g HB), normal DPG (13 μ mole/g HB), and low DPG (2 μ mole/g HB) indicate that in low concentrations DPG has a direct effect on the rate of oxygen dissociation, whereas at normal or high levels of DPG, the increased rate of oxygen dissociation is due entirely to the proton effect of DPG in reducing erythrocyte pH. Moreover, with normal or high DPG concentrations, there is a pH effect on the dissociation constants that is not present at low DPG levels. In the past, this "kinetic Bohr effect" has often been ignored when correcting in vitro measurements of P50 in erythrocytes with low DPG levels.

The metabolism of DPG has received considerable study since the discovery of its influence in mammalian oxygen transport.[25-27] Its concentration in the erythrocyte depends upon a balance of synthesis from 1,3-DPG and of degradation to 3-phosphoglycerate (Fig. 4). In most mammalian cells, glycolysis is associated with dephosphorylation of 1,3-DPG directly to 3-phosphoglycerate. In human erythrocytes, this reaction can be bypassed by the intermediate formation of 2,3-DPG through the Rapoport-Luebering cycle. The synthesis of 2,3-DPG is determined primarily by the amount of its substrate, 1,3-DPG, and by product inhibition of its synthetic enzyme, DPG mutase. Under normal conditions of glycolysis and oxygenation, increases in 2,3-DPG result from increased 1,3-DPG formation as a result of activation of glycolysis. Increased erythrocyte pH is a strong stimulus of the enzyme, phosphofructokinase, which results in increased concentrations of 1,3-DPG and 2,3-DPG. The synthesis of 2,3-DPG is also self-regulated, since concentrations of the unbound form inhibit DPG mutase activity. Degradation of 2,3-DPG is controlled by the activity of its phosphatase and by the concentration of its product, 3-phosphoglycerate. In normal human erythrocytes, the concentration of DPG is 17 μ mole/g of hemoglobin with a normal mean corpuscular hemoglobin concentration of 34%. In terms of the volume of erythrocytes in blood, the normal DPG concentration is 5.1 μ mole/ml RBC. Infants, children, and

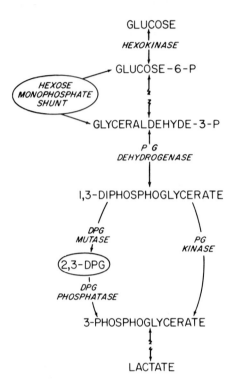

GLUCOSE

HEXOKINASE

GLUCOSE - 6 - P

HEXOSE MONOPHOSPHATE SHUNT

GLYCERALDEHYDE - 3 - P

P G DEHYDROGENASE

1,3-DIPHOSPHOGLYCERATE

DPG MUTASE

PG KINASE

2,3-DPG

DPG PHOSPHATASE

3-PHOSPHOGLYCERATE

LACTATE

Fig. 4.   Schema of erythrocyte glycolysis with the 2, 3-diphosphoglycerate cycle.

adults have essentially the same DPG concentrations, and small differences are largely due to concentration changes related to erythrocyte age.[28]

Fetal Hemoglobin

A fetal form of hemoglobin is found in nearly all mammalian species. In human newborns, hemoglobin F makes up 80% of the total hemoglobin mass, and physiologically significant levels persist until 2 or 3 mo of age.[29] The affinity for oxygen is significantly greater in newborn blood than in blood from the older infant, child, or adult.[30] Although these marked differences in oxygen affinity can be shown for intact erythrocytes from newborns and adults, when solutions of the isolated molecules of hemoglobin F and hemoglobin A are oxygenated, the equilibrium curves demonstrate identical oxygen affinities. These different characteristics are accounted for by differences in the oxygen affinity of deoxyhemoglobin F and deoxyhemoglobin A in the presence of DPG.[19,31] When equal amounts of DPG are added to solutions of hemoglobin F and hemoglobin A, the position of the curve illustrating oxygenation of hemoglobin F is significantly to the left of the curve, representing hemoglobin A oxygenation. The leftward oxygen-hemoglobin equilibrium curve of normal newborns appears to be the consequence of this significant diminution in DPG-hemoglobin F binding in comparison to DPG-hemoglobin A binding.

Normal Fetal–Newborn Transitions in Erythrocyte Oxygen Transport

The affinity for oxygen is widely different in maternal and fetal blood.[32] During human pregnancy, a significant decrease in oxygen affinity occurs as a consequence of increased erythrocyte DPG concentration.[33] During the last month of normal pregnancy, the oxygen-hemoglobin equilibrium curve is shifted to the right of normal (P50 27–28 mm Hg). This decrease in affinity provides a greater oxygen unloading capacity to all tissues, including the placenta. During this same period of gestation the position of the oxygen-hemoglobin equilibrium curve of fetal blood is shifted markedly to the left of normal (P50 20 mm Hg). The significantly greater oxygen affinity of fetal blood provides for greater oxygen loading capacity as deoxygenated fetal blood flows to the maternal placenta. The wide difference in oxygen affinity between fetal and maternal blood allows for significant advantages in transplacental maternal-to-fetal oxygenation.

As organs of respiration, the human placenta and lung have several similarities, but there are important differences in the determinants of end-capillary oxygen tension.[34] The oxygen loading and unloading characteristics of fetal and maternal bloodstreams play a major role in placental respiration. Placental end-capillary oxygen tension, the oxygen tension supplied to the fetus, can be diminished significantly and rapidly by reductions in the oxygen tension of blood entering the placenta from fetal or maternal arteries. Because of this dependence, the oxygen loading capacity of fetal blood (hemoglobin concentration) is the dominant factor in adaptations to oxygen stresses before birth and especially during labor. After placental separation, birth, and respiration by alveolar gas exchange, the oxygen unloading characteristics (oxygen-hemoglobin equilibrium) become dominant. Except during conditions of extreme alveolar underventilation or underperfusion, oxygen loading is seldom a limitation after birth. Unlike placental gas transfer, alveolar oxygenation is independent of the oxygenation state of pulmonary arterial blood, since alveolar oxygen tension remains stable during blood flow through the pulmonary gas exchange area. Adaptations in the production, structure, and metabolism of the erythrocyte play an important role in the postnatal change from reserves for fetal oxygen loading in the placenta to the reserves for newborn oxygen unloading to the tissues.

In normal human infants, the adaptive erythrocyte response to air breathing develops during the first 6 mo of life.[35] Two basically different mechanisms operate (Table 1). During the first mo after birth, the primary change is an increase in oxygen loading of blood as a result of elevated hemoglobin concen-

Table 1. Maturation of Erythrocyte Structure and Function in Healthy Full-term Infants

Age	Total HB (g/100 ml)	O_2 Loading Capacity (ml/100 ml)	P_{50} (mm Hg)	DPG (μ mole/ml RBC)	Fetal HB (% Total)	FF DPG* (μ mole/ml RBC)	O_2 Unloading Capacity† (ml/100 ml)
1 day	17.8 ± 2.0	24.7 ± 2.8	19.4 ± 1.8	5.4 ± 1.0	77.0 ± 7.3	1.2 ± 0.6	1.8
3 wk	12.0 ± 1.3	16.7 ± 1.9	22.7 ± 1.0	5.4 ± 0.7	70.0 ± 7.3	1.6 ± 0.3	2.4
6–9 wk	10.5 ± 1.2	14.7 ± 1.6	24.4 ± 1.4	5.6 ± 0.7	52.1 ± 11.0	2.7 ± 0.6	2.5
3–4 mo	10.2 ± 0.8	14.3 ± 1.2	26.5 ± 2.0	5.8 ± 1.2	23.2 ± 16.0	4.5 ± 1.4	4.6
6 mo	11.3 ± 0.9	14.7 ± 0.6	27.8 ± 1.0	5.1 ± 1.6	4.7 ± 2.2	4.8 ± 1.5	3.1

* Functioning Fraction of 2.3-diphosphoglycerate = DPG × HB A%.

† O_2 Unloading capacity = theoretical systemic arteriovenous oxygen content differences assuming venous PO_2 40 mm Hg and arterial PO_2 that gives 95% oxyhemoglobin saturation.

By permission.[35]

trations. An increase in hemoglobin concentration occurs immediately after birth, but, thereafter, throughout the first mo of life, there is a progressive drop in the number of erythrocytes and in hemoglobin concentration. However, a concurrent reduction in erythrocyte volume operates to maintain mean erythrocyte hemoglobin concentration at a remarkably constant level from birth (MCHC 30%–35%) to adulthood (MCHC 32%–36%).[36]

After the first mo of life, a progressive fall in oxygen loading capacity is compensated for by an increase in oxygen unloading capacity, due entirely to the postnatal transition from fetal to adult hemoglobin production. The relative percentage of fetal hemoglobin diminishes from 70%–80% at birth to 5% at 6 mo of age.[29] During this same time, the affinity of blood for oxygen diminishes progressively, as demonstrated by the rightward shift in oxygen-hemoglobin equilibrium curves from a P50 of 19 mm Hg at birth to the adult value of 28 mm Hg at 6 mo (Table 1 and Fig. 5). This increase in systemic oxygen unloading capacity is the result of relatively constant concentrations of newborn erythrocyte DPG acting upon increasingly large amounts of deoxyhemoglobin A. The product of DPG concentration and hemoglobin A percentage has been referred to as the Functioning Fraction of DPG (FF DPG). In premature infants without other abnormalities, fetal hemoglobin persists for longer periods of time, and, consequently, the adult capacity for oxygen unloading is obtained at a later age in development.

Abnormal Cardiovascular Function in Infants

In infants with cogential cardiac defects, the most common abnormalities of oxygen transport are hypoxemia and heart failure. In each of these conditions, alterations in erythrocyte function operate as homeostatic mechanisms.

Erythrocytosis is an important compensatory mechanism for chronic hypoxemia.[37] In infants with cyanotic forms of congenital cardiac disease, increased plasma erythropoietin has been measured throughout the first several mo of life.[2] Although the erythropoietin response can be demonstrated as rapidly as 8 hr after an hypoxic stimulus, the effects upon marrow erythropoiesis require several days.[38] Moreover, the availability of erythrocyte substrates, especially

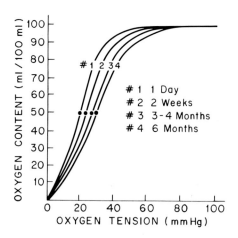

Fig. 5.   Normal shifts in oxygen-hemoglobin equilibrium curves and P50 (closed circles) in healthy, full-term infants from 1 day to 6 mo of age. (By permission.[35])

iron, determines both the time and the rate of the polycythemic response to hypoxemia.[39] In infants with severe cyanosis from birth, the postnatal reduction in erythrocyte number and hemoglobin concentration is less pronounced than in normal infants, and significant polycythemia can be found by 3 or 4 mo of age if iron intake has been adequate. Several natural biologic abnormalities of oxygen supply indicate that the secretion of erythropoietin by the kidney is due to diminished oxygen flow, rather than reductions in the rate or amount of blood or hemoglobin flow.[40-42] Increased levels of erythropoietin and resultant polycythemia have been found among adults with severe degrees of heart failure, but not in those with only moderate reductions in cardiac output.[43] Reliable studies in infants with heart failure have not been reported. In summary, polycythemia, or increased oxygen loading capacity, is an effective, delayed homeostatic response in patients with chronic cyanosis, but evidently it is seldom a mechanism of compensation for heart failure.

Increased oxygen unloading capacity is a second major adaptive response to oxygen transport deficiencies. Shifts in the oxygen-hemoglobin equilibrium curve represent a more rapid and more sensitive adaptation to hypoxemia than does polycythemia. The oxygen affinity response is particularly important during neonatal life, since it becomes operational immediately after birth. Among patients with congential cardiac diseases, significant rightward shifts in the oxygen-hemoglobin equilibrium curve are found in those with significant cyanosis (arterial oxygen saturations less than 85%) and in others with measurable heart failure (cardiac output less than 70% of normal).[44-47] Under these circumstances, the increase in oxygen unloading capacity, proportional to the degree of cyanosis or the reduction of cardiac output, is accounted for by increases in erythrocyte DPG.[48-52] At all ages, there is a significant correlation between the values for P50 and for the Functioning Fraction of DPG. Even during the first postnatal days, when levels of DPG-insensitive hemoglobin F remain high, the concentration of erythrocyte DPG is elevated in patients with severe hypoxemia or heart failure, and the oxygen-hemoglobin equilibrium curve is shifted to the right of normal for that age.

The quantitative significance of adaptations in oxygen loading and unloading can be demonstrated by studies performed in two patients with congenital cardiac dysfunction. Measurements of arteriovenous oxygen difference were made in a 6-mo-old infant with intractable heart failure from large arteriovenous shunts through a ventricular septal defect and a patent ductus arteriosus (Fig. 6). Before ductal ligation and pulmonary artery banding, a marked reduction in oxygen affinity was demonstrated, as shown by the abnormal shift of the equilibrium curve to the right (P50 33.2 mm Hg). Erythrocyte DPG concentration was elevated (6.6 μ mole/ml RBC) and cardiac output was 60% of normal for height and weight (1.2 liter/min). The infant was markedly improved 3 mo after surgery. Cardiac output was normal (1.8 liter/min), erythrocyte DPG was normal (4.9 μ mole/ml RBC) and the oxygen-equilibrium curve had returned to a normal position (P50 25.8 mm Hg). During the period of severe heart failure, the rightward-shifted oxygen-hemoglobin equilibrium curve provided for significant amounts of systemic oxygen transport. Without such a change in oxygen unloading capacity, a large, probably intolerable,

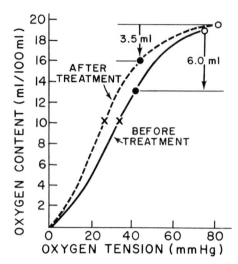

Fig. 6. Measurements of differences in arterial (open circles) and mixed venous (closed circles) oxygen content and oxygen tension in an infant before and after effective surgical palliation of severe congestive heart failure.

demand for additional cardiac output of blood would have been required to meet the same tissue oxygen flow.

In patients with cyanotic congenital cardiac defects, both oxygen loading and unloading operate as homeostatic responses. In an infant with significant hypoxemia from pulmonary atresia and ventricular septal defect, studies were performed at 7 mo of age, immediately before systemic artery-pulmonary artery anastomosis, and they were repeated several mo later (Fig. 7). Before surgical palliation, the infant demonstrated moderate cyanosis and polycythemia. An abnormally large arteriovenous oxygen difference (6.2 ml/100 ml blood) was due to the combined effects of an increase in oxygen loading capacity (HB 19 g/100 ml) and a rightward-shifted oxygen-hemoglobin equilibrium curve (P50 37.6 mm Hg). Cardiac output was 70% of normal for height and weight (1.3 liter/min) and erythrocyte DPG was elevated (7.9 μ moles/ml RBC). Surgery resulted in excellent palliation of hypoxemia, and 6 mo later

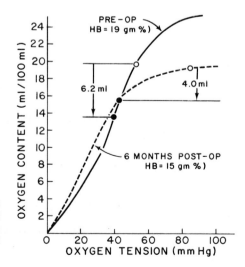

Fig. 7. Measurements of differences in arterial (open circles) and mixed venous (closed circles) oxygen content and oxygen tension in an infant before and after effective surgical palliation of hypoxemia and polycythemia.

the infant had a normal oxygen loading capacity (HB 15 g/100 ml), normal P50 (26.3 mm Hg), and erythrocyte DPG (5.2 μ mole/ml RBC). Cardiac output and arteriovenous oxygen difference were normal. In this patient, both polycythemia and increased DPG provided greater tissue oxygen delivery. With the elimination of hypoxemia by surgery, cardiac output increased, probably as a result of reduced viscosity with the correction of polycythemia.

With tissue hypoxemia, the adaptive increase in erythrocyte DPG appears to be due primarily to an elevation of erythrocytic pH and to an increase in the amount of deoxyhemoglobin.[25-27] In certain conditions of hypoxemia associated with respiratory alkalemia as a result of hyperventilation, the resultant increase in erythrocyte pH stimulates glycolysis by activation of phosphofructakinase. This results in an increase in 1,3-DPG and 2,3-DPG. The increased erythrocyte pH also diminishes DPG degradation by slight depression of DPG phosphatase activity. Increased concentrations of deoxyhemoglobin also increase DPG synthesis, because the cationic charge of deoxyhemoglobin is smaller than that of oxyhemoglobin, i.e., the deoxy-form of hemoglobin is less acidic than the oxy-form. According to Gibbs-Donnan equilibrium, the fewer negative charges characteristic of hypoxemic accumulations of deoxyhemoglobin are associated with a redistribution of ions across the erythrocyte membrane, resulting in elevated erythrocyte pH. At a plasma pH of 7.40, oxygenated erythrocytes are at pH 7.20 and deoxygenated erythrocytes are at pH 7.27.[24] Thus, the relative alkalemia of deoxygenated erythrocytes increases 2,3-DPG synthesis through stimulation of phosphofructakinase. Changes in pH are of additional importance in limiting the DPG response to hypoxemia. With increased levels of DPG, there is a build-up of nonpenetrating, highly charged anions within the erythrocyte. According to Gibbs-Donnan equilibrium, the resultant decrease in erythrocyte pH diminishes further DPG synthesis and counterbalances the hypoxic stimulation of synthesis.

Miscellaneous Oxygen Transport Disorders of Infancy

Changes in oxygen-hemoglobin equilibrium due to altered DPG concentrations are found in a variety of conditions during infancy. The intracellular effects of acidemia operate upon erythrocyte glycolysis to reduce DPG concentration, probably over a period of several hr. The sudden neutralization of acidemia by the i.v. administration of alkali results in significant immediate shifts in the oxygen-hemoglobin equilibrium curve to the left. It seems likely that further study will indicate that this rapid temporary increase in oxygen-hemoglobin affinity may be a significant disadvantage in conditions with limited oxygen transport reserves.[53] Several forms of anemia are associated with DPG increases in oxygen unloading capacity.[54-56] The degree of rightward shift in the equilibrium curve is generally proportional to the severity of the anemia. Rightward shifts in oxygen-hemoglobin equilibrium curves and increased erythrocyte DPG have been measured in patients with pulmonary insufficiency, hyperthyroidism, and uremia.[49,57-60] Leftward shifts in the equilibrium curve and subnormal erythrocyte DPG concentrations have been found in patients with septic shock, hyperoxic exposures, and hypophosphatemia from intravenous hyperalimentation.[61-63]

Blood Storage and Transfusion

In infancy, relatively large quantities of blood are required in the treatment of serious hemolytic disease by exchange transfusion and for blood replacement during major surgical operations. The value of using only fresh blood for all transfusions to infants has been emphasized by the demonstration that storage of blood in ACD medium at 4°C is associated with rapid and profound reductions in the oxygen unloading capacity as a consequence of decreased erythrocyte DPG (Fig. 8).[64] Under ordinary conditions of blood banking, the hemoglobin affinity for oxygen is markedly increased after only 5 days of storage. The infusion of blood stored beyond this time produces decreases in circulating erythrocyte DPG concentration and in whole blood P50.[65] Since the in vivo half-recovery time for DPG is 4 hr, the use of large amounts of such blood, especially in small infants, may be associated with significant limitations in tissue oxygen delivery. The awareness of gross deficiencies of DPG in blood stored beyond 5 days provides a strong additional indication for the use of fresh whole blood or of packed red cells in all transfusions to infants and in most instances in older children where more than two or three units are needed. The requirement for blood with adequate DPG levels may be particularly important during infant surgery in which cardiopulmonary bypass or deep hypothermia techniques are used.[66] In open heart operations in older children, the use of fresh blood and the maintenance of normal acid–base balance is not associated with significant changes in circulating DPG or in whole blood P50.[51,67,68]

Modification of Oxygen-Hemoglobin Equilibrium

Except under extreme conditions of inadequate alveolar gas exchange, an increase in the capacity for unloading oxygen appears to be a major beneficial homeostatic response to relative tissue hypoxemia. If further in vivo study verifies this theory, the induction of rightward shifts in the oxygen-hemoglobin equilibrium curve can be a useful technique in the acute management of severe

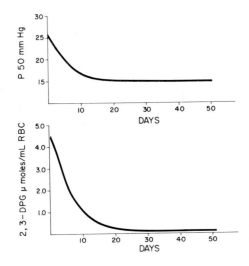

Fig. 8.   Changes in oxygen affinity (P50) and erythrocyte DPG concentration during storage of whole blood at 4°C preserved in acid citrate dextrose solution.

hypoxemia. The administration of fresh blood with normal levels of DPG and P50 represents the simplest form of this therapy.[69] In newborns with severe hemolytic disease, blood with high concentrations of fetal hemoglobin and markedly leftward P50 position (20 mm Hg) is replaced by fresh adult blood with a significantly higher P50 (26 mm Hg).[70] Such a transfusion increases the unloading capacity of blood 50%–60% by a change in oxygen-releasing capacity from 1.6 ml to 2.5 ml/100 ml blood exchange.

In patients with intractable heart failure, DPG-rich erythrocytes may be useful in the early treatment of pulmonary edema or during critical periods of low cardiac output following cardiac surgery. Such blood also may be useful in the acute management of patients, especially newborns, with severe hypoxemia from intracardiac or intrapulmonary venoarterial shunts, and in patients with shock, cold exposure, or certain forms of accidental poisoning. Acute elevations of erythrocyte DPG may be indicated to modify the extent of tissue ischemia in myocardial or cerebrovascular infarctions.

Since the erythrocyte membrane is impermeable to DPG, changes of intracellular DPG concentration require the use of metabolic modifiers that can enter the erythrocyte. Several chemicals and drugs alter the hemoglobin affinity for oxygen either by direct action as protons or through indirect effects on DPG metabolism. Increased P50 has been demonstrated in vitro in blood incubated with methylprednisolone, thyroid hormone, methylene blue, dipyridamole, propranalol, sulfate, and a combination of inosine, pyruvate, and inorganic phosphate.[58,69,71–76] "Super cells," erythrocytes with abnormally high DPG and P50 values, have been induced in vivo by the direct administration of thyroid hormone, methylene blue, sulfate, propranalol, cortisol, aldosterone, and the inosine, pyruvate, and phosphate combination.[57,71,72,74,77–80] In the temporary treatment of patients with severe localized or generalized tissue hypoxemia, the use of such nontoxic modulators of oxygen release may prove to be as logical and useful as the administration of oxygen itself.

REFERENCES

1. Finne, P. H.: Erythropoietin production in fetal hypoxia and in anemic uremic patients. Ann. N. Y. Acad. Sci. 194:497, 1968.

2. Halversen, S.: Plasma erythropoietin levels in cord blood during the first weeks of life. Acta Paediatr. 52:425, 1963.

3. Perutz, M. F.: The haemoglobin molecule. Proc. R. Soc. Lond. (Biol.) 173:113, 1969.

4. Schroeder, W. A., Shelton, J. R., Shelton, J. B., Cormick, J., and Jones, R. T.: The amino acid sequence of the γ chain of human fetal hemoglobin. Biochemistry 2:992, 1963.

5. Cooper, H. A., and Hoagland, H. C.: Fetal hemoglobin. Mayo Clin. Proc. 47:402, 1972.

6. Bohr, C., Hasselbalch, K., and Krogh, A.: Ueber einen in biologischer Beziehung wichtigen Einfluss, den die Kohlensäurespannung des Blutes auf dessen Sauerstoffbindung übt. Skand. Arch. Physiol. 16:402, 1904.

7. Severinghaus, J. W.: Blood gas calculator. J. Appl. Physiol. 21:1108, 1966.

8. Gibson, Q. H.: The reaction of oxygen with hemoglobin and the kinetic basis of the effect of salt on binding of oxygen. J. Biol. Chem. 245:3285, 1970.

9. Naeraa, N., Petersen, E. S., Boye, E., and Severinghaus, J. W.: pH and molecular CO_2 components of the Bohr effect in human blood. Scand. J. Clin. Lab. Invest. 18:96, 1966.

10. Bellingham, A. J., Detter, J. C., and Lenfant, C.: Regulatory mechanisms of hemoglobin oxygen affinity in acidosis and alkalosis. J. Clin. Invest. 50:700, 1971.

11. Roughton, F. J. W.: Some recent work on the interactions of oxygen, carbon dioxide and hemoglobin. Biochemistry 117:801, 1970.

12. Benesch, R. E., Benesch, R., and Yu, C. I.: The oxygenation of hemoglobin in the presence of 2,3-diphosphoglycerate. Effect of

temperature, pH, ionic strength, and hemoglobin concentration. Biochemistry 8:2567, 1969.

13. Kilmartin, J. V., and Rossi-Bernardi, L.: Inhibition of CO_2 combination and reduction of the Bohr effect in haemoglobin chemically modified at its α-amino groups. Nature (London) 222:1243, 1969.

14. Wranne, B., Woodson, R. D., and Detter, J. C.: Bohr effect: interaction between H^+, CO_2, and 2,3-DPG in fresh and stored blood. J. Appl. Physiol. 32:749, 1972.

15. Bauer, C.: Reduction of the carbon dioxide affinity of human haemoglobin solutions by 2,3-diphosphoglycerate. Resp. Physiol. 10: 10, 1970.

16. Benesch, R., and Benesch, R. E.: The effect of organic phosphates from the human erythrocyte on the allosteric properties of hemoglobin. Biochem. Biophys. Res. Commun. 26:162, 1967.

17. Chanutin, A., and Curnish, R. R.: Effect of organic and inorganic phosphates on the oxygen equilibrium of human erythrocytes. Arch. Biochem. Biophys. 121:96, 1967.

18. Bishop, C.: In Bishop, C. and Surgenor, D. M. (Eds.): The Red Blood Cell. New York, Academic Press, 1964, p. 163.

19. Bauer, C., Ludwig, M., Ludwig, I., and Bartels, H.: Factors governing the oxygen affinity of human adult and foetal blood. Resp. Physiol. 7:271, 1969.

20. Shappell, S. D., and Lenfant, C. J. M.: Adaptive, genetic, and iatrogenic alternations of the oxyhemoglobin-dissociation curve. Anesthesiology 37:127, 1972.

21. Valeri, C. R., Zaroulis, C. G., and Fortier, N. L.: Peripheral red cells as a functional biopsy to determine tissue oxygen tension. In Alfred Benzon Symposium IV: Oxygen Affinity of Hemoglobin and Red-cell Acid Base Status. New York, Academic Press, 1972.

22. Lenfant, C., Torrance, J. D., Woodson, R. D., Jacobs, P., and Finch, C. A.: Role of organic phosphate in the adaptation of man to hypoxia. Fed. Proc. 129:1115, 1970.

23. Battaglia, F. C., McGaughey, H., Makowski, E. L., and Moschia, G.: Postnatal changes in oxygen affinity of sheep red cells: A dual role of diphosphoglyceric acid. Am. J. Physiol. 219:217, 1970.

24. Salhany, J. M., Keitt, A. S. and Eliot, R. S.: The rate of deoxygenation of red blood cells: effect of intracellular 2,3-diphosphoglycerate and pH. FEBS Letters 16:257, 1971.

25. Gerlach, E., and Duhm, J.: 2,3-DPG metabolism of red cells: Regulation and adaptive changes during hypoxia. In Alfred Benzon Symposium IV: Oxygen Affinity of Hemoglobin and Red-cell Acid Base Status. New York, Academic Press, 1972.

26. Duhm, J.: The effect of 2,3-DPG and other organic phosphates on the Donnan equilibrium and the oxygen affinity of human blood. In Alfred Benzon Symposium IV: Oxygen affinity of Hemoglobin and Red-cell Acid Base Status. New York, Academic Press, 1972.

27. Rörth, M. R., Nygaard, S. F., and Parving, H. H.: Red cell metabolism and oxygen affinity of healthy individuals during exposure to high altitude. Advances in Experimental Medicine and Biology, Vol. 28. Hemoglobin and Red Cell Structure and Function. New York, Plenum Press, 1972.

28. Haidas, S., Labie, D., and Kaplan, J. C.: 2,3-diphosphoglycerate content and oxygen affinity as a function of red cell age in normal individuals. Blood 38:463, 1971.

29. Garby, L., Sjölin, S., and Vuille, J.-C.: Studies of erythrokinetics in infancy. II. The relative rate of synthesis of haemoglobin F and haemoglobin A during the first months of life. Acta Paediatr. Scand. 51:245, 1962.

30. Allen, D. W., Wyman, J., Jr., and Smith, C. A.: The oxygen equilibrium of fetal and adult hemoglobin. J. Biol. Chem. 203:81, 1953.

31. de Verdier, C. H., and Garby, L.: Low binding of 2,3-diphosphoglycerate to haemoglobin F. A contribution to the knowledge of the binding site and an explanation for the high oxygen affinity of foetal blood. Scand. J. Clin. Lab. Invest. 23:149, 1969.

32. Anselmino, K. T., and Hoffman, F.: Die ursachen des icterus neonatorum. Arch. Gynaekol. 143:477, 1930.

33. Rörth, M., and Bille Brahe, N. E.: 2,3- diphosphoglycerate and creatine in the red cell during human pregnancy. Scand. J. Clin. Lab. Invest. 28:271, 1971.

34. Novy, M. J., Frigoletto, F. D., Easterday, C. L., Umansky, I., and Nelson, N. M.: Changes in umbilical-cord blood oxygen affinity after intrauterine transfusions for erythroblastosis. N. Engl. J. Med. 285:589, 1971.

35. Delivoria-Papadopoulos, M., Roncevic, N. P., and Oski, F. A.: Postnatal changes in oxygen transport of term, premature and sick infants: The role of red cell 2,3-diphosphoglycerate and adult hemoglobin. Pediatr. Res. 5:235, 1971.

36. Matoth, Y., Zaizov, R., and Varsano, I.: Postnatal changes in some red cell parameters. Acta Paediatr. Scand. 60:317, 1971.

37. Rosenthal, A., Button, L. N., Nathan, D. G., Miettinen, O. S., and Nadas, A. S.:

Blood volume changes in cyanotic congenital heart disease. Am. J. Cardiol. 27:162, 1971.

38. Faura, J., Ramos, J., Reynafarje, C., English, E., Finne, P., and Finch, C. A.: Effect of altitude on erythropoiesis. Blood 33:668, 1969.

39. Hillman, R. S.: Characteristics of marrow production and reticulocyte maturation in normal man in response to anemia. J. Clin. Invest. 48:443, 1969.

40. Schmid, R., and Gilbertson, A. S.: Fundamental observations on the production of compensatory polycythemia in a case of patent ductus arteriosus with unusual blood flow. Blood 10:247, 1955.

41. Stohlman, F., Jr., Rath, C. E., and Rose, J. C.: Evidence for a humoral regulation of erythropoiesis. Studies on a patient with polycythemia secondary to regional hypoxia. Blood 9:721, 1954.

42. Rosenthal, A., Nathan, D. G., and Nadas, A. S.: Observations on the compensatory response to hypoxemia in a case of reversed differential cyanosis. Pediatrics 49:910, 1972.

43. Finch, C. A.: Erythropoietin. Triangle 9:127, 1969.

44. Morse, M., Cassels, D. E., and Holder, M.: The position of the oxygen dissociation curve of the blood in cyanotic congenital heart disease. J. Clin. Invest. 29:1098, 1950.

45. Edwards, M. J., Novy, M. J., Walters, C.-L., and Metcalfe, J.: Improved oxygen release: An adaptation of mature red cells to hypoxia. J. Clin. Invest. 47:1851, 1968.

46. Mulhausen, R., Astrup, P., and Kjeldsen, K.: Oxygen affinity of hemoglobin in patients with cardiovascular diseases, anemia, and cirrhosis of the liver. Scand. J. Clin. Lab. Invest. 19:291, 1967.

47. Metcalfe, J., Dhindsa, D. S., Edwards, M. J., and Mourdjinis, A.: Decreased affinity of blood for oxygen in patients with low-output heart failure. Circ. Res. 25:47, 1969.

48. Oski, F. A., Gottlieb, A. J., Delivoria-Papadopoulos, M., and Miller, W. W.: Red cell 2,3-diphosphoglycerate levels in subjects with chronic hypoxemia. N. Engl. J. Med. 280:1165, 1969.

49. Lenfant, C., Ways, P., Aucutt, C., and Cruz, J.: Effect of chronic hypoxic hypoxia on the O_2-Hb dissociation curve and respiratory gas transport in man. Resp. Physiol. 7:7, 1969.

50. Oski, F. A., Gottlieb, A. J., Miller, W. W., and Delivoria-Papadopoulos, M.: The effects of deoxygenation of adult and fetal hemoglobin on the synthesis of red cell 2,3-diphosphoglycerate and its in vivo consequences. J. Clin. Invest. 49:400, 1970.

51. Rosenthal, A., Mentzer, W. C., Eisenstein, E. B., Nathan, D. G., Nelson, N. M., and Nadas, A. S.: The role of red blood cell organic phosphates in adaptation to congenital heart disease. Pediatrics 47:537, 1971.

52. Woodson, R. D., Torrance, J. D., Shappell, S. D., and Lenfant, C.: The effect of cardiac disease on hemoglobin-oxygen binding. J. Clin. Invest. 49:1349, 1970.

53. Bellingham, A. J., Detter, J. C., and Lenfant, C.: The role of hemoglobin affinity for oxygen and red cell 2,3-diphosphoglycerate in the management of diabetic ketoacidosis. Trans. Assoc. Am. Physicians 83:113, 1970.

54. Torrance, J., Jacous, P., Restrepo, A., Eschbach, J., Lenfant, C., and Finch, C. A.: Intraerythrocytic adaptation to anemia. N. Engl. J. Med. 283:165, 1970.

55. Edwards, M. J., and Canon, B.: Oxygen transport during erythropoietic response to moderate blood loss. N. Engl. J. Med. 287:115, 1972.

56. Oelshlegel, F. J., Brewer, G. J., Penner, J. A., and Schoomaker, E. B.: Enzymatic mechanisms of red cell adaptation to anemia. Advances in Experimental Medicine and Biology, Vol. 28. Hemoglobin and Red Cell Structure and Function. New York, Plenum Press, 1972.

57. Miller, W. W., Delivoria-Papadopoulos, M., Miller, L., and Oski, F. A.: Oxygen releasing factor in hyperthyroidism. JAMA 211:1824, 1970.

58. Snyder, L. M., and Reddy, W. J.: Mechanism of action of thyroid hormones on erythrocyte 2,3-diphosphoglyceric acid synthesis. J. Clin. Invest. 49:1993, 1970.

59. Miller, L. D., et al.: Increased peripheral oxygen delivery in thyrotoxicosis: Role of red cell 2,3-diphosphoglycerate. Ann. Surg. 172:1051, 1970.

60. Lichtman, M. A., and Miller, D. R.: Erythrocyte glycolysis, 2,3-diphosphoglycerate and adenosine triphosphate concentration in uremic subjects: Relationship to extracellular phosphate concentration. J. Lab. Clin. Med. 76:267, 1970.

61. Miller, L. D., et al., The affinity of hemoglobin for oxygen: Its control and in vivo significance. Surgery 68:187, 1970.

62. Duhm, J., and Gerlach, E.: On the mechanisms of the hypoxia-induced increase of 2,3-diphosphoglycerate in erythrocytes. Pfluegers Arch. 326:254, 1971.

63. Travis, S. F., et al.: Alterations of red cell

glycolytic intermediates and oxygen transport as a consequence of hypophosphatemia in patients receiving intravenous hyperalimentation. N. Engl. J. Med. 285:763, 1971.

64. Bunn, H. F., May, M. H., Kocholaty, W. F., and Shields, C. E.: Hemoglobin function in stored blood. J. Clin. Invest. 48:311, 1969.

65. Valeri, C. R., and Hirsch, N. M.: Restoration in vivo of erythrocyte adenosine triphosphate, 2,3-diphosphoglycerate, potassium ion, and sodium concentrations following the transfusion of acid-citrate-dextrose-stored human red blood cells. J. Lab. Clin. Med. 73: 722, 1969.

66. Baum, D., Dillard, D. H., Mohri, H., and Crawford, E. W.: Metabolic aspects of deep surgical hypothermia in infancy. Pediatrics 42:93, 1968.

67. Ecker, R. R., Rea, W. J., Sugg, W. L., and Miller, W. W.: Changes in 2,3-diphosphoglycerate after cardiopulmonary bypass. Ann. Thorac. Surg. 13:364, 1972.

68. Bordiuk, J. M., McKenna, P. J., Giannelli, S., and Ayres, S. M.: Alterations in 2,3-diphosphoglycerate and O_2 hemoglobin affinity in patients undergoing open-heart surgery. Circulation 43 (Suppl.):I-141, 1971.

69. Sugarman, H. J., Davidson, D. T., Vileul, S., Delivoria-Papadopoulos, M., Miller, L. D., and Oski, F. A.: The basis of defective oxygen delivery from stored blood. Surg. Gynecol. Obstet. 131:733, 1970.

70. Delivoria-Papadopoulos, M., Morrow, G., III, and Oski, F. A.: Exchange transfusion in the newborn infant with fresh and "old" blood: The role of storage on 2,3-diphosphoglycerate, hemoglobin-oxygen affinity, and oxygen release. J. Pediatr. 79:898, 1971.

71. McConn, R., and Del Guercio, L. R. M.: Respiratory function of blood in the acutely ill patient and the effect of steroids. Ann. Surg. 174:436, 1971.

72. Mills, G. C.: The physiologic regulation of erythrocyte metabolism. Tex. Rep. Biol. Med. 27:773, 1969.

73. Duhm, J., Deuticke, B., and Gerlach, E.: Metabolism of 2,3-diphosphoglycerate and glycolysis in human red blood cells under the influence of dipyridamole and inorganic sulfur compounds. Biochim. Biophys. Acta 170:452, 1968.

74. Oski, F. A., Travis, S. F., Miller, L. D., Delivoria-Papadopoulos, M., and Cannon, E.: The in vitro restoration of red cell 2,3-diphosphoglycerate levels in banked blood. Blood 37: 53, 1971.

75. Duhm, J., Deuticke, B., and Gerlach, E.: Complete restoration of oxygen transport function and 2,3-diphosphoglycerate concentration in stored blood. Transfusion 11:147, 1971.

76. Keitt, A. S.: Metabolic characteristics of 2,3-DPG-rich red cells. Clin. Res. 19:40, 1971.

77. Oski, F. A., Miller, L. D., Delivoria-Papadopoulos, M., Manchester, J. H., and Shelburne, J. C.: Oxygen affinity in red cells: Changes induced in vivo by propranolol. Science 175:1372, 1972.

78. Bauer, C. H., and Ratschlag-Schaefer, A. M.: The influence of aldosterone and cortisol on oxygen affinity and cation concentration of the blood. Resp. Physiol. 5:360, 1968.

79. Pollock, T. W., Sugarman, H. J., and Oski, F. A.: In vivo effect of inosine, pyruvate, and phosphate (IPP) on oxygen-hemoglobin affinity. Fed. Proc. 30:546, 1971.

80. Proctor, H. J., and Parker, J. C.: Treatment of severe hypoxia by transfusion with red cells high in 2,3-diphosphoglycerate (2,3-DPG). Clin. Res. 20:497, 1972.

Etiologic Aspects of Cardiovascular Disease and Predisposition Detectable in the Infant and Child

James J. Nora, Robert R. Wolfe, and Vincent N. Miles

IN THE PEDIATRIC PATIENT, there are four categories of cardiovascular disease with which we may be justifiably concerned from the point of view of etiology: congenital heart disease, coronary artery disease, rheumatic fever, and hypertension. The newborn patient presents for diagnosis in only one of these categories, congenital heart disease, but a significant portion of these patients go unrecognized well beyond the newborn period, and sometimes beyond the pediatric period. For the other three categories, etiologic interest focuses on identifying predisposition in the newborn, older infant, and child. Where actual presentation of disease in these three categories is concerned, rheumatic fever occurs mainly in childhood, while essential hypertension and coronary artery disease occur predominantly in adult life.

Etiologic information has been obtained in varying quantities and qualities for all four of these categories. Two of these categories will be developed in moderate detail. We will discuss congenital heart diseases most extensively, since we have a considerable amount of personal etiologic data, and since it is clinically the most important cardiovascular disease of the infant and child. We will then devote a sizable portion of this presentation to atherosclerosis, specifically coronary artery disease, not so much because we have personal data, but because it is the most important disease of Western society and its recognition and prophylactic treatment in the pediatric patient may offer real therapeutic hope. Essential hypertension and rheumatic fever will be considered only briefly.

CONGENITAL HEART DISEASES

Congenital heart diseases are familial. Environmental teratogens, such as rubella, thalidomide, and dextroamphetamine have also been implicated as causes of cardiovascular malformations. These are not necessarily two mutually exclusive etiologic modes. We hope to show that the concept of multifactorial inheritance encompasses a genetic predisposition and an environmental trigger. A genetic–environmental interaction appears to be responsible for the production of the majority of congenital heart diseases.[1]

Genetic Aspects

Single Mutant Genes: Table 1 displays the authors' findings as to the etiology of congenital cardiovascular diseases in children being followed in our pediatric

From the Department of Pediatrics, Division of Pediatric Cardiology, University of Colorado Medical Center, Denver, Col. 80220.

Supported by NIH Grant HL 5981-01 and American Heart Association Grant 70-708.

James J. Nora, M.D.: *Associate Professor of Pediatrics and Director of Pediatric Cardiology, University of Colorado Medical Center and affiliated hospitals, Denver, Col.* Robert R. Wolfe, M.D.: *Assistant Professor of Pediatrics and Associate Director of Pediatric Cardiology, University of Colorado Medical Center and affiliated hospitals, Denver, Col.* Vincent N. Miles, M.D.: *Fellow in Pediatric Cardiology, University of Colorado Medical Center and affiliated hospitals, Denver, Col.*

Table 1. Etiologic Categories of Congenital Heart Lesions as Seen in a Pediatric Cardiology Clinic

Category	Per cent	Examples
Single mutant gene	2	Holt-Oram syndrome
Chromosomal	4	Down syndrome
Multifactorial	94	"Nonsyndrome" VSD

heart clinics. Single mutant gene syndromes account for about 2% of congenital cardiovascular diseases. The Ullrich-Noonan syndrome (Turner phenotype) is by far the most common single mutant gene syndrome in our heart clinic. Table 2 lists single mutant gene causes of congenital heart diseases.

The point to be made here is that single mutant genes of large effect cause congenital cardiac malformations *as part of a syndrome.* There is little evidence for single mutant genes causing discrete heart lesions, such as ventricular septal defect. A single mutant gene may cause ventricular septal defect as part of the Holt-Oram syndrome, but not ventricular septal defect alone. The only discrete heart lesion that clearly appears to exceed the expectations of multifactorial inheritance and to satisfy the predictions of Mendelian inheritance in a signifi-cant percentage of families studied is idiopathic hypertrophic subaortic stenosis (IHSS). In the strictest sense, however, this is not a congenital heart lesion, but is an abiotrophy, as is the aortic and mitral disease of Marfan's syndrome. Abiotrophic Mendelizing heart lesions are, for simplicity, classified with the congenital heart lesions in Table 2.

Chromosomes: Our experience and the experience of others suggest that gross chromosomal anomalies account for about 4% of congenital heart de-fects.[1,2] Again, as with single mutant gene etiology, congenital heart defects caused by chromosomal anomalies are seen as a part of a syndrome. We and others[1,2,4] have studied families with more than one first-degree relative with discrete congenital heart defects unassociated with syndromes, such as 21 trisomy, and have found no gross chromosomal anomalies.

Table 2. Selected Single Mutant Gene Syndromes and Cardiovascular Disease Other Than Coronary Artery

Autosomal Dominant	Autosomal Recessive	X-linked
Apert	Adrenogenital syndrome	Incontinentia pigmenti
Crouzon	Alkaptonuria	Mucopolysaccharidosis II
Ehlers-Danlos	Carpenter	Muscular dystrophy
Forney	Conradi	
Holt-Oram	Cutis-laxa	
IHSS (not strictly a syndrome)	Ellis-van Creveld	
Leopard	Friedreich's ataxia	
Marfan	Glycogenosis IIa, IIIa, IV	
Myotonic dystrophy	Jervell-Lange Nielsen	
Neurofibromatosis	Laurence-Moon-Biedl	
Osteogenesis imperfecta	Mucolipidosis III	
Romano-Ward	Mucopolysaccharidosis IH, IV, V, VI	
Treacher Collins	Osteogenesis imperfecta	
Tuberous sclerosis	Refsum	
Ullrich-Noonan	Seckel	
	Smith-Lemli-Opitz	
	Thrombocytopenia absent radius (TAR)	
	Weill-Marchesani	

With the new chromosomal banding techniques and the increased discrimination they add to karyotyping,[5] it is worth reevaluating these earlier findings in the light of recent technologic advances. We are in the process of obtaining new data in this area.

Table 3 shows the incidence of and the most common congenital heart diseases in the chromosomal syndromes, in which there is clearly a higher frequency of heart defects than in the general population. It should be noted that syndromes such as Klinefelter, XYY, and XXX, while they are common chromosomal disorders, do not have significant increase in cardiovascular maldevelopment. (Small series suggest that there is a slightly higher frequency of congenital heart disease in these syndromes, but this is equivocal.)

Multifactorial Inheritance: Multifactorial inheritance does *not* mean simply many factors, and should not be regarded as a vague, ill-defined, genetic category. This is a specific mode of inheritance, for which there are mathematical models. In the simplest terms, multifactorial inheritance means that there is a genetic predisposition caused by many genes, and there is usually an important interaction with an environmental influence—a genetic–environmental interaction.

An experimental model may first be used to illustrate how this mode of inheritance operates. The C57 BL/6 mouse has a hereditary predisposition to ventricular septal defect. About 1% of C57 BL/6 mice are born with ventricular septal defects. If on day 8 of gestation one shot of dextroamphetamine is given to the C57 BL/6 dam, 11% of the offspring will have congenital heart anomalies, two-thirds of which will be ventricular septal defects.[7] If an injection of anti-heart antibody is given at the same time to the C57 dam, 22% of the offspring will have cardiac malformations, three-fourths of which will be ventricular septal defects. Thus, it appears that ventricular septal defect is the congenital heart lesion "running in the family" of C57 mice, just as ventricular septal defect is the heart lesion running in the human families whose pedigrees are shown in Figs. 1 and 2. (These family pedigrees will serve as focal points for our subsequent discussion of Type B and Type C familial predisposition.)

Table 3. Congenital Heart Diseases (CHD) in Selected Chromosomal Aberrations

Population Studied	Incidence of CHD	Most Common Lesions		
		1	2	3
General Population	1%	VSD	PDA	ASD
4p-	40%	VSD	ASD	PDA
5p- (Cri-du-chat)	25%	VSD	PDA	ASD
C Mosaic	50%	VSD		
13 trisomy	90%	VSD	PDA	DEX
13q-	50%	VSD		
18 trisomy	99+%	VSD	PDA	PS
18q-	50%	VSD		
21 trisomy	50%	VSD	A-V canal	ASD
XO Turner	35%	COARC	AS	ASD

Abbreviations: VSD, ventricular septal defect; PDA, patent ductus arteriosus; ASD, atrial septal defect; DEX, dextrocardia; PS, pulmonic stenosis; A-V, atrioventricular; COARC, coarctation of aorta; and AS, aortic stenosis.

By permission.[6]

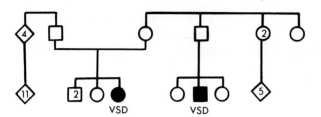

Fig. 1. Pedigree of a Type B family with VSD. This is the usual low risk-of-recurrence situation that one sees in the majority of families with congenital heart lesions. Actual risk of recurrence in either sibship (since there is only one affected first-degree relative) is 4.4%.

An environmental trigger (e.g., dextroamphetamine) acts upon the developing heart of the predisposed individual and "brings out" the heart defect running in the family (i.e., increases the chance of its occurrence). Environmental triggers act upon developmental thresholds. Visualize, in an overly simplistic way, that it requires the products of a lot of different genes to build a ventricular septum—genes specifying structural proteins, genes specifying enzymes—and that there is a rather precise timetable that must be followed. The right building blocks must be laid in the right sequence and at the right speed. The contribution from the endocardial cushions, conus, and ventricular septum must arrive at precisely the right time for the ventricular septum to close. If the contribution from the endocardial cushion is a little late in arriving due to several minor deficiencies of building blocks and a few minor delays in timing, the ventricular septum will not close completely. The threshold from normal to abnormal development has been crossed. This is probably what happens in cardiac maldevelopment of the multifactorial inheritance mode. A number of *normal genes* are affected by environmental triggers to the extent that many delays or accelerations in the delivery of primary gene products occur, and the orderly sequence of development is thrown enough off schedule so that the date of completion of the job cannot be met.

To continue with the over-simplification of the construction metaphor—and suggest why a single mutant gene of large effect will cause a ventricular septal defect but will also, at the same time, cause other malformations (a syndrome)—let us think of ventricular septal defect in the Holt-Oram syndrome. In a dominantly inherited syndrome, the abnormal primary gene product is often a structural protein. Thus, for the entire body, a "building block of the wrong size and/or shape" has been made. This is such a major error in design that many minor errors are not required before a ventricular septal defect is produced, since this single major error, the wrong building blocks, affects other parts of the overall structure (e.g., the arms).

Now to return to developmental thresholds. Figure 3 shows three hypothetical distribution curves of polygenic hereditary predisposition. A Type A family is not predisposed to congenital heart disease; their genetic make-up has a wide

Fig. 2. Pedigree of a Type C family. In the sibship, which already has three affected individuals, the risk of recurrence is extremely high. For genetic counseling, the risk may well approach what has already been experienced in the family (i.e., potentially 100% recurrence risk).

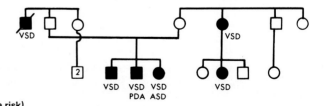

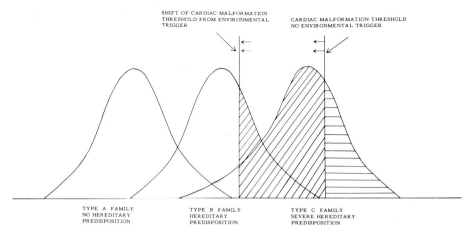

Fig. 3.   Three hypothetical distribution curves of predisposition to congenital heart disease. The Type A family has no predisposition, and even the addition of an environmental trigger does not push the threshold of cardiac maldevelopment far enough to the left (or curve of predisposition far enough to the right) to produce a congenital heart lesion. The Type B family represents the usual family in which a congenital heart lesion occurs. The curve of polygenic predisposition is to the right and the addition of an environmental trigger produces a congenital heart lesion in portion of those predisposed. A Type C family has such a polygenic predisposition that "spontaneous" cardiovascular malformation may occur, and the addition of environmental triggers may produce a very high frequency of malformation. (By permission.[6])

range of tolerance, so that minor delays and shortages cannot alter the time-table sufficiently to delay the schedule. Historically, no one in the family has ever had a congenital heart lesion.

The Type B family is the typical family with a predisposition to a congenital heart disease. Their genetic make-up is such that they cannot tolerate many delays and deficiencies in building material and still complete the job on time. If dextroamphetamine is added at the vulnerable period of cardiac development (in this example, at time the ventricular septum is being constructed) and throws the project off schedule, a ventricular septal defect will result. This may be visualized in Fig. 3 as moving the threshold to the left (or the curve to the right). What is important is the relationship of the threshold to the curve.

A Type C family has such a profound predisposition (the polygenic curve is so far to the right that some offspring are born with VSD without having a significant environmental insult). Add an environmental insult, however, and the relationship of the threshold to the curve is so altered that the risk becomes very great.

Environmental Aspects

This is the place to note some basic principles of teratology. There are probably few environmental triggers that have the widespread teratogenic effects of rubella and thalidomide, although there are probably a large number of teratogens, taken singly or in combination, that act as environmental triggers. We use dextroamphetamine as an example of a teratogen, which, under the proper circumstances, produces cardiovascular malformations. The proper circumstances are: (1) The subject is predisposed to the malformation;

(2) the subject is predisposed to the effects of the environmental agent; and (3) The teratogenic effect is at the vulnerable period of organogenesis.

Predisposition to the Malformation: The subject would have a ventricular septal defect resulting from the administration of dextroamphetamine, and according to our example, he would be from a Type B or a Type C family predisposed to VSD. We will leave the question open as to whether hereditary predisposition to VSD may be necessary for a teratogen as potent as thalidomide to cause the defect. There is evidence of such a predisposition to VSD even in patients who develop this lesion in rubella syndrome (although no predisposition to patent ductus arteriosus can be documented by positive family history in rubella syndrome patients). In any case, since thalidomide and rubella are exceptional teratogens, our attention is better directed toward exploring mechanisms of teratogenesic environmental triggers that may better reflect the genetic–environmental interaction.

Predisposition to the Effects of the Environmental Agent: There are clearly species and individual differences in response to the teratogenic effects of an environmental agent. The malformations that thalidomide so readily produced in humans could not be duplicated in common laboratory animal models (but were induced without difficulty in certain subhuman primates). In addition, not all pregnant women who ingested thalidomide during vulnerable periods of embryogenesis produced malformed infants. There is considerable experimental evidence of genetic differences that influence the embryo's response to a given teratogen.

Teratogenic Effect at the Vulnerable Period of Organogenesis: Thalidomide given to a mother after trunco-conal development is completed will not cause a trunco-conal malformation, and, in the case of thalidomide and cardiac development, exposure to the drug had to occur about 2 wk before the completion of the developmental event. Extrapolating from mouse work and utilizing a modest quantity of human data, it appears that dextroamphetamine exposure must also occur about 2 wk before the completion of a cardiac development event (i.e., for VSD, the dextroamphetamine must be given by the end of the fifth week of gestation).

There are a number of other principles of teratology: Usually a single or short-term exposure to a drug is likely to be teratogenic, and a long-term exposure is more likely to cause fetal death or be tolerated without ill effect (frequently only one dose of thalidomide resulted in malformation); teratogens in combination may produce malformations when the agents taken singly would have no adverse effect on development; certain drug and viral teratogens may produce characteristic patterns of malformation (e.g., phocomelia from thalidomide; patent ductus arteriosus, pulmonary branch stenosis, deafness and cataracts from rubella virus).

Finally, the most important principle of teratology is such a simple one that it is hard to understand how physicians prescribing medications for pregnant women can so often appear to be unaware of it. *The developing embryo is not a little adult.* The requirements for building a heart are quite different from those for maintaining a heart. One dose of thalidomide, which most effectively tranquilizes a mother without any damaging effect on her, may have disastrous effects on the developing heart of her unborn child. The same could probably be said of a large number of drugs as yet unidentified or only unsubstantially suspected at this time.

Prevention of Congenital Heart Disease

That the goal of etiologic studies is prevention is self-evident. The more we know about the genetic predisposition and the environmental interaction, the better will be our opportunity to reduce the incidence of congenital heart disease, which approximates 1% of live births in North America.

Genetic Risk: Identifying individuals and families at risk of the majority of congenital heart defects, those that are determined by multifactorial inheritance, is at the moment almost exclusively *ex post facto.* After a child with a congenital heart disease is born into a family, the family is identified as being predisposed to congenital heart disease, and empiric and theoretic risks can be applied to offer counseling regarding subsequent pregnancies. Empiric and theoretic risks will be discussed in a later section.

For the single mutant gene syndromes with associated congenital heart defects, the genetic risk is appreciated by recognition of the syndrome. For example, observing that a child with pulmonic stenosis has phenotypic features of the Ullrich-Noonan syndrome and has a mother with a similar phenotype immediately places the risk of recurrence of the syndrome at 50% and recurrence of heart disease in those with the syndrome at 35%. Such a family is identified as having a substantially higher risk of recurrence of congenital heart disease than in the simple multifactorial inheritance situation. (The risk of congenital heart disease occurring in the next offspring would be 50% × 35%, or 17.5%). Counseling and, when applicable, antenatal diagnosis by amniocentesis become relevant in these situations.

The vast majority of chromosomal aberrations do not recur, thus, the congenital heart defects associated with these chromosomal syndromes also do not recur. There is some increased risk in familial translocations in which the syndrome with its cardiovascular anomalies recur at a much higher frequency than the sporadic chromosomal aberrations. However, familial translocations are relatively rare. It is possible that anomalies of chromosomes not detectable by earlier methods will be disclosed by the newer chromosomal banding techniques, and that a number of familial cases of cardiovascular malformations will be identified. This area of potential increase in genetic risk is being investigated. Again, counseling and antenatal diagnosis become relevant options in these families.

This brings us back to the main genetic category of congenital heart etiology—multifactorial inheritance. Here the risks of recurrence may be stated in a slightly over-simplified manner or obfuscated by mathematical jargon. We opt for the over-simplified:

(1) The risk of a congenital heart lesion recurring in a family that already has one first-degree relative with a congenital heart lesion is 1%–5% depending on how common the lesion is in the general population. The more common the lesion, the higher the frequency of recurrence. Note in Table 4 that VSD has a recurrence risk of 4.4% and Ebstein's anomaly 1.1%. The empiric recurrence

**Table 4. Observed and Expected Recurrence Risks in Siblings
of 1,478 Probands With Congenital Heart Lesions**

Anomaly	Probands	Affected Siblings		
		No.	Per cent	Exp. ($\sqrt{p}$)
Ventricular septal defect	212	24/543	4.4	5.0
Patent ductus arteriosus	204	17/505	3.4	3.5
Tetralogy of Fallot	157	9/338	2.7	3.2
Atrial septal defect	152	11/342	3.2	3.2
Pulmonic stenosis	146	10/345	2.9	2.9
Aortic stenosis	135	7/317	2.2	2.1
Coarctation of aorta	128	5/272	1.8	2.4
Transposition of great vessels	103	4/209	1.9	2.2
Atrioventricular canal	73	4/151	2.6	2.0
Tricuspid atresia	51	1/96	1.0	1.4
Ebstein's anomaly	42	1/96	1.1	0.7
Truncus arteriosus	41	1/86	1.2	0.7
Pulmonic atresia	34	1/77	1.3	1.0
Total	1,478	95/3,376		

By permission.[8]

risks for the 13 heart lesions in Table 4 may be used in genetic counseling specifically. Without having the table handy, or when dealing with a lesion for which there are no empiric data staring risk of recurrence, the only thing to remember is that the frequency of recurrence is 1%–5% *if there is only one affected first-degree relative.* This would be an example of a Type B family, the typical congenital heart family with low recurrence risk.

(2) If there are two affected first-degree relatives, the recurrence risk is tripled. For VSD, the recurrence risk for the next offspring would become 13%. In these families one must be cautious, since, in multifactorial inheritance, the risk rises precipitously with each affected individual. In an autosomal recessive disorder, the redurrence risk is fixed at 25% for the next child, but in multi-factorial inheritance, the risk can go as high as 100%. We characterize these high-risk families as Type C families. Our present policy is to counsel that a family that has three affected first-degree relatives with a congenital heart disease has a prohibitive recurrence risk of the order of 60%–100%.

(3) If there is no affected first-degree relative (only a cousin or uncle or other distant relative) with a congenital heart defect, the risk of recurrence is the same as for the general population. All of us have a risk of the order of 1%.

What would be extremely useful would be to find genetic markers to identify the family at risk before a congenital heart defect is experienced. Biochemical tests would be most useful, and one can speculate that at some future date the premarital blood test required by law to look for syphilis could be used to screen rapidly for a large number of single gene, chromosomal, and multi-factorial inheritance predipsositions (or, if it is not taken as being too Orwellian or Skinnerian, these tests could be taken from the newborn and the profile be made available to each individual long before the occasion arises for premarital blood tests). It is also possible to consider even the potential for genetic engineering in this context. At the present time, however, our identification of the family at risk is mainly limited to the positive family history.

Environmental Risk: While genetic engineering may appear somewhat removed from our present capacity (and the philosophy of many), environmental engineering is readily achievable at this time. An immediate attack on environmental risks such as thalidomide and rubella is possible only after identifying the risks as such. We do not visualize that teratogens comparable to thalidomide and rubella are abroad in our environment at the present time, even though they may be introduced at some future time. Careful surveillance will be required to identify promptly any new "super-teratogens." However, thoughtful studies today based on sound clinical observations and innovative laboratory investigation could uncover many agents, which individually are environmental triggers producing small percentages of congenital cardiovascular disease but collectively may account for a significant proportion of congenital malformations of all types, not just cardiovascular.

Studies in the etiology of congenital heart diseases are no longer across uncharted expanses. The maps are still rather crude, but they are available now.

CORONARY ARTERY DISEASE AND ATHEROSCLEROSIS

The heritability of coronary artery disease has long been recognized and has received varying amounts of etiologic emphasis. Levine, following observations made in the 1920s, stated through successive editions of his textbook, *Clinical Heart Disease,* that the most important etiologic factor in coronary thrombosis was heredity.

Given the familial predisposition to coronary artery disease and the available knowledge regarding therapeutic intervention, what can be done about the leading cause of death in the United States? It has become apparent that recognition of the predisposition and initiation of therapy in the fourth and fifth decades severely limits therapeutic options and influences outcome much less than had been anticipated. In fact, a conclusion of the recently terminated Framingham study on coronary artery disease is that atherosclerosis is a pediatric problem.

Looking at the prevention of atherosclerosis as a pediatric problem would appear to offer an opportunity for innovative research by geneticists and biochemists and a therapeutic thrust by pediatricians, whose traditional orientation is that of prevention. There is reason for optimism. However, before the data are in, some rather far-reaching conclusions are being made, more on preliminary findings and hopeful speculation than one would like.

The question that is far from being answered is: What is the etiology of coronary artery diseases? Granted that there is good evidence of hereditary predisposition, what is the precise genetic nature? One approach that has offered promise is the effort to get a biochemical handle on a significant proportion of coronary artery diseases: the Fredrickson schema for hyperlipoproteinemia phenotyping. There is a certain amount of dissatisfaction with present phenotyping, which may or may not be relieved by increasing the precision of the tests. It may be that entirely different tests will eventually be required, but at the moment biochemical phenotyping offers the best approach to investigating etiology and identifying the infant and child at risk.

Below is our current assessment of the genetics of the hyperlipoproteinemias which is based on data from the literature and data of our own, both of which would have to be considered inadequate at this time: (1) Type I, autosomal recessive; (2) Type IIa, some cases autosomal dominant with severe disease in the homozygote; some cases multifactorial; (3) Type IIb, multifactorial; (4) Type III, multifactorial; (5) Type IV, multifactorial; and (6) Type V, multifactorial.

The phenotypic characteristics of the blood of patients having the basic six types have been investigated almost entirely in adults and are displayed in Table 5. It has been assumed, correctly or incorrectly, that the six phenotypes may be identified in the infant and child by applying these criteria (or variants thereof), although clear statements have been made that at least some of the phenotypes have only been recognized in adults.

If it appears that undue emphasis is being placed on biochemical phenotyping (with positive family history) as the primary method of identifying infants at risk, one only needs to review other risk factors that are useful in the adult, such as cigarette smoking, inadequate exercise, stress, striving, obesity, and hypertension, to see how poorly applicable they are to the infant (although they become progressively more applicable to the child).

We now must ask the next question: Can we identify the infant and child predisposed to coronary artery disease? (And we must add: at a level of confidence comparable to the experience in the adult.) We find we have already appreciated the irrelevancy in the infant of a number of risk factors useful in the adult. So now we are required to rely more heavily on biochemical phenotyping. But do we really have the data from the infant and child? The answer to this question is no. Although a number of groups, including our own, are presently working on the problem, there are more pitfalls than milestones.

Current Status of Phenotyping Pediatric Patients

Without giving undue emphasis to the pitfalls, or unjustified optimism to the positive findings, we can offer a current status report. Our experience leads us to believe that we can identify the six Fredrickson phenotypes in the child and probably in the infant. We also have recognized that the phenotype is a long way from the genotype, and that there is a great deal more heterogeneity and less specificity than the simple enumeration of six phenotypes would imply.

For example, we have seen as many as four of the six phenotypes among the first-degree relatives of the same family. We have also identified families

Table 5. Classification of Hyperlipidemias and Hyperlipoproteinemias

Type	↑Cholesterol	↑Triglyceride	Electrophoresis	Ultracentrifugation	Chylomicron
I	+			±VLDL[*]	+
IIa	+		β	LDL[†]	
IIb	+	+	β and pre-β	LDL & VLDL	
III	+	+	Broad β		
IV	+	+	pre-β	VLDL	
V	+	+	pre-β	VLDL	+

[*]Very low density lipoprotein.
[†]Low density lipoprotein.
By permission.[6]

in which both biologic parents of a so-called "homozygous" Type II child were without phenotypic manifestations of the "heterozygous" form of Type II disease. (And we have recently seen a mother of a "homozygous" Type II child who manifested no biochemical abnormality of a hyperlipidemia prior to sustaining a myocardial infarction at 30 yr of age). We have noted individuals to change from one phenotype to another, depending on diet or physiologic state (e.g., pregnancy). It is also well recognized that phenotypic lipid abnormalities appear and disappear during a variety of pathologic as well as physiologic conditions. Clearly, there is room for the development of methods offering greater precision in biochemical phenotyping of patients of every age.

But what of the infant and child? Does a cord blood cholesterol really identify Type II newborns? There are an enormous number of methodologic problems that we will not amplify in this limited space. Longitudinal studies of sufficient duration, precision, and magnitude are lacking. However, short-duration, longitudinal studies suggest little correlation between cord blood cholesterol with subsequent studies during the first year of life.[11] Figure 4 reveals that, although serum cholesterol values are generally higher in heel stick specimens (taken after the initiation of feeding for the Guthrie test), this trend is by no means consistent. The role of the placenta, nutritional states of mother and newborn, and gestational age may all require evaluation.

The generally (although inconsistently) higher levels of serum cholesterol after institution of feeding suggest that screening tests following dietary challenge may be informative, since correlation between cord blood and subsequent

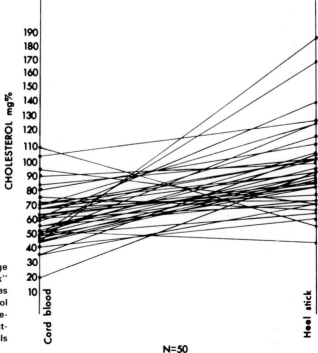

Fig. 4. A dietary challenge before obtaining a "heel stick" serum cholesterol produces generally higher cholesterol levels, but the relationship between cord blood and post-feeding heel-stick cholesterols is far from consistent.

N=50

290   NORA ET AL.

cholesterol values has proved to be unsatisfactory in some hands. The point is
that adequate longitudinal studies of various screening methods are lacking.

However, since there are approximately three adults with Type IV disease
for every adult with Type II disease, is cholesterol screening enough? While
significantly elevated serum cholesterol suggests Type IIa disease, what about
Type IV and even Type IIb? The great majority of pediatric patients predisposed to coronary artery disease are not going to be recognized (even if cholesterol screening is valid) by cholesterol screening alone.

Our screening test, therefore, is for both cholesterol and triglyceride abnormalities. Figure 5 reveals the general trend toward higher triglycerides after
a feeding challenge, with a number of exceptions. Again, longitudinal studies
will be required to see if cord-blood or heel-stick values (after dietary challenge) correlate better with subsequent evaluations during childhood. Although
screening tests in the newborn are sound logistically and from the point of view
of being able to initiate therapy at the earliest possible time, it may become
evident that they are of no value in that we cannot identify the infant at risk.
It may be that the 5- or 10-yr-old child will prove to be the pediatric patient
in whom risk may be recognized.

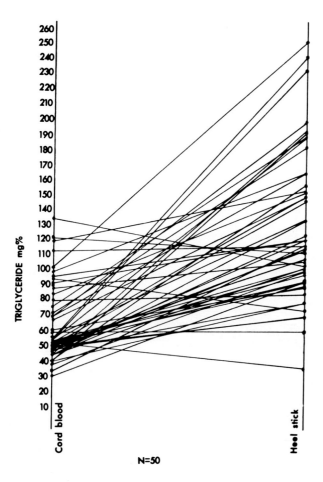

Fig. 5. Heel-stick triglyceride values show an inconsistent, but generally upward,
trend when compared with
cord-blood levels.

N=50

Beyond the screening test is the need to phenotype accurately the proband and all first-degree relatives. This is not only to provide a feedback loop regarding probabilities that the proband does have a predisposition but also to develop pedigree data for much-needed etiologic studies, to develop risk data that correlates with the specific phenotypes, and to identify other first-degree relatives at risk. (Although preventive therapy in the adult in the fourth and fifth decades has been unsatisfactory, perhaps identification of some 25-yr-old fathers will be early enough to afford meaningful intervention.)

In summary, the etiology of coronary artery disease seems to be consistent with multifactorial inheritance in the majority of cases, including those that have been characterized by biochemical phenotyping. The exceptions to this would be the rare Type I disease and some Type IIa patients. The genetic input clearly requires considerable amplification and refinement. The less than satisfactory results of medical intervention at the fourth and fifth decades of the life of the patient predisposed to coronary artery disease has led many investigators to a new emphasis on atherosclerotic predisposition as a pediatric problem. The problem now is that much must be learned about the pediatric patient. It is not even certain that we can accurately identify the child (much less the infant at risk) because of lack of basic genetic information, lack of longitudinal studies, lack of precision in phenotyping, and a variety of methodologic pitfalls.

It is certainly premature to talk about treatment until these diagnostic deficiencies are corrected. (Who should you really treat?) And when one finally gets to the point of treatment, a great deal of other information will be necessary. For example, perhaps it will prove more efficacious, in producing lower serum cholesterol in adults, to introduce an early *high* cholesterol diet (to "induce enzymes"?) than an early low cholesterol diet.

RHEUMATIC FEVER

Familial aspects of rheumatic fever have been recognized for decades. The National Danish Twin Study reveals a significantly higher concordance in monozygotic than in dizygotic twins. As in the other cardiovascular disorders of a multifactorial mode of inheritance, the genetic-environmental interaction obtains. However, in rheumatic fever, the environmental determinant is of greater importance (see Fig. 6).

ESSENTIAL HYPERTENSION

Our review of the subject strongly favors a multifactorial mode of inheritance in the majority of cases of essential hypertension, but does not exclude that a minority of patients (as in congenital heart diseases) may have hypertension at-

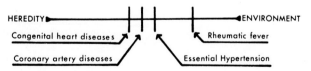

Fig. 6. The relative roles of heredity and environment (as visualized by the authors) in the etiology of the four major categories of cardiovascular disease place congenital heart disease, coronary artery disease, and essential hypertension in the middle of the continuum, suggesting that genetic and environmental determinations are of approximately equal importance. The role of the streptococcus acting on predisposed individuals places greater emphasis on the environmental determination of rheumatic fever.

tributed to single mutant genes. Plasma renin determinations may prove to be a step toward defining usable risk factors.[12]

CONCLUSION

Etiologic information concerning major cardiovascular diseases is relevant to the pediatric patient, including the newborn. It is realistic to believe that meaningful risk factors will be identified for all cardiovascular disease in the not-too-distant future and will be applicable to the newborn and, as yet, unborn. The goal of prevention is not beyond reach.

REFERENCES

1. Nora, J. J.: Multifactorial inheritance hypothesis for the etiology of congenital heart diseases: The genetic-environmental interaction. Circulation 38:604, 1968.

2. Emerit, I., et al.: Chromosomal abnormalities and congenital heart disease. Circulation 36:886, 1967.

3. Anders, J. M., Moores, E. C., and Emanuel, R.: Chromosome studies in 157 patients with congenital heart disease. Br. Heart J. 27:756, 1965.

4. Rohde, R. A.: Chromosomes in heart disease: Clinical and cytogenetic studies of 68 cases. Circulation 34:484, 1966.

5. Caspersson, T., Lamakka, G., and Zech, L.: The 24 fluorescence patterns of the human metaphase chromosomes—distinguishing characters and variability. Hereditas 67:89, 1971.

6. Nora, J. J., and Fraser, F. C.: Pediatric Genetics. Philadelphia, Lea & Febiger, 1973.

7. —, Sommerville, R. J., and Fraser, F. C.: Homologies for congenital heart diseases: Murine models influenced by dextroamphetamine. Teratology 1:413, 1968.

8. —: Etiologic factors in congenital heart diseases. Pediatr. Clin. N. Am. 18:1059, 1971.

9. Kannel, W. B., and Dawber, T. R.: Atherosclerosis as a pediatric problem. J. Pediatr. 80:544, 1972.

10. Fredrickson, D. S., and Lees, R. S.: A system for phenotyping hyperlipoproteinemia. Circulation 31:321, 1965.

11. Darmady, J.: Serum lipids during first four months. Arch. Dis. Child. 80:398, 1971.

12. Brunner, H. R., et al.: Essential hypertension: Renin and aldosterone, heart attack and stroke. N. Engl. J. Med. 286:441, 1972.

Index

3
4 b
5 c
6 d
7 e
8 f
9 g
0 h
1 i
8 2 j